1

This informative and fully illustrated new textbook covers all aspects of cancer biology, from the cellular processes underlying tumorigenesis, all the way through to the development of new agents and strategies to improve cancer treatment and prevention. No prior medical knowledge is assumed, and each chapter provides an authoritative self-contained account. Uniquely, this book extends a broad net over the whole subject, and is not restricted only to the ferociously advancing field of cancer genetics. It describes how cancer is diagnosed and classified, how causes are identified, how tumours behave and how flawed fundamental biological processes drive them. It explains how clinicians assess tumours, it explores well-established therapeutic options and evaluates the potential for innovative new treatments in the future. The text concludes with a helpful glossary of terminology. Every detail of information is clearly described from first principles and the book will thus provide an ideal introductory account for students of medicine, cell biology and pathology, as well as healthcare professionals working on cancer and drug development.

Understanding cancer

POSTGRADUATE MEDICAL SCIENCE

This important new series is based on the successful and internationally well-regarded specialist training programme at the Royal Postgraduate Medical School in London. Each volume provides an integrated and self-contained account of a key area of medical science, developed in conjunction with the course organisers and including contributions from specially invited authorities.

The aim of the series is to provide biomedical and clinical scientists with a reliable introduction to the theory and to the technical and clinical applications of each topic.

The volumes will be a valuable resource and guide for trainees in the medical and biomedical sciences and for laboratory-based scientists.

In the series:

Radiation protection of patients by R. Wootton

Image analysis in histology: conventional and confocal microscopy by D. Springall, R. Wootton and J. Polak

Monoclonal antibodies edited by M.A. Ritter and H.M. Ladyman.

Molecular neuropathology edited by G.W. Roberts and J.M. Polak

Clinical gene analysis and manipulation by J.A.Z. Jankowski and J.M. Polak

Understanding cancer

From basic science to clinical practice

MALCOLM R. ALISON BSc, PhD, MRCPath

and

CATHERINE E. SARRAF BSc, PhD

Royal Postgraduate Medical School, London

Published in association with the Royal Postgraduate Medical School
University of London by

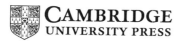

4|9|97
M

PUBLISHED BY THE PRESS SYNDICATE OF THE UNIVERSITY OF CAMBRIDGE
The Pitt Building, Trumpington Street, Cambridge CB2 1RP, United Kingdom

CAMBRIDGE UNIVERSITY PRESS
The Edinburgh Building, Cambridge CB2 2RU, United Kingdom
40 West 20th Street, New York, NY 10011–4211, USA
10 Stamford Road, Oakleigh, Melbourne 3166, Australia

First published 1997

Printed in the United Kingdom at the University Press, Cambridge

Typeset in Linotype Times 10/13 pt

*A catalogue record for this book is available from
the British Library*

Library of Congress Cataloguing in Publication data

Alison, Malcolm.
    Understanding cancer : from basic science to clinical practice /
Malcolm R. Alison and Catherine E. Sarraf.
        p.   cm. – (Postgraduate medical science)
    Includes bibliographical references and index.
    ISBN 0 521 56154 X (hardback). – ISBN 0 521 56751 3 (pbk.)
    1. Cancer.   I. Sarraf, Catherine E. (Catherine Elizabeth), 1945–
    II. Title.   III. Series.
    [DNLM: 1. Neoplasms.   QZ 200A414u 1997]
    RC261.A655   1997
    616.99′4–dc20   96–32623 CIP
    DNLM/DLC
    for Library of Congress

ISBN 0 521 56154 X hardback
ISBN 0 521 56751 3 paperback

Contents

1

Introduction to cancer

1.1 Introductory note

Cancer is a common and widely publicized disease, and in spite of ever increasing efforts to understand it as a process, its incidence in the population is rising. The main reason for this is the close correlation of the number of cancer cases with increasing age of patients, and the number of more aged people, in Western society at least, is rising. It used to be suggested that some aspect of the ageing process increased the susceptibility to cancer, perhaps by impairing immune surveillance, however, it is now generally accepted that the relationship of many cancers to increasing age is rather a reflection of the time required to accumulate a critical number of genetic abnormalities for a cancer to arise. Cancer may affect any organ or tissue, but while some cancers are common, e.g. lung, breast, skin, gut and prostate, others are very rare; those affecting young people often being amongst the rarest.

As a cause of mortality overall in the Western World, cancer is second only to cardiovascular disease. In particular, cancer affects epithelial tissues and over 90% of tumours are derived from this tissue. This is not surprising since many of the known cancer-causing agents (*carcinogens*) are from natural radiation, in the air we breath and from the foodstuffs we ingest, and epithelial cells are the first line of defence to the outside world in the skin, lungs and gastrointestinal tract. Although a great deal of effort has been devoted to defining the optimum protocols for eradicating each type of *primary tumour*, there are often two confounding factors conspiring against a successful outcome: metastatic spread and the unwanted toxicity of the treatment to normal tissue. The most important cause of mortality is spread of the original tumour to a distant site, a process called *metastasis*. If the site of that spread is to a vital organ, e.g. the liver, then death is likely to be significantly hastened.

As metastases have often developed *before* diagnosis, it is widely believed that the greatest single advancement in cancer management (thus improving prognosis) would be gained through more effective methods of early detection – i.e. an *efficient cancer screening programme*. This is not as simple as it sounds, apart from being able to detect a reliable marker of an asymptomatic tumour mass, the test needs to be relatively non-invasive to ensure high patient compliance and, in these so-called recessionary times, seen to be cost-effective. A number of screening programmes are already in operation, with cervical screening and mammography probably being the most widely adopted; so-called cost-effectiveness can be improved by actively encouraging participation of the group thought to be at the greatest risk of a particular disease, e.g. mammography for women in the 50–64 age group. Colorectal cancer seems an ideal disease for screening because there is a recognized preinvasive state (the adenoma), and the prognosis for invasive lesions classified as Dukes' A stage (see Fig. 6.6) is good, whereas the more invasive stages have a poor prognosis. However, the screening methods of sigmoidoscopy or faecal occult blood tests do not exactly encourage patient compliance. Likewise, there is poor compliance from workers, particularly those retired, in the rubber and dye industries who are at greatest risk from bladder cancer, where six-monthly urine samples to detect haematuria (blood in the urine caused by the haemorrhage of exophytic growths) could be of use. For many types of cancer it could be argued that the most spectacular reductions in incidence could be achieved through *simply* changing lifestyle – e.g. encouraging people to stop smoking and reduce their intake of dietary fat!

The greatest obstacle to the effective eradication of disseminated malignant disease by cytotoxic drugs is the inflicted life-threatening toxicity to normal tissues. The drugs currently in use are perfectly good at killing proliferative cells in tumours, but unfortunately they also kill proliferative cells elsewhere, e.g. in the bone marrow, gut and hair follicles. Thus the treatment of the tumour is limited by the amount of damage which can be tolerated by the normal tissues, particularly the bone marrow, and suitable treatment-free intervals must be scheduled to allow for recovery of the normal tissue. In the case of the bone marrow these intervals may be shortened by courses of recombinant growth factors to correct the induced myelosuppression. The rapid advancements in knowledge of the molecular mechanisms underlying the neoplastic process certainly promise radically new approaches to cancer treatment (see Chapter 7, section 7.4), superseding the relatively crude sledgehammer approaches currently adopted.

Oncology is that branch of medicine that deals with *tumours*, and is literally the science of new growths (Gr. *ogkos*, a swelling; *logos*, science). A tumour (L. *tumor*, swelling) is a swelling caused by excessive continued growth of cells in a tissue, which may be *benign* or *malignant*, while the term *neoplasm* means a new and diseased form of tissue growth. In clinical practice, the words 'neoplasm' and 'tumour' are often used interchangeably. However, the term *cancer* is loosely used to mean any malignant growth, being derived from the Latin meaning 'crab', since the general outline of many malignant growths resembles a crab with the body being the main tumour mass and the claws being the invasive tumour margins. Tumours have been defined as 'masses of tissue whose growth exceeds and is uncoordinated with that of normal tissues, and which persist in the same excessive manner after cessation of the stimuli that evoked the change' (R.A. Willis, *Pathology of Tumours*, 1948). This latter point highlights an important distinction between neoplasia and hyperplasia; neoplasia persists after the removal of the stimulus because of heritable genetic defects in the affected cells, but the elevated cell proliferation rate seen in hyperplastic tissue *ceases* after removal of the stimulus that evoked the change, e.g. after skin wounding the excessive epidermal proliferation ceases once the tissue defect is healed. Of course, cell proliferation is a normal property of all tissues during embryological development, and it continues throughout adult life in some of them, e.g. bone marrow, gut and skin. These tissues and the glandular epithelia (e.g. liver, kidney and adrenal) can all become hyperplastic to effect wound healing, while in the immune system there is continuous selection of newly derived T- and B-cell clones. All these proliferative reactions are precisely controlled, but it is worth remembering that tumour growth *is not uncontrolled*, for if it were any tumour might soon overwhelm its host in size. Of course, Willis' definition is not by any means complete since excessive growth is not the only behavioural abnormality exhibited by the affected cells: local invasion and the capacity for colonization at distant sites being the most obvious. Furthermore, tumour cell populations are not totally anarchic. They often exhibit patterns of differentiation which to a greater or lesser degree resemble their tissue of origin. In summary, all facets of tumour behaviour, *viz.* cell proliferation, cell death, differentiation, invasion and metastasis appear to be the result of the inappropriate or aberrant expression of probably many genes regulating the cell phenotype.

1.2   Identifying tumours

Imaging techniques

The presence of a tumour at or near the surface of the body provides no problem of accessibility to the clinician, and, for example, testicular and prostate cancer and even lymph node metastases are initially investigated by palpation. Other tumours such as those of the bladder, cervix and rectum are often diagnosed by the clinician by endoscopy before referral to the Radiology Department. However, tumours within the body mass are better revealed by more sophisticated imaging methods. The most widely available investigative procedure is *diagnostic radiography*. The simple radiograph or the use of X-irradiation after the administration of radio-opaque dyes provides information of the extent of local growth of a tumour (Fig. 1.1A, B). Conventional radiology provides the highest spatial resolution, and is therefore best suited to the gastrointestinal tract and bone where fine detail can be shown.

X-rays are produced whenever high speed electrons are brought abruptly to a halt, commonly by a block of tungsten. A high voltage is applied so that the electrons are attracted to the 'target' (positive electrode), and upon striking the target the acquired kinetic energy is surrendered and converted into other forms, one being X-irradiation. In diagnostic radiology, a beam of X-rays is directed at the patient, some are stopped (absorbed), some are deflected (scattered) and some pass through unaffected (transmitted). The X-ray beam emerging from the patient is the result of these events, but the human eye is not visually sensitive to X-irradiation. However, photographic film exposed to X-rays and then developed will be found to be blackened – the irradiation has affected the emulsion of silver salts so that after development, metallic silver is released and the film or paper appears dark. The amount of silver released obviously depends on the level of radiation to which the film is subjected, 'the expo-

(A)

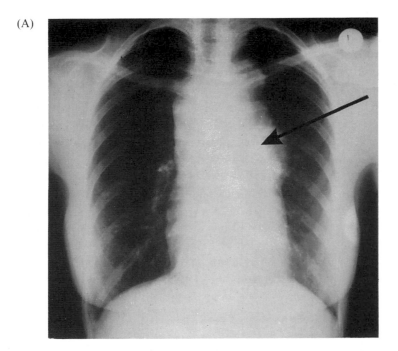

(B)

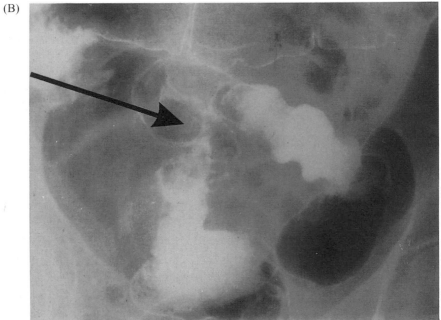

Fig. 1.1 (A) Plain chest radiograph of a patient with tumour involvement of mediastinal lymph nodes as indicated by increased opacity (arrow) and (B) a tumour of the large intestine indicated by an irregular defect (arrow) in the lumen which is highlighted by an opaque contrast medium.

sure', thus regions of the film exposed to a lot of X-rays are black, while regions exposed to few X-rays appear relatively light – hence bones which are very dense, absorb X-rays and are outlined as light-coloured structures (Fig. 1.1A). The final film is therefore in the form of a negative, dark where there is little X-ray shadow, and bright where the film has been shaded by dense tissue, e.g. bone.

A three-dimensional image of the subject can be formed with the aid of *computed tomography* (CT), in which the information from numerous small X-ray beams is digitally integrated. CT has in fact been one of the most spectacular advances in medicine over the last few years, and since the installation of the first prototype in 1972 the technology has swiftly advanced. X-ray CT scanning relies on the principle of reconstruction from projections, and a three-dimensional (3-D) image of the patient in cross-section can be obtained (Fig. 1.2); 3-D images may be thought of as a set of stacked 2-D tomograms. Basically the X-ray tube rotates around the patient, and the images are collected either by detectors which rotate synchronously with the X-ray tube round the patient through 360°, or by a complete ring of stationary detectors (Fig. 1.3). CT has a higher tissue density discrimination than conventional radiology and is, therefore, useful for the diagnosis of tumours of the abdominal organs and

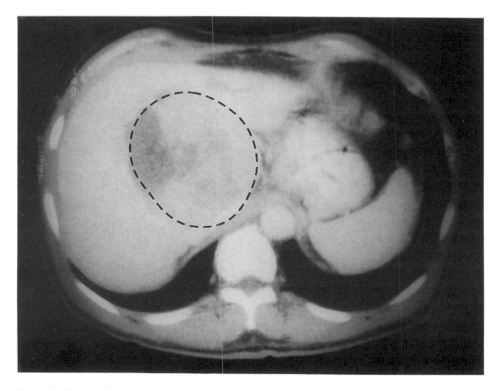

Fig. 1.2 CT scan through the abdomen showing the presence of a hepatocellular carcinoma as an area of diminished density (encircled), here more X-rays have been transmitted through this area and the film is more blackened. (Image kindly supplied by Dr. Pat Price, Department of Clinical Oncology, Hammersmith Hospital.)

(A)   (B)

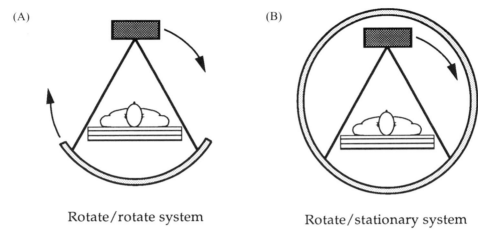

Rotate/rotate system   Rotate/stationary system

Fig. 1.3 Schematic diagram illustrating the two basic types of CT scanner: (A) either the X-ray tube and the detectors rotate synchronously round the patient through 360° – the *rotate/rotate* system, or (B) there is a complete ring of stationary detectors and the X-ray tube rotates around the patient within the ring – the *rotate/stationary* system.

brain (see Figs. 1.2 and 1.4) where small differences in density between soft tissue, fluid, fat and other structures can be discerned.

Magnetic resonance imaging (MRI) is another technique for producing high-resolution fully 3-D tomographic data sets, and therefore like CT, is useful for planning radiotherapy geometrically tailored to the target – *conformal therapy*. Like X-ray CT, MRI is highly suitable for displaying soft tissue detail. The method employs radiofrequency radiation in the presence of carefully controlled magnetic fields, and basically portrays the distribution of hydrogen nuclei and parameters relating to their motion in water and lipids. Any nuclei with a net charge are suitable for MRI, but most data have been on the nuclear magnetism of the hydrogen nucleus (or proton) because of its ubiquitous distribution in biological material.

Nuclear medicine techniques assess organ and tissue function by observing the distribution of an injected radiopharmaceutical. It is hoped that the kinetics and/or distribution of the pharmaceutical are different between the normal and tumour tissue, and this can be detected by localizing the radioactivity emitted from the radiopharmaceutical. This radioactivity can be imaged by a gamma-camera, a process called *scintigraphy*. Obviously a pharmaceutical with appropriate biological behaviour must be chosen, the bound radionuclide must not affect the biological behaviour, while the half-life of the radionuclide should be sufficiently long to complete the imaging process without presenting the patient with an unnecessary radiation burden. So, for example, technetium-99m (^{99m}Tc) is widely used for scintigraphic studies because of its short half-life (six hours), and in the search for skeletal metastases ^{99m}Tc-diphosphonate is used since bony metastases are associated with increased blood flow and osteoblastic (bone-forming) activity – hence increased radiopharmaceutical uptake (Fig. 1.5).

Positron emission tomography (PET) is a nuclear medicine procedure that is a form of sectional imaging of a radiopharmaceutical in which the radionuclide is a positron emitter, and is based on the coincidence detection of high energy photons from positron emission. Unlike CT and MRI, which provide images of precise anatomical localization, PET aims to provide information on metabolic differences between normal and neoplastic tissue (see Fig. 1.4). A positron emitted during radionuclide decay is very rapidly 'captured' by an electron, and results in a burst of radiation in the form of two 511 KeV photons travelling at 180° to each other. By encircling the patient with a ring of radiation detectors, it is possible to record these pairs of photons emerging from the body in opposite directions, using coincidence circuitry which thus defines the line along which the decay must have occurred (Fig. 1.6). If enough coincidental counts are made then a complete tomographical representation of the distribution of radioactivity can be obtained by computer reconstruction in much the same way as in CT.

Ultrasonography relies on the differing echo patterns which tissues create when bombarded by sound from an ultrasonic generator. Echoes are generated at interfaces of tissues whose density differs, but they cannot be obtained if the organ is shielded by bone, since bone reflects all the sound from the beam. Additionally, ultrasound is unable to cross a tissue–gas boundary, so bowel gas is another barrier to adequate

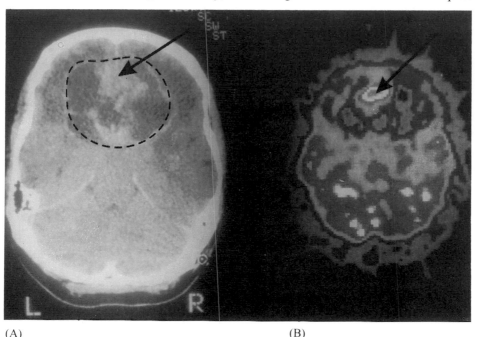

(A)   (B)

Fig. 1.4 Imaging of a brain tumour by CT scan (A) and the same tumour imaged by positron emission tomography (PET) (B) after administration of ^{18}F-labelled 2-fluoro-2-deoxyglucose (^{18}F-FDG). The CT scan shows a cystic tumour in the frontal lobe (encircled) with a solid component anteriorly (arrow) which corresponds to the hot spot in the PET ^{18}F-FDG scan (arrow) indicating an area of high glucose uptake – a recognized marker of neoplastic growth. (Images kindly supplied by Dr. Pat Price, Department of Clinical Oncology, Hammersmith Hospital.)

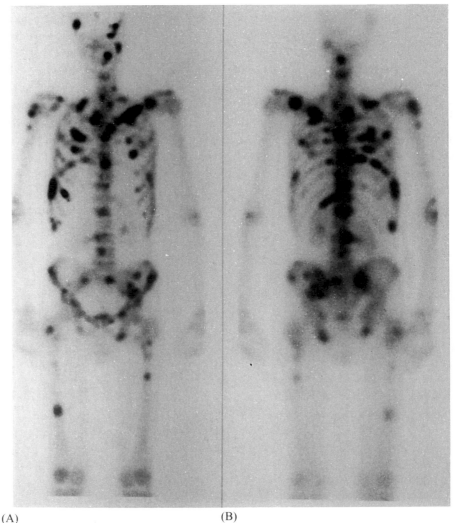

(A)   (B)

Fig. 1.5 Whole-body bone scintigraphy, four hours after injection with 550 MBq of ^{99m}Tc-diphosphonate. Focal increased activity in all areas of the skeleton is compatible with multiple skeletal metastases. (A) Shows the anterior view and (B) shows the posterior view. (Kindly supplied by Daphne Glass, Radiology Department, Hammersmith Hospital.)

visualization. Ultrasound is an excellent technique for imaging in the liver, and metastases down to 1 cm diameter can be reliably detected (Fig. 1.7).

Histological techniques

The investigations mentioned above reveal the space occupying properties of a tumour, which might provide an indication of *stage* (see Chapter 6, section 6.3) of tumour development, however, the *histogenesis* and *grade* (see below and Chapter 6, section 6.2) of the tumour are determined after surgical removal and microscopical

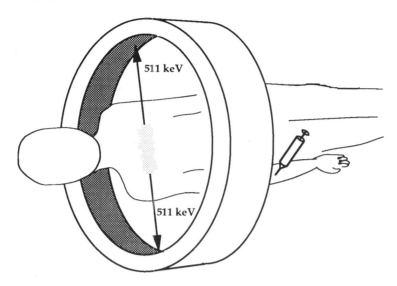

Fig. 1.6 Schematic representation of the positron emission tomography (PET) scanner, showing the recording, by coincidence circuitry, of pairs of photons of similar energy emerging from the body in opposite directions.

assessment. This morphological diagnosis takes the form of an examination of either cells (*cytological* diagnosis) or of tissue sections (*histopathological* diagnosis). In practical terms, clinical cytology is divided into two types (*exfoliative* and *aspiration*) depending upon the means used to collect the material. Exfoliative cytology comprises all examinations carried out on cells which are normally desquamated from surfaces or dislodged from them by mechanical means such as by spatulae or brushes, while aspiration cytology is the examination of cells collected by a thin needle attached to a syringe. Exfoliative cytology can be used in the diagnosis of tumours of the respiratory and urinary tracts by simply looking at sputum and urine samples, though the exact location of the tumour cannot be identified. Probably the most important use of exfoliative cytology is in the mass screening programme to detect cervical intra-epithelial neoplasia (Fig. 1.8A, B), a well recognized preinvasive lesion (see Chapter 4, section 4.3 and Fig. 4.2). Fine needle aspiration cytology can be used in the diagnosis of palpable suspect lesions in tissues such as breast, prostate and lymph node, and with the advent of accurate imaging techniques it can also be applied to the examination of non-palpable deep-seated lesions in all parts of the body (Fig. 1.9).

When tissue is used for histopathological diagnosis, a biopsy may be obtained by a variety of means. In the respiratory, gastrointestinal and genitourinary tracts a variety of fibre optic-guided endoscopy instruments can be used for sampling, while often the diagnosis is made after complete resection of the tumour (excision biopsy). As discussed above, to observe tissues at the cellular level one has to use a microscope, and for the commonest modes of observation including bright field microscopy and transmission electron microscopy, the illumination needs to pass through the tissue, thus requiring the tissue to be in the form of thin sections. Clearly, cutting sections

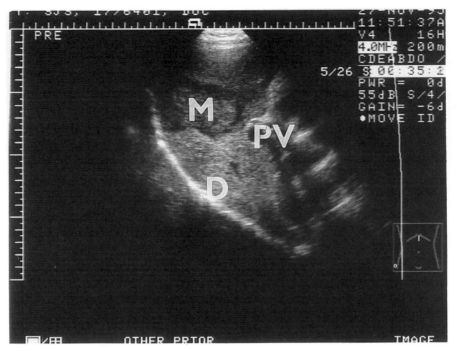

Fig. 1.7 A typical pie-shaped field of view obtained by a sector plan ultrasound sweep. Here a large liver metastasis (M) from an oesophageal carcinoma is seen as a heterogeneous lesion of generally lower reflectivity than the surrounding liver. Conventionally the strength of echoes is represented by degrees of brightness in a grey scale image, the brighter the image the stronger the reflection. This is a longitudinal section through the liver as depicted by the plane of section (small vertical line) in the body icon in the bottom right. D, diaphragm; PV, portal vein. (Kindly supplied by Dr David Cosgrove, Department of Diagnostic Radiology, Hammersmith Hospital.)

of tissue thin enough to be transparent is not possible without prior preparation of the tissue. These considerations are served either by *fixing* then *embedding* the tissue in a rigid medium, or by *rapid freezing* followed by cutting frozen sections. Fixation is the term used to describe chemical preservation of tissue, by cross-linking and/or precipitation of proteins, so that the architecture it had while viable is retained. Samples, therefore, need to be fixed immediately they are removed to preserve the tissue in its original form; this requires killing of bacteria and moulds, inhibition of the activity of autolytic enzymes and prevention of decomposition, as well as main-tainance of osmotic differentials. Tissue also needs to be given a texture which permits easy sectioning – not brittle, not soft, and it must be robust enough to avoid damage in subsequent processing. Sectioned tissue is finally counterstained for observation, so the fixation methods need to render the tissue receptive to the proposed stains. All fixatives cause tissue shrinkage to a greater or lesser extent, and with the removal of water in later stages of processing there can be as much as a 50% reduction in volume; this needs to be borne in mind when measurements are made on processed tissue.

Several fixative mixtures are based on formaldehyde, which is a colourless gas, very

(A)

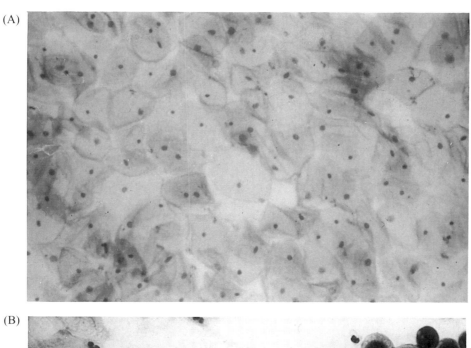

(B)

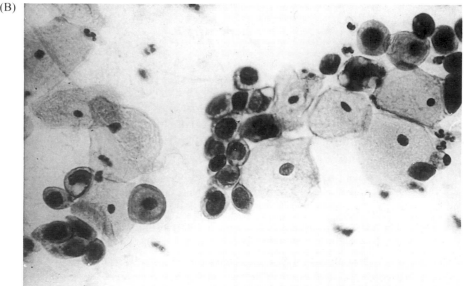

Fig. 1.8 (A) Superficial squamous (scale-like) cells from a cervical smear of normal uterine cervix having typical pyknotic (shrunken) nuclei and a very low nuclear:cytoplasmic ratio. By contrast (B) in a case of cervical intraepithelial neoplasia (see also Fig. 4.2) many of the cells have not differentiated into squamous cells, but have remained small with a high nuclear: cytoplasmic ratio, often with irregular nuclear shapes (nuclear pleomorphism) – features of neoplastic cells. (See Chapter 4, section 4.7 and Fig. 4.18.)

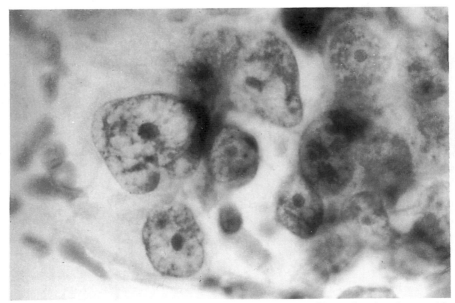

Fig. 1.9 A fine needle aspiration cytology specimen of lung tissue, illustrating the pleomorphic nuclei of a large cell anaplastic lung carcinoma. (Kindly supplied by Ian Phillips, Cytology Department, Hammersmith Hospital.)

soluble in water and generally used as a 4% aqueous solution. The word 'formalin' is used for the commercial saturated solution of formaldehyde in water which is approximately 40% weight/volume (w/v); the working solution is thus 10% formalin. Neutral buffered formalin is the most commonly used fixative in pathology laboratories because of its wide-range applicability and low cost. Tissue from archives very many years old can always be referred back to, and because formalin is cheap, reference material as big as whole organs (or bodies) can be preserved for museums. The chemical properties of neutral buffered formalin mean that treated tissue is suitable for dissection even after fixation and it is the only fixative that will accept many of the silver impregnation stains so useful, for example, for neurones and their processes.

Except for frozen samples (see below), fixed tissue needs to be embedded in a rigid block to render it amenable to sectioning. For light microscopy the most common medium is paraffin wax, although some synthetic resins, such as the methacrylates, are commonly employed. Whichever medium is to form the block, the tissue has to be *dehydrated* to accept impregnation by the liquid embedding medium, which then solidifies into its final form. Tissue sections are cut on a microtome and the sections are collected on glass slides – wax sections usually have a thickness of 5 μm.

In certain circumstances instead of fixing and embedding tissue, preservation and sectioning can be achieved by freezing tissue blocks. This is the method of choice for very rapid assessment of biopsies during surgery, and also for the preservation of labile antigens. Frozen sections are cut on a cryotome, essentially a microtome permanently mounted inside a freezing cabinet. Although excellent preservation can be obtained with care, frozen sections are generally of poorer quality than those from fixed and embedded tissue.

To examine the tissue microscopically it has to be stained. Tissue staining is performed in stages, first involving removal of wax from the section on the glass slide by an appropriate solvent. This is necessary because wax is immiscible with aqueous solutions. Then water is introduced gently into the sections through a series of graded alcohols, without this, tissue architecture would become distorted. The process of tissue rehydration is generally referred to as 'taking down to water'. The routine examination of sections is normally accomplished after staining with the combination of *haematoxylin* and *eosin* dyes (H&E).

Haematoxylin is a cationic dye, behaving as positively charged dye ions and reacting with negatively charged tissue groups, imparting a blue/purple colouration to the 'basophilic' components. Nucleic acids, both DNA and RNA, are the principal basophilic cell constituents, hence nuclei and ribosome-rich areas are prominently stained (Fig. 1.10 A, B, C). Eosin, however, is an anionic dye acting as negatively charged dye ions which react with positively charged tissue constituents. 'Acidophilic' components stain varying shades of orange to red, and include cytoplasmic proteins, abundant extracellular proteins like collagen, the haemoglobin in red blood cells and mitochondria; hence the strong staining of muscle cells (Fig. 1.10B).

Though much of diagnostic histopathology requires only H&E stained tissue sections, the science of *immunocytochemistry*, developed over the past 50 years, has revolutionized the field. Immunocytochemistry is the use of labelled antibodies as specific reagents for the localization of tissue constituents, and its application has removed much of the uncertainty from diagnosis which relied on special stains and 'educated guesswork'; antigen–antibody reactions are absolutely specific so positive identification of tissue constituents can be achieved. Of course, like any technique, false negatives and false positives through inadequate precautions must be guarded against.

Immunocytochemistry plays a vital role in diagnostic tumour pathology in circumstances where morphology alone cannot reliably be used to infer the tissue of origin, or, for example, where the identity of a secreted hormone is unknown. In addition, immunocytochemistry plays a vital role in understanding the biology of neoplastic growth, and the technique has been applied to examining all facets of cell behaviour: the expression of transcription factors, growth factors and their receptors, cell adhesion molecules and measurement of proliferation.

The use of immunocytochemistry enables the localization of the antigen of interest in cytological material as well as in histological sections at both light and electron microscope levels. Antigens are usually demonstrated by an *indirect technique* (Fig. 1.11), the simplest of which involves the use of a *primary antibody* to detect the antigen of interest, and then a labelled *secondary antibody* to detect the primary. The label conjugated to the secondary antibody can be a fluorescent marker such as fluorescein isothiocyanate, which can then be visualized by fluorescence microscopy. More commonly, the label is an enzyme, usually horseradish peroxidase, which is demonstrable by its ability to reduce H_2O_2 to water in the presence of an electron donor.

The electron donor is commonly diaminobenzidine, which is oxidized to a coloured final reaction product which is an insoluble precipitate that survives long-term storage (Fig. 1.12).

Many modifications to these relatively simple procedures have evolved in order to improve the sensitivity of the immunostaining, i.e. bind more marker enzyme to each primary antigen site. Avidin/biotin techniques are the most sensitive methods of this genre. These substances are both naturally occurring components of egg which have a great affinity for each other, with avidin, a large basic glycoprotein from egg white, having four high affinity biotin binding sites, biotin being a vitamin found in egg yolk,

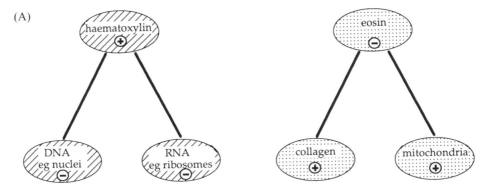

Fig. 1.10 (A) The principle of haematoxylin and eosin staining resulting from electrostatic binding. (B) Nucleic acids are basophilic, staining blue/purple (dark staining) as seen in nuclei, whereas muscle cells (M) and red blood cells (RBC) are intensely eosinophilic staining orange/red. (C) *opposite* The RNA-rich perinuclear cytoplasm (arrows) of neurones is also intensely basophilic.

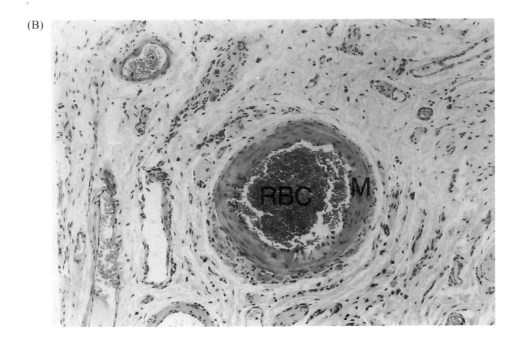

thus adding greater sensitivity over simple indirect methods. Both can be conjugated to antibodies, peroxidase or fluorescent markers but the most common technique is that of the ABC technique (*a*vidin/*b*iotin *c*omplex) in which the secondary antibody is labelled with biotin and this is recognized by an avidin/peroxidase complex final layer (Fig. 1.13). Streptavidin, a 60 kDa protein (also with four biotin-binding sites) from the bacterium *Streptomyces avidinii* is often used in place of avidin. Streptavidin reduces background staining because its near neutral isoelectric point eliminates electrostatic binding, and in addition, its absence of carbohydrate side-chains ensures it does not bind to tissue lectins.

At electron microscope level simple indirect techniques are generally used. The primary antibody is applied and this is followed by either a peroxidase conjugate (which is then rendered electron dense by osmication) or a colloidal gold conjugated secondary antibody. Colloidal gold is available in a variety of particle sizes from 1 nm to 40 nm, the most convenient being in the 10–20 nm range. Colloidal gold is preferred to peroxidase when the antigen of interest is localized to already electron-dense structures such as the endocrine granules of endocrine cell tumours (Fig. 1.14).

Lectins are proteins or glycoproteins frequently of plant origin, used to localize carbohydrates; in nature they may be concerned with the recognition of host plant roots by symbiotic bacteria. Specificity and binding of lectins is not an immune process, but because each lectin specifically recognizes a certain carbohydrate moiety they can be used as accurate markers. A lectin in common use is *Ulex europaeus* agglutinin (UEA 1), which recognizes α-L-fructose and binds to terminal fucosyl groups linked to certain oligosaccharides. It agglutinates erythrocytes of blood group

(C)

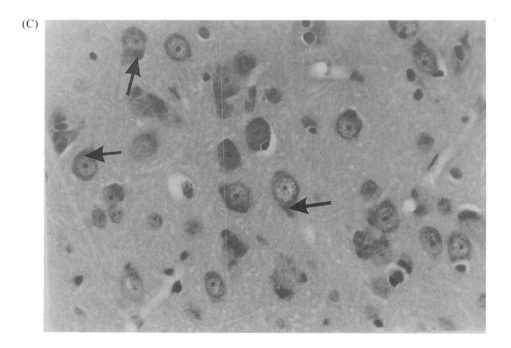

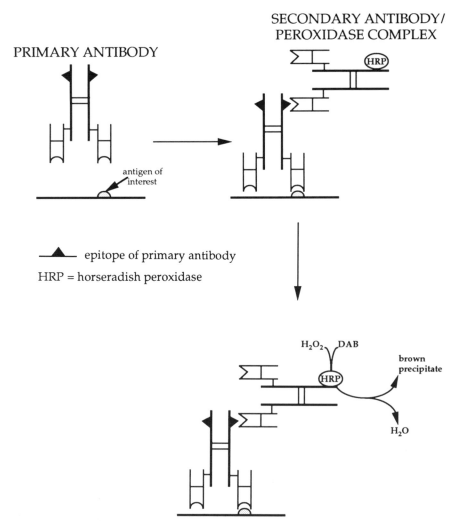

Fig. 1.11 The principle of immunocytochemistry using a simple indirect technique, with the secondary antibody conjugated to horseradish peroxidase (HRP). HRP has the ability to reduce hydrogen peroxide to water in the presence of an electron donor such as diaminobenzidine (DAB), forming a brown-coloured final reaction product.

O as they contain α-fucosyl groups, and similarly has an affinity for such carbohydrates associated with endothelial cells and some tumours, particularly those associated with the vascular endothelium such as angiosarcomas. Lectins are multivalent, so in addition to the carbohydrate they identify, they can be bound to a label such as biotin which can then be visualized by an avidin–biotin–peroxidase complex.

The demonstration of the presence of a polypeptide antigen in a tissue or cell by immunocytochemistry imparts no definitive information about the processes that have lead to its synthesis. Hybridization is the technique by which specific sequences of DNA and RNA can be identified by matching them up to complementary labelled 'probes'. In fact

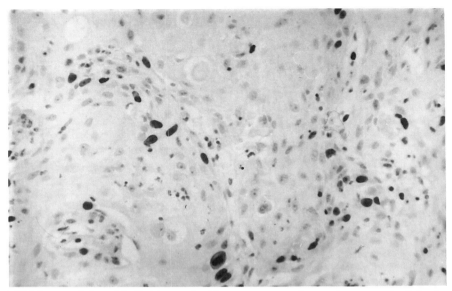

Fig. 1.12 Many nuclei are labelled brown in this squamous carcinoma, immunostained for the presence of the proliferation-associated Ki-67 antigen using the MIB1 (Molecular Immunology Borstel) antibody. (See Chapter 5, section 5.1.)

each type of macromolecule (DNA, RNA and protein) can be analyzed in two ways, either directly in tissue sections (immunocytochemistry or *in situ* hybridization) or after extraction from the tissues. In the latter, tissue can be homogenized, macromolecules extracted and then separated according to molecular weight by electrophoresis through a gel. Genomic DNA is much too large to migrate through an agarose gel, and is therefore cleaved with restriction enzymes before separation. The size-fractionated material is then transferred to a membrane support, often by capillary action, hence the term 'blotting', and finally the target molecule is detected by exposing the membrane to the labelled probe, or antibody if proteins are being analyzed. Analysis of DNA in this way is called *Southern* blotting (after its inventor, see Fig. 3.12), while detection of RNA and protein are referred to as Northern and Western blotting respectively. We have already discussed the localization of proteins in tissue sections using immunocytochemistry, while the procedure for the detection of DNA or RNA in tissue sections is termed *in situ* hybridization. In this way gene sequences, particularly viral DNA sequences, and gene expression can be assessed and related to their protein products and other topographical information. A 'hybridization probe' is the general term for a complementary nucleic acid; they are commonly radiolabelled with ^{32}P or ^{35}S and detected by autoradiography (Fig. 1.15A, B). Alternatively, probes can be 'non-isotopically' labelled with substances such as digoxigenin, which is then detected using typical immunocytochemical procedures beginning with an anti-digoxigenin antibody. The methodology is considerably more technically demanding than immunocytochemistry, particularly because mRNA is notoriously labile, being easily degraded through fixation delay and the ubiquity of RNases. Thus its application to the study of neoplasia has so far been more at the level

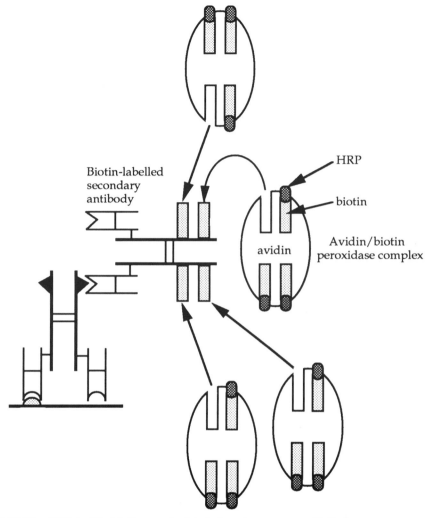

Fig. 1.13 The ABC (avidin/biotin complex) technique improves sensitivity because many more molecules of peroxidase can be bound for each bound antibody molecule. The second layer antibody has a number of attached biotin molecules (in this case four), while each avidin molecule has three of its four biotin binding sites already taken up with horseradish peroxidase (HRP)-labelled biotin. The biotin of the second layer antibody fills the vacancy.

of tumour behaviour (synthesis of growth factors, cell adhesion molecules, etc.) rather than in diagnosis.

So far we have discussed imaging techniques, in which, after suitable processing, the results are visible to either the naked eye or through light microscopy. To be able to see subcellular detail of tissues one has to use an *electron microscope (EM)*; the important property of the electron microscope is the vast improvement possible in *resolution* of detail, over that of the light microscope. When a structure is illuminated by light, the smallest resolvable detail is governed by the wavelength of the illuminat-

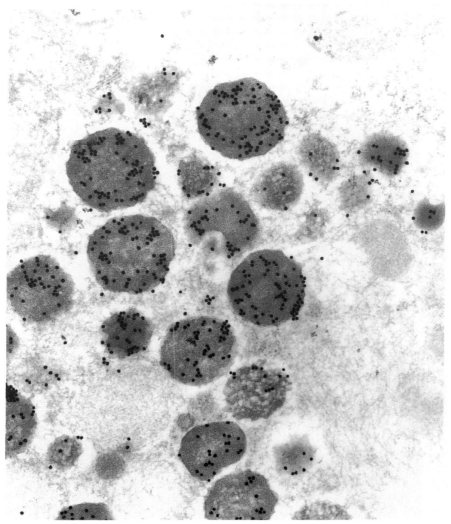

Fig. 1.14 Immunolabelling at the electron microscope level – a gold-labelled secondary antibody pinpoints the localization of somatostatin immunoreactivity in the cytoplasmic granules of this somatostatinoma.

ing beam and the refractive index of the medium that the beam has to pass through from the specimen. Clearly, for normal light microscopy the beam is white light from an element and the medium is air: even at light microscope level improved resolution is commonly obtained by using shorter wavelength ultraviolet light and/or changing the medium to oil. By extrapolation, the shortest possible wavelength will be the most advantageous one to use. Electrons are negatively charged particles, but when travelling in a beam their properties approximate those of electromagnetic waves, with their equivalent wavelength inversely proportional to the energy of the electrons (the higher the voltage at which the electrons are produced, the higher their energy). Electrons produced at high voltage are equivalent to very short wavelength irradiation, thus,

(A)

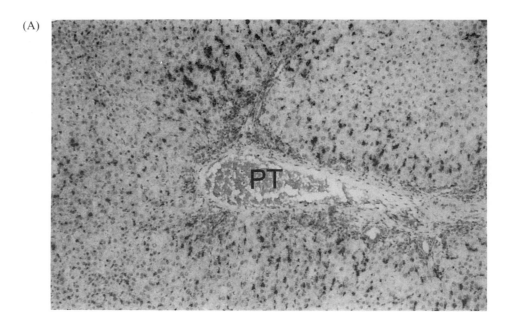

(B)

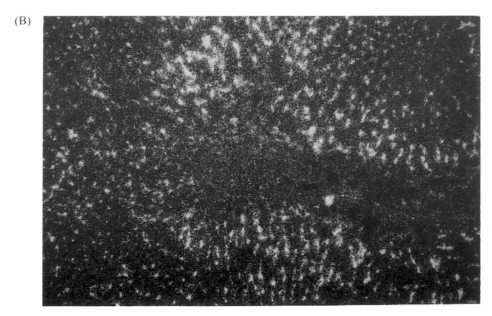

Fig. 1.15 Expression of hepatocyte growth factor (HGF) mRNA by sinusoid-lining cells in the liver detected by *in situ* hybridization and autoradiography after incubation of the tissue section with a ^{35}S-labelled RNA probe complementary to HGF mRNA. The autoradiograph can be viewed by either bright-field illumination (A) in which case the light source illuminates the section from beneath and the silver grains in the emulsion appear black, or, alternatively (B) by dark-field illumination, for which the light source shines down on the autoradiograph and the black silver grains reflect light towards the observer (camera). The labelled cells in (A) are sinusoidal-lining cells crowded around a portal tract (PT).

when they are used as the source of illumination very fine structures are resolvable. The wave-like properties of an electron beam plus their propagation across an evacuated medium are both used to produce high resolution images in the electron microscope.

Broadly, there are two types of EM, the scanning electron microscope (SEM) and the transmission electron microscope (TEM), though only the TEM is used in tumour diagnosis. Figure 1.16 (C) illustrates how electron microscopy improves on light microscopy (Fig 1.16A, B) for the observation of fine, subcellular detail. In the case of undifferentiated tumours, a distinction has to be made between tumours of epithelial origin (*carcinomas*) and those of connective tissue origin (*sarcomas*): the characteristic cell junction of epithelial cells is the desmosome, and these are not found on connective tissue cells (Fig. 1.17A, B). Desmosomes are not the only plasma membrane adaptations that aid in diagnosis of tumours. Mesotheliomas, for example are tumours, often occurring in the lung, that arise in response to asbestos damage; at light microscope level or low power EM they also tend to look rather undifferentiated (Fig. 1.18A), but at higher magnification (Fig. 1.18B) it can be seen that these tumour cells bear characteristic long surface microvilli which are diagnostic of this tumour type. Normal cells have organelles that are morphologically recognizable and are fundamentally related to the cells‘ function; in tumours, typical organelles may be retained to some extent even when other features are lost. In the case of the frequently very aggressive malignant tumour of skeletal muscle, the rhabdomyosarcoma, cells may bear little resemblance to skeletal muscle, but subcellularly the vestiges of ‘thick and thin’ cytoplasmic filaments can remain (Fig. 1.18C). The oncocytoma is a benign tumour, frequently of the kidney. Cells are typically packed with mitochondria but at light microscope level these are not visible, although they render cytoplasm highly eosinophilic. At EM level the organelles are easily distinguishable (Fig. 1.18D), and thus the diagnosis can be made. These are two examples where the presence of specific organelles can be diagnostic; tumours of many other specific organelle-bearing cells can be identified in this way, for example melanomas (melanocytes), angiosarcomas (Weibel-Palade bodies), and histiocytomas (Birbeck granules).

Cells of the neuroendocrine system store their hormones in granules; tumours of this system tend to retain this ability to some extent. Some granules have specific shapes which may be of help in diagnosis (Fig. 1.19A, B), but in other cases immunocytochemistry is required to reach a diagnosis (see Fig. 1.14).

1.3 Tumour classification

Introduction

Why do we bother to classify tumours? Well, if all tumours behaved in the same way, were equally life-threatening and could all be treated by the same cocktail of drugs and/or irradiation, then there would, indeed, be little purpose to the exercise. However, tumours from one tissue behave patently differently from those arising in another. Patients with liver and pancreatic cancers unfortunately have a grim outlook;

(A)

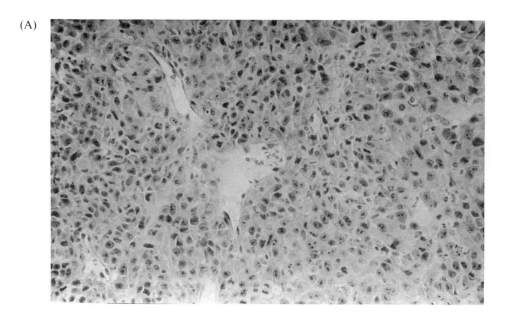

(B)

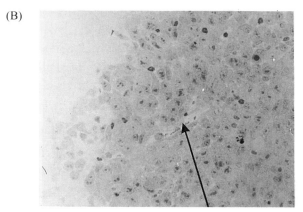

even in the USA less then 5% of sufferers of these are alive 5 years after diagnosis. However, the *relative 5-year survival rate* for thyroid and testicular cancers is in excess of 90%. Such a spectacular difference highlights the need to pinpoint the origin of the primary tumour, but we must add the caveat that differences are not solely attributable to the relative aggressiveness (local growth and metastatic ability) of the tumour types. Sensitivity to the various treatment modalities will vary, and more importantly, some deep-seated cancers will have reached an advanced stage of growth when they are detected clinically, whereas superficial cancers, e.g. those of the skin, have a much better chance of being detected during their earliest stages of development. Survival figures for most cancers are greatly affected by the extent of disease

(C)

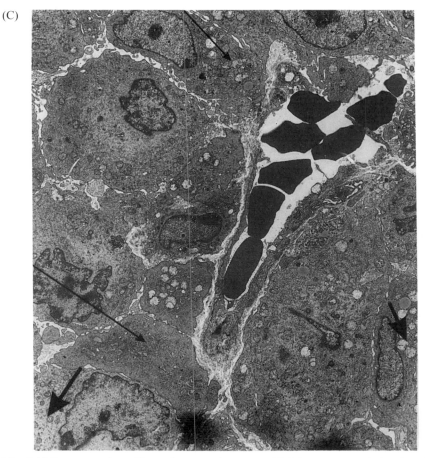

Fig. 1.16 Demonstration of how electron microscopy (EM) improves resolution in microscopy and thus enables more information to be gleaned from higher magnification micrographs. (A) Is a light microscopic view of a round cell sarcoma in which little cytoplasmic detail can be discerned, whereas (B) is a light microscopic view of a resin-embedded section from an EM block of the same tumour. The blood vessel (arrowed) is the same as that featured in (C). (C) An electron micrograph of the same cells as illustrated in (B), showing a wealth of subcellular detail such as mitochondria (thick arrows) and endoplasmic reticulum (thin arrows).

at the time of detection, suggesting major improvements in overall cancer survival can be achieved through developing techniques enabling earlier detection.

Identification of common properties between individual tumours is invaluable in being able to predict future development and *prognosis* – patient survival. Aetiology, behaviour, histology and immunophenotype *superficially* would all seem equally helpful. Aetiological considerations (concerning the causative agent of the neoplasm) however, are not appropriate means of classification, as identical lesions can be caused by

(A)

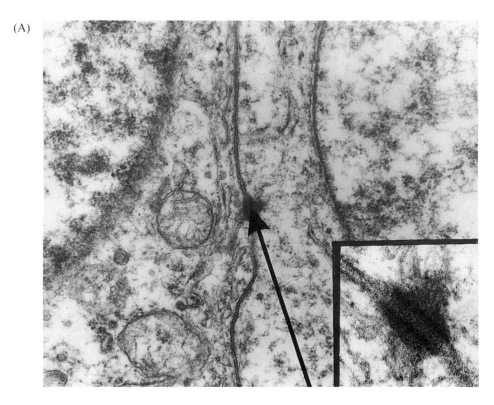

different means. For example, squamous carcinoma of the skin can arise after exposure to agents as varied as UV light, X-rays, contact with arsenic, contact with certain hydrocarbons and a wide range of other chemicals.

Behaviouristic classification

Broadly speaking the greatest distinction of tumour types is between benign and malignant tumours; this is a fundamental difference in tumour state. Benign tumours are generally slow growing expansive masses, often with a 'pushing margin', and enclosed within a fibrous capsule. Malignant tumours, are usually rapidly growing, invading local tissue (infiltrative growth pattern) and spreading to distant sites – metastasizing. Truly benign tumours exist (e.g. papillomas – benign surface epithelial tumours), as do incontrovertibly malignant ones (e.g. carcinomas – malignant tumours of epithelial tissues). However, there are benign tumours that predispose to malignancy (e.g. adenomas of the large intestine), and there are some *in situ* carcinomas that progress so slowly that they may never achieve malignancy (e.g. some *in situ* carcinomas of the uterine cervix); thus, a spectrum of types of tumour behaviour exists. The ability of a tumour to metastasize from its site of origin (the primary tumour) to form a tumour (the secondary tumour) at a distant site, is unequivocal evidence of malignancy.

(B)

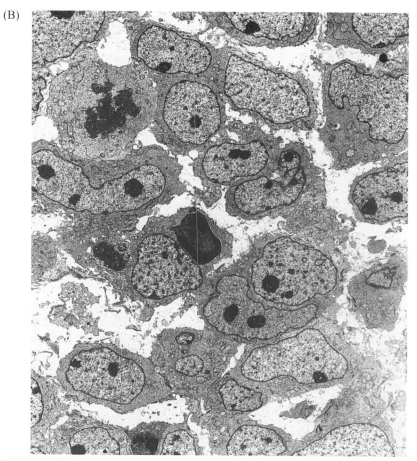

Fig. 1.17 (A) Electron micrograph illustrating an anaplastic (see Chapter 6, section 6.2) carcinoma of the pancreas indicating its epithelial origin by the presence of a desmosome (arrow). Inset: a higher power view of a single desmosome. (B) Low power electron micrograph of a sarcoma. Although the cells are closely apposed there are no junctional complexes.

Histogenetic classification

The most useful way of classifying tumours is according to the tissue of origin and cell type involved. A tumour forming thyroid-like vesicles and secreting thyroglobulin presents no problems and can be recognized as derived from thyroid tissue, and can be expected to produce characteristic symptoms and behave in a predictable fashion. Alternatively, some tumour cells grow in such a way that they bear no resemblance to any structure or cell type. Such *anaplastic* tumours require more detailed investigation to discover their histogenesis. A further problem is that sometimes a tumour resembles tissue which is not normally present at the site of origin. A classical example of this is squamous carcinoma of the lung, which probably arises from metaplastic squamous epithelia in the conducting airways.

The suffix *-oma* usually indicates a benign tumour, but there are exceptions to this rule. For example, myelomas and lymphomas are malignant tumours of plasma cells

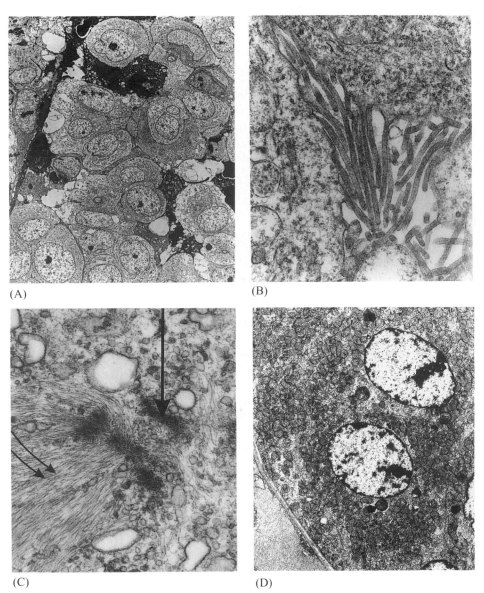

Fig. 1.18 The value of organelle identification in tumour diagnosis. (A) Low power electron micrograph of a mesothelioma in which the cells appear to have few distinguishing (diagnostic) features, but at higher power (B) it can be seen that the cells have the long microvilli diagnostic of mesothelioma. (C) High power electron micrograph of the cytoplasm of a rhabdomyosarcoma cell showing the disorganized thick (thick arrow) and thin (thin arrows) filaments which are diagnostic for skeletal muscle tumours. (D) Low power electron micrograph of an oncocytoma illustrating that the cells are packed with mitochondria.

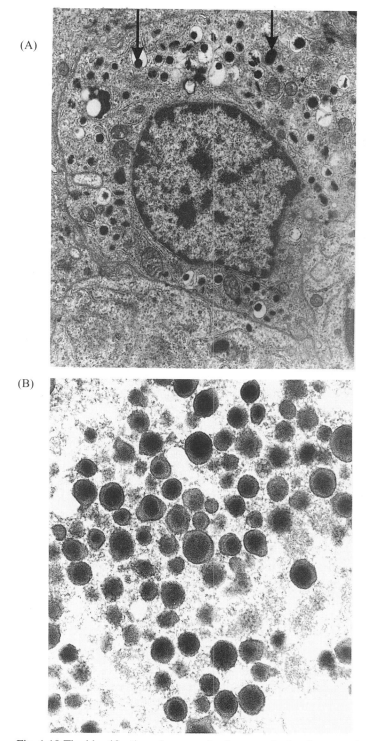

Fig. 1.19 The identification of neuroendocrine granules by electron microscopy. (A) Low power electron micrograph of an insulinoma cell with typical membrane-bound granules which have an eccentric dense core (arrows). (B) High power electron micrograph of the cytoplasm of a glucagonoma cell illustrating the granules with a large dense core surrounded by a penumbra.

Table 1.1. *Histogenetic classification of benign tumours*

Normal tissue	Benign tumour arising
Glandular epithelium	Adenoma
Surface epithelium	Papilloma
Fibroblasts	Fibroma
Cartilage	Chondroma
Striated muscle	Rhabdomyoma
Smooth muscle	Leiomyoma
Blood vessels	Haemangioma
Fat	Lipoma
Bone	Osteoma
Liver	Hepatoma

and lymphoid tissue, respectively, while other lesions ending in the suffix -oma, e.g. granulomas, are not tumours at all but are collections of macrophages formed in response to certain infectious agents. Examples of benign tumour nomenclature are given above in Table 1.1.

The names of malignant tumours, with several notable exceptions, are compiled by the name of the tissue with the suffix of the appropriate malignant tumour, e.g. malignant tumours of bone are *osteo*sarcomas and malignant tumours of the colonic epithelium are colonic *adeno*carcinomas (Table 1.2).

As one can readily appreciate, the status of tumour classification is hardly satisfactory, with a collection of eponymous (Hodgkin's disease), archaic (phaeochromocytoma – adrenal medulla) and downright misleading terms (a myeloma is malignant and not from granulocytes) tacked on to the histogenetic framework. Further problems occur, for example, in the classification of tumours of the neuroendocrine system. The neuroendocrine system comprises all those cells which store polypeptide hormones, biogenic amines (adrenaline and noradrenaline) or serotonin (5-hydroxytryptamine) in granules, and includes the endocrine cells of the pituitary gland, thyroid (parafollicular cells), pancreas and adrenal medulla. Also included in this system are the cells of the *diffuse neuroendocrine system* (DNES) which is a network of scattered endocrine cells chiefly found throughout the gastrointestinal, respiratory and genitourinary tracts, and cardiovascular systems. All of these cells probably have the potential for malignant behaviour, but their lack of cellular atypia (when viewed under the light microscope) and little mitotic activity makes the distinction between benign and malignant difficult to determine on purely histopathological grounds. Of course, the assessment of malignancy is straightforward if there is clearcut evidence of tumour infiltration into neighbouring tissue, or with the presence of metastases. Neuroendocrine tumours are usually classified in a functional manner according to the major active regulatory peptide which is responsible for their clinical manifestation (Table 1.3).

Most tumours of the diffuse neuroendocrine system originate in the gastrointestinal tract, pancreas and tracheo-bronchial tree, but also included in this group are the

Table 1.2. *Histogenetic classification of malignant tumours*

Normal tissue	Malignant tumour arising
Epithelium	Carcinoma
Connective tissue	Sarcoma
Bone marrow	Leukaemia
More specifically:	
Glandular epithelium	Adenocarcinoma
Squamous epithelium	Squamous carcinoma
Fibroblasts	Fibrosarcoma
Cartilage	Chondrosarcoma
Striated muscle	Rhabdomyosarcoma
Smooth muscle	Leiomyosarcoma
Endothelium	Angiosarcoma
Fat	Liposarcoma
Bone	Osteosarcoma
Liver	Hepatocellular carcinoma
Some malignant tumours with atypical names:	
Skin – melanocytes	Malignant melanoma
Fibroblast/histiocyte	Malignant fibrous histiocytoma
Myeloid stem cells	Myeloid leukaemia
Plasma cells	Multiple myeloma
Lymphoid tissue	Lymphoma/Hodgkin's disease
Sympathetic neurones (neuroblasts)	Neuroblastoma
? Endothelium	Kaposi's sarcoma
Embryonal kidney	Nephroblastoma
Embryonal retina	Retinoblastoma
Gonad (male germ cells)	Seminoma
Gonad (female germ cells)	Dysgerminoma
Germ cells	Malignant teratoma

carcinoid tumours, a term originally used to describe tumours with a 'carcinoma-like' (i.e. sheets of cells) structure. However, the name then became associated with tumours producing and releasing serotonin, which was responsible for the clinical features of tachycardia, sweating, skin flushing and diarrhoea. Not all tumours with this morphology, though, produce serotonin, so they are better simply placed under the general umbrella of neuroendocrine tumours. It is also worth remembering that circulating levels of active peptides can be elevated due to other causes, e.g. hyper-gastrinaemia can result from a drug-induced blockade of gastric acid secretion in the treatment of peptic ulcer disease.

Tumours of a mixed cell phenotype have, in the past, been difficult to classify histogenetically. Pleomorphic tumours of salivary glands contain an admixture of ductal epithelial cells and myoepithelial cells, but are now believed to arise from a single cell type, the intercalated duct cell which is probably a multipotential stem cell for the salivary gland, and not from two independent cell types. Teratomas can be composed of tissues typical of ectoderm, mesoderm and endoderm, but are now

Table 1.3. *Classification of some neuroendocrine tumours*

Neuroendocrine tumour	A common clinical symptom
Pituitary adenomas	
GH-producing	Acromegaly
Prolactinoma	Amenorrhea
Corticotrophic adenoma	Cushing's syndrome
Thyrotrophic cell adenoma	Hyperthyroidism
Null tumours (endocrinologically silent)	Space occupying, e.g. compression of optic nerve
Plurihormonal tumours	Often GH and prolactin
Thyroid C cells	
Medullary carcinoma	Hypercalcitoninaemia
Adrenal medulla	
Phaeochromocytoma (usually benign)	Sustained hypertension with paroxysms
Gastrointestinal tract and pancreas	
	Commonly hypersecretion of active regulatory peptide
Insulinoma	Hypoglycaemia
Gastrinoma	Extensive peptic ulceration of the upper gastrointestinal tract
Somatostatinoma	Diabetes mellitus
VIPoma	Watery diarrhoea
Glucagonoma	Skin rash (necrolytic migratory erythema)
Carcinoids	Skin flushing

considered to be of germ cell origin rather than from a totipotent stem cell which has escaped the influence of organizers in the embryo.

Immunocytochemistry in tumour diagnosis

Presentation of certain antigens (immunophenotype) can be indicative of histogenesis and when a tumour is poorly differentiated it may be essential to correctly determine the tumour's origin. It is of particular use, for example, when a poorly differentiated metastasis is the only symptom of a cryptic primary tumour. Recognition of immuno-phenotypes depends on the preservation of immuno-characteristics of the progenitor tissue in the neoplastic one. The presence of specific antigens can be revealed both at light and electron microscope levels with the powerful techniques of immunocytoch-emistry. In the purest sense, *tumour markers* do not exist for histopathological use, but a wide range of monoclonal and polyclonal antibodies is commercially available which react with antigens which are products of embryonic and adult tissue differen-tiation. Perhaps the most obvious examples are the hormones produced by endocrine tumours, thus secondary tumours having either immunoreactive thyroglobulin or calci-tonin could reasonably be expected to have originated in the thyroid gland. Even the presence of hormone has to be interpreted with caution, since some tumours, e.g. small cell lung carcinoma, produce a hormone (adrenocorticotrophic hormone, ACTH)

Table 1.4. *Products of cell differentiation that can be detected by immunocytochemistry and which are useful in tumour diagnosis*

Product	Cell type recognized	Often markers for
Intermediate filament		
Cytokeratins	Epithelial cells	Carcinomas, mesotheliomas
Vimentin	Mesenchymal cells	Mesenchymal tumours, lymphomas
Desmin	Muscle cells	Smooth and striated muscle tumours
Neurofilaments	Neural cells	Neural tumours
Glial fibrillary acidic protein	Glial cells	Gliomas
Tissue specific proteins		
S-100	Ubiquitous	Gliomas, schwannomas melanomas
Prostatic acid phosphatase	Prostatic epithelia	Prostate tumours
Factor VIII-related antigen	Endothelial cells	Angiosarcoma
Alpha-foetoprotein	Foetal or regenerating hepatocytes	Hepatocellular carcinoma
Myoglobin	Striated muscle	Striated muscle tumours
CEA	Various epithelia	? colonic adenocarcinomas
hCG	Syncytiotrophoblastic cells	Trophoblastic tumours and tumours of germ cells
Neurone-specific enolase	Various, especially endrocine cells	Endocrine neoplasms
Chromogranin	Endocrine cells	Endocrine neoplasms
Thyroglobulin	Thyroid follicular cells	Thyroid carcinomas
Calcitonin	C cells of thyroid	Medullary carcinoma of thyroid
Leukocyte common antigen	All leukocytes	Most leukocyte malignancies
Pituitary hormones	Appropriate pituitary cell	Corresponding adenoma
Hormones of DNES	Appropriate cell	Corresponding tumour

Table 1.4 lists some of the more common tumour markers. They are, of course, expressed by normal cells as well as by their benign or malignant counterparts. In addition, each indicated tumour may or may not express the particular antigen.

not normally associated with the tissue of origin of the tumour – this is called *ectopic hormone production*. Some of the cell products (antigens) which can be detected immunocytochemically and are useful in the diagnosis of hitherto unclassifiable tumours are listed in Table 1.4.

The intermediate filaments are a group of intracellular proteins visible as cytoskeletal elements, approximately 10 nm in diameter and midway in size between microtubules and the actin and myosin microfilaments, that illustrate clearly the problems in the use of differentiation markers for the classification of tumours. It was originally hoped that neoplasms would maintain the intermediate filament type of their tissue of origin, regardless of the degree of differentiation of the tumour. Unfortunately this is not the case, with much overlap of intermediate filament types, some cells co-expressing two different types. Thus, intermediate filament typing alone is not a reliable way of determining histogenesis, particularly in the very area it is needed, the differential diagnosis of anaplastic tumours. Having said this, *cytokeratins* are almost exclusive to epithelial cell tumours, thus tumours such as undifferentiated carcinomas and large cell lymphomas, which might bear a superficial resemblance, can be distinguished from each other. The commonest tumours in the liver are derived from either hepatocytes or biliary cells, however, though both cell types express cytokeratins 8 and 18, biliary cells additionally express cytokeratins 7 and 19 and this property can be exploited to distinguish cholangiocarcinomas from hepatocellular carcinomas (Fig. 1.20A). Vimentin is found in mesenchymal cells such as fibroblasts and macrophages and in endothelial cells, melanocytes and lymphocytes. It is thus, the major intermediate filament seen in most sarcomas and lymphomas. Once again, the diagnostic value of anti-vimentin antibodies is reduced by the expression of vimentin in other cell types; vimentin and cytokeratins are co-expressed in many epithelial lesions, including carcinomas. Desmin characterizes adult smooth as well as cardiac and skeletal muscle. In both types of striated muscle it is located in the Z-line, near the plasma membrane/cell junctions. The use of desmin as a tumour marker is greatest in conjunction with other markers such as vimentin – to distinguish between myogenic (Fig. 1.20B) and non-myogenic sarcomas – and with S-100 (see below) to distinguish between myogenic and neural tumours (often used in the gastrointestinal tract). Glial fibrillary acidic protein (GFAP) and neurofilament proteins are found in glial cells and neurones respectively. In the peripheral nervous system, GFAP has been demonstrated in Schwann cells, enteric glial cells and the satellite cells of sensory ganglia. In neoplasms, GFAP is not specific to glial cells, but in conjunction with other diagnostic information available, it is the most common marker used to identify astrocytes and glial-related neoplasms – astrocytomas and ependymomas.

S-100 protein is a soluble protein widely distributed in different tissues, though it was originally thought to be localized to the nervous system since it was first isolated from bovine brain. It may function as a calcium-binding protein and be involved in cell growth. Despite its broad tissue distribution it does have a use in the differential diagnosis of tumours. One of the most notable applications of S-100 immunostaining is in the evaluation of lesions of melanocytic origin where staining intensity of S-100 is inversely related to the pigmentation of the cells.

Prostatic acid phosphatases (APs) are a family of enzymes catalysing the hydrolysis of monophosphate esters in an acid environment. Blood levels of APs appear to correlate well with disseminated prostatic tumour burden, though non-prostatic sources of AP decrease the specificity of serum AP as a marker for both detecting and assessing prostatic tumour mass. The sites of synthesis of von Willebrand factor, also called factor VIII-related antigen (VIIIR:Ag) are almost exclusively in endothelial cells and megakaryocytes. VIIIR:Ag staining is useful in the diagnosis of angiosarcomas. Another useful marker of angiosarcomas is the antibody to CD31, otherwise known as platelet endothelial cell adhesion molecule-1; some angiosarcomas present no prob-

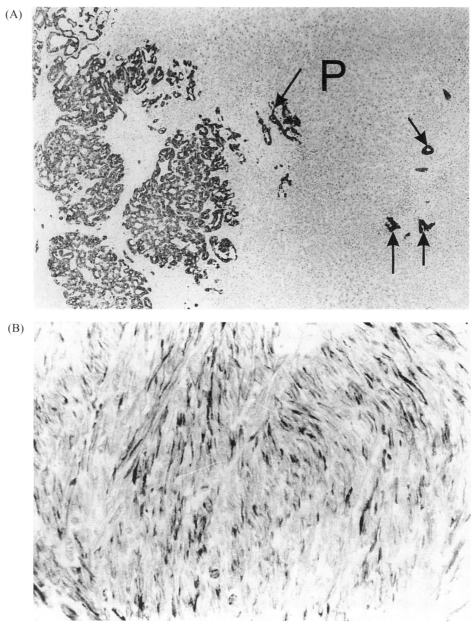

Fig. 1.20 The use of immunocytochemistry in tumour diagnosis. (A) Cytokeratin 19 expression identifies a tumour of biliary epithelium in the liver, where the ribbons of stained cells are in sharp contrast to the unstained parenchymal (P) cells – note staining of normal bile ducts (arrows) in the portal areas. (B) Desmin expression in the cytoplasm of these spindle-shaped cells identifies this as a smooth muscle tumour. *Overleaf* (C) This angiosarcoma is easily recognized by large dysplastic endothelial cells lining vascular channels (arrows), but the tumour cells featured in (D) resemble epithelial cells in that they are closely apposed to each other in a sheet. Some of these cells formed primitive channels and along with prominent membranous expression of CD31 (E) a diagnosis of epithelioid (epithelial-like) angiosarcoma could be made. (Kindly supplied by Dr. Thomas Krausz.) (F) Chromogranin expression (arrows) highlights endocrine cells in a benign biliary tumour.

(C)

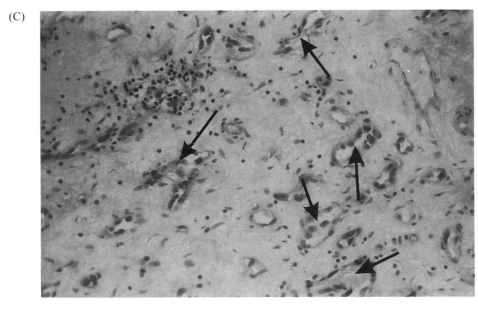

(D)

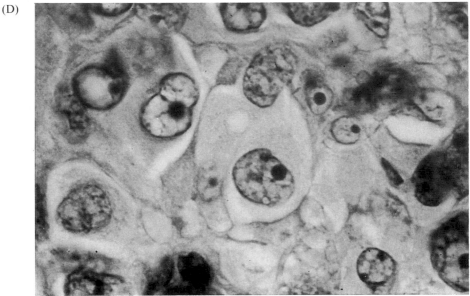

Fig. 1.20 (*cont.*)

lems in recognition (Fig. 1.20C), but some tumours mimic epithelial cells (Fig. 1.20D) and the diagnosis of angiosarcoma is aided by CD31 staining (Fig. 1.20E).

Structurally related to albumin is alpha-foetoprotein (AFP), serum AFP levels are greatest in the foetus and decline with gestational age, being essentially undetectable in adults. Its synthesis is strongly linked to rapid cell turnover, e.g. foetal liver and regenerating liver after injury, and it is heterogeneously expressed by hepatocellular

(E)

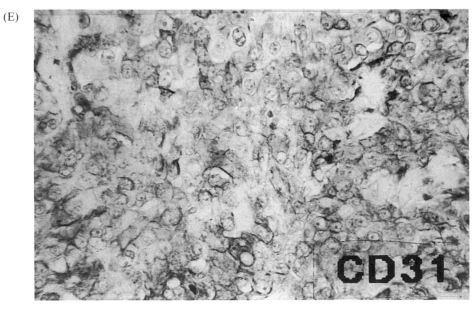

(F)

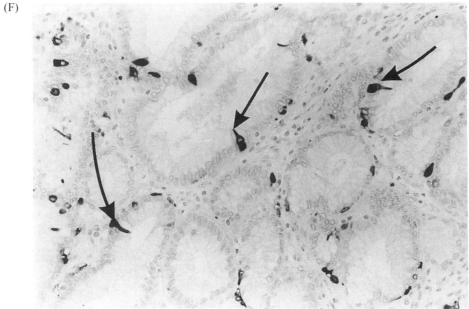

carcinoma cells. Myoglobin is an oxygen transport protein, found exclusively in skeletal muscle, and myoglobin immunoreactivity can confirm skeletal muscle differentiation in otherwise anaplastic tumours.

The pituitary gland, gastrointestinal tract and pancreas have a variety of endocrine cells that can be the progenitor tissues of tumours. Many of these tumours display little cellular atypia and scarce mitotic activity. However, at light microscope level such tumours can be classified by using immunocytochemical methods with antibodies raised to the hormones that the tumours are suspected of producing, although on occasion the tumour cells can in fact produce more than one hormone. For example, ACTH-producing tumours can also synthesize β-lipotropin, α-melanocyte stimulating hormone (α-MSH), endorphins and enkephalins, and this is not really surprising since all these peptides are derived from a common precursor, proopiomelanocortin. There are some other more general markers of endocrine differentiation useful in tumour diagnosis. Neurone specific enolase (NSE) is operationally a family of homodimeric and heterodimeric isoenzymes, which are expressed by many cells, particularly endo-crine cells. Likewise, chromogranins, a group of acidic glycoproteins, implicated in endocrine granule packaging and calcium homeostasis, are useful in highlighting endo-crine cells (Fig. 1.20F).

Carcinoembryonic antigen (CEA) is another diagnostically helpful although not necessarily pathognomonic marker, being one of a family of epithelial cell membrane glycoproteins, belonging to the Ig superfamily of cell adhesion molecules (see Fig. 4.7), and was initially identified in colonic carcinomas. However, CEA has been shown to be produced at various sites, and to be present in the serum of patients who do not have cancer. It can be of use when assessed with caution in people with a high risk of developing gastrointestinal and related cancers. Human chorionic gonado-trophin is normally found in plasma during pregnancy, but otherwise is associated with the presence of trophoblastic tumours and tumours of germ cells, and is of par-ticular value in monitoring the success of therapy in these conditions. One of the most widely employed immunocytochemical markers is leukocyte common antigen (CD45), and this recognizes about 95% of all lymphomas.

1.4   Further reading

Filipe, M. I. & Lake, B. D. (1990). *Histochemistry in Pathology*, 2nd edn. Edinburgh: Churchill Livingstone.

Ghadially, F. N. (1982). *Ultrastructural Pathology of the Cell and Matrix*, 2nd edn. London: Butterworths.

Grainger, R.G., Allison, D.J., Margulis, A.R. & Steiner, R.E. (1992). *Diagnostic Radiology. An Anglo-American Textbook of Imaging*. Edinburgh: Churchill Livingstone.

Meredith, W.J. & Massey, J.B. (1977). *Fundamental Physics of Radiobiology*. Bristol: John Wright & Sons Ltd.

Polak, J.M. & Van Noorden, S. (1992). *An Introduction to Immunocytochemistry: Current Techniques and Problems*. Oxford: Oxford Science Publications.

Souhami, R. & Tobias, J. (1995). *Cancer and its Management*, 2nd edn. Oxford: Blackwells Science Ltd.

True, D.L. (1990). *Atlas of Diagnostic Immunopathology*. New York: Gower Medical Publishing.

2

The causes of cancer

2.1 Age distribution

There is now overwhelming proof that cancer is basically a genetic disease, but there are two key differences between it and the other genetic diseases. First, cancer is generally caused by *somatic* mutations, whereas other genetic diseases arise as a result of *germ-line* mutations, although a sizeable minority (~5%) of cancers do arise because of germ-line mutations (see Chapter 3). Second, each individual cancer appears to arise, not from a single mutation, but from several sequential mutations. This latter fact has crystallized into the *multi-hit* or *multi-stage* theory of carcinogenesis.

A common general feature of carcinogenesis in both humans and experimental studies is that a relatively long time period elapses between the application of a carcinogenic stimulus and the emergence of clinically recognizable cancer. This is known as the latent period and can be anything from a few months to many years. The most likely reason for the latent period is that the carcinogenic agent does not cause cancer in one step, but rather genetically alters a normal cell(s) so that it enjoys a proliferative advantage over its normal neighbours. This altered cell then undergoes clonal expansion driven by mutation, and the resultant cells could in some way be more susceptible to further changes. Accordingly, *one* of these cells later acquires a further mutation allowing its progeny to overgrow its neighbours and perhaps form a small benign tumour. Further phases of clonal expansion and mutation will eventually give rise to a cell with a sufficient number of mutations ('hits') to bestow the malignant phenotype upon cells arising from it, so that they invade surrounding tissue and metastasize to other organs – thus multi-stage carcinogenesis (Fig. 2.1).

If one plots, on a semilog scale, the age distribution of some of the most important cancers (Fig. 2.2A, B, C), then most carcinomas are rare under the age of 30, but then the incidence rate increases dramatically (10^3–10^4 times) with age. The most attractive explanation for this exponential relationship is that three to seven 'hits' (mutations) are required for a cancer to form. As we shall see, there is compelling evidence for an accumulation of mutations in growth-regulating genes being responsible for the evolution of colorectal cancer. Inspection of Fig. 2.2 (A, B, C) shows that the recorded rate of increase in many cancers diminishes after about 75 years of

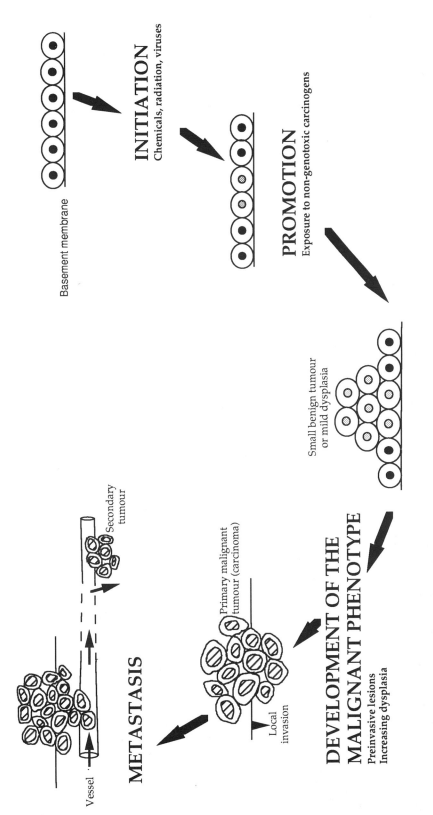

Fig. 2.1 Schematic diagram illustrating the multi-stage model of carcinogenesis for a simple epithelium.

age, but this is likely to be a statistical artefact, due to incomplete investigation of the terminal illnesses of old people. Of course, not all cancers show a sharp rise in incidence rate with age (Fig. 2.2C); testicular cancer shows a peak incidence between the second and fifth decades and then declines, while the peak incidences for leukaemia and nervous system cancers occur not only at greater ages but also in early childhood, suggesting the influence of prenatal factors.

2.2 Initiators and promoters

The foundations of the theory of multi-stage carcinogenesis are largely based on the classical experiments carried out by Berenblum and associates in the 1940s on skin carcinogenesis in the mouse. They recognized that there were two types of chemical involved in causing cancer, *initiators* and *promoters*. Initiating agents like polycyclic hydrocarbons were 'genotoxic agents', binding to DNA and causing mutations. Painting them on to mouse skin at high doses caused the development of carcinomas, but lower doses did not give rise to carcinomas, even after a long period of time. However, if skin treated with a subthreshold dose of the initiating agent was then treated with a 'promoting agent' (e.g. a phorbol ester, such as 12-o-tetradecanoyl phorbol-13-acetate, TPA), then benign tumours (papillomas) and carcinomas were eventually produced (Fig. 2.3). The promoting agent was ineffective in producing cancer on its own, or when given before the initiator. Equally important was the observation that the effects of the initiator were irreversible, suggesting that the mutations were probably caused in cells which permanently resided in this continually renewing epithelium, i.e. in the *stem cells* (see Chapter 4, section 4.8).

Thus the processes of chemical and irradiation-induced carcinogenesis are thought to initially involve genotoxic events which irreversibly damage DNA (initiation), followed by circumstances which 'promote' the expansion of the altered cells. Such progeny could then be 'at risk' of further initiation, leading to cycles of initiation and promotion before emergence of the malignant phenotype (Fig 2.1). According to the nomenclature, promoting agents do not damage DNA, they are non-mutagenic in short-term bacterial mutagenicity tests (e.g. the Ames test), and appear to do little more than selectively stimulate cells already initiated by another agent. Agents which fall into this category include TPA, organochlorine pesticides, bile acids and many hormones.

2.3 The environment

There is no doubt that the common fatal cancers mainly occur as a result of lifestyle and other environmental factors, and are, in principle, preventable: in the UK, probably 80–90% of cancers can be attributed to the environment. The evidence that much of human cancer is avoidable can be summarized as follows:

- Differences in the incidence of various types of cancer among different settled communities.

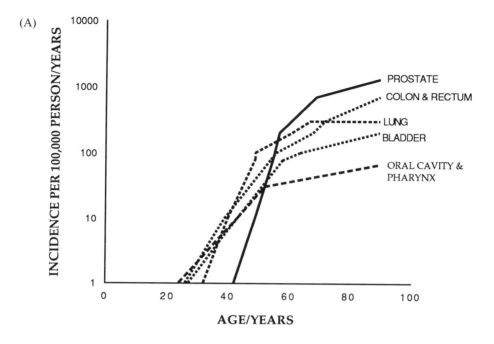

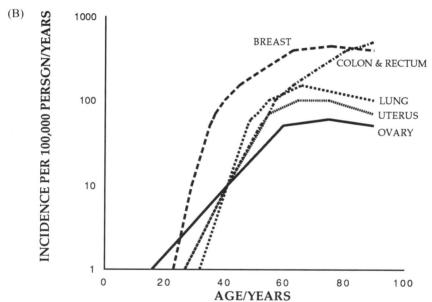

- Differences between migrants from a community and those who remained behind.
- Actual identification of many specific causes or preventative factors.

The environmental risk factors fall into three categories: (i) physical agents such as X-rays and UV light, (ii) chemical agents, and (iii) infectious agents such as bacteria, fungi, parasitic animals, but most importantly viruses.

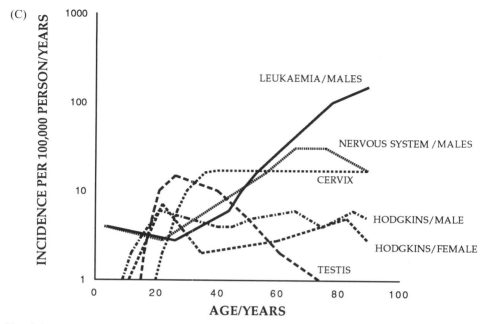

Fig. 2.2 Age-specific incidence patterns for selected cancers in the USA white population. Epithelial cancers among males (A) and females (B), and (C) for certain other cancers. (Source: Surveillance, Epidemiology, and End Results (SEER) program, 1984 to 1988.)

It is not surprising that the environment is implicated in carcinogenesis, as the vast majority of tumours are carcinomas arising from epithelium in direct contact with the environment. The gut is simply an invagination of the exterior body surface and it has intimate contact with a very wide variety of chemicals in the shape of food, drinks and all other ingested material; the lungs too are an interface between gaseous and airborne moieties and the body. However, some habits and situations more than others expose people to events able to initiate carcinogenesis; the most notable of these are diet, industrial and environmental exposure to chemicals and radiation, and their involvement can be inferred by epidemiological evidence even when the exact carcinogen is difficult to pin-point. Such questions as racial susceptibility to certain forms of cancer, for example, are particularly complex as certain races are often inseparable from their geographical location and cultural habits. Light may be thrown on the situation when there are large movements of population, for example, from an area of low susceptibility to a particular type of cancer to an area of high incidence of that form of the disease. Cancer of the stomach is relatively uncommon in Africa, but in the USA the incidence in its black population is as high as in its population of European origin. Americans of Japanese descent also tend to show an incidence of stomach cancer similar to that of their compatriots of European extraction, which is lower than that in Japan. So, in this case at least, it seems to be the adoption of the same diet that has evened out the risk of stomach cancer.

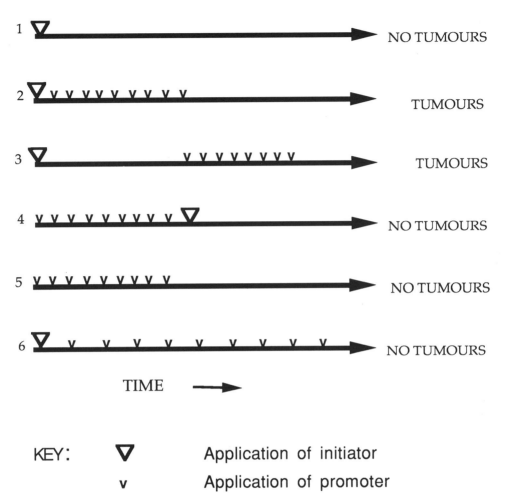

KEY: ▽   Application of initiator
         v   Application of promoter

Fig. 2.3 Protocols for demonstrating the principles of initiation and promotion in mouse skin.

2.4 Epidemiological studies

Epidemiology is the study of the incidence of disease in groups of people who share defined characteristics (e.g. from a particular geographical location or with a particular diet), and has been one of the principle means of obtaining knowledge about the causes of cancer. It is worth remembering that it is just 30 years since Richard Doll and Richard Peto (*British Medical Journal*, 1976; 2: 1525–36) provided conclusive epidemiological evidence that cigarette smoking was a direct cause of lung cancer. Epidemiologists frequently gather information from large numbers of cases. In the collection of mortality rates resulting from different types of cancer, for example, the wide net cast for the statistical sample minimizes the influence of errors due to misdiagnosis or variations in the efficacy of treatment. The appropriate collection of incidence (rate) data depends on the total number of new cases of a particular cancer per year, and is subject to the inaccuracies due to differences in age distribution of the

Table 2.1. *Common human cancers in males which vary dramatically in incidence in different parts of the world*

Cancer	Incidence	Community
Oesophagus	High	N.E. Iran
	Low	UK, USA
Stomach	High	Japan
	Low	Africa
Colon	High	UK
	Low	Nigeria
Liver	High	Tropical Africa, S.E. Asia
	Low	England
Bronchus	High	UK
	Low	Nigeria

populations or the prevalence of other diseases. Whether or not these variables are controlled, it seems quite clear that the incidence of some cancers amongst people at a given age in different parts of the world can vary by at least ten – or possibly a hundred fold. Table 2.1 lists some of common causes of cancer in males which have marked disparities in incidence in different areas of the world.

In these extreme cases the identification of a link (if not the causal mechanism) has been reasonably straightforward, backed up by scientific experiment in which a particular action leads to a reduction in the incidence of the disease. Cancers of the digestive tract would seem to be associated with components of the diet. Oesophageal cancer has been linked to the intake of tannic acid and certain dietary deficiencies, stomach cancer with smoked foodstuffs and a lack of fruit and vegetables, while large bowel cancer is associated with high fat, low fibre diets and inextricably linked to heavy meat consumption (Fig. 2.4A); likewise breast cancer appears to be linked to fat consumption (Fig. 2.4B). These epidemiological studies do not necessarily imply a causal relation between, say, dietary fat intake and breast cancer, but they do suggest that decreasing the former might reduce the latter. However, more recent epidemiological studies in the USA do not support a relationship between dietary fat intake and breast cancer either in premenopausal or post postmenopausal women; clearly any existing link between these factors is multifactorial and complex.

Most primary cancers of the liver are hepatocellular carcinomas and usually arise in a cirrhotic liver caused either by hepatitis B virus (HBV) infection and the consequent hepatitis (in high incidence areas) or alcohol consumption (in low incidence areas). Bronchial carcinoma became the most common cause of death from cancer in the early 1980s, and has been clearly linked to the inhalation of tobacco smoke.

Even tissues which give rise to hormone-dependent tumours can show marked differences in incidence across the world (Table 2.2). Differences in occurrence of prostate cancer may have something to do with genetic susceptibility, but this is not the whole reason since in the USA, black and Japanese ethnic groups both have higher rates of this tumour than in Africa and Japan. It is likely that the great majority of

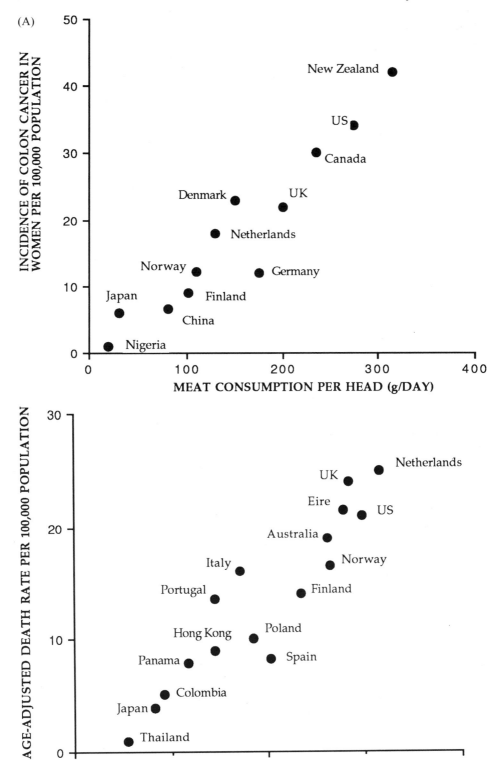

Table 2.2. *Tumours derived from hormone-dependent tissues that vary dramatically in incidence in different parts of the world*

Cancer	Incidence	Community
Prostate	High	USA (blacks)
	Low	Japan
Uterine cervix	Common	Hindu, Christian
	Low	Jewish, Moslem
Breast	High	USA, W. Europe
	Low	Asia
Endometrium	High	Developed countries
	Low	Poor countries

cervical carcinomas owe their origin to infection by human papillomaviruses (HPV), presumably spread during sexual intercourse; male circumcision seems to reduce the hazard. Breast cancer is the most common fatal cancer in women throughout most of the developed world, being responsible for 20% of all female cancer deaths. No clear cause has been established, but hormonal factors are indicated since early menarche, late menopause and late age of first full-term pregnancy are all associated with increased risk. Endometrial cancer is very definitely linked to oestrogen unopposed by progesterone, it can be associated with oestrogen-secreting ovarian tumours, the use of oestrogens post-menopausally and adiposity.

Evidence of a change in the incidence of cancer in a migrant group from that of the population of the country they have left towards that of their new country of residence, provides good evidence of the importance of environmental factors in the production of disease. Black Americans, for example, have cancer incidence rates more like those of white Americans than those of the black population of West Africa from which the large majority were originally drawn. Thus, black Americans have ten-fold higher incidences in colorectal cancer and equally dramatic lower incidences in liver cancer compared to the Nigerian population. Similar comparisons can be made between Japanese settlers in Hawaii and the Japanese in Japan; the incidence of stomach cancer in ethnically Japanese people in Hawaii is very similar to that in the Caucasian residents, and much less like that of the Japanese in Japan.

Fig. 2.4 (A) Correlation between colon cancer incidence in various countries and meat consumption. (Redrawn from B. Armstrong & R. Doll, 1975 *British Journal of Preventative and Social Medicine*, 30, 151–7.) (B) Correlation between breast cancer incidence in various countries and fat consumption. (Redrawn from K. K. Carrol, 1975, *Cancer Research*, 35, 3374–83). Note that more recent studies have shown no simplistic link between dietary fat intake and breast cancer.

2.5   Identifying the causes

Introduction

Through a combination of epidemiological and experimental studies it has been possible, with a reasonable degree of certainty, to identify certain agents which have something to do with the carcinogenic process. Some of these agents linked through either
occupational, medicinal or social contact are listed in Table 2.3.

Doll and Peto (1981) suggested that there were three determinants for cancer
development:

- Nature
- Nurture
- Luck

Nature relates to a person's genetic make-up at conception. For example, all else
being equal, a white-skinned person is more likely to develop skin cancer in response
to sunlight than a black person. Similarly, people who have inherited xeroderma pigmentosum, a rare genetically determined inability to carry out excision repair of sun-
light-damaged DNA, are likely to develop multiple skin carcinomas. *Nurture* relates
to what people do (e.g. the type of food they eat and what they drink) or have done
to them (e.g. through their occupational environment) during the course of their lives,
and even while still in the womb. Having apparently taken both nature and nurture
into account, which affect the probability that any individual will develop cancer, *luck*
perhaps determines exactly who will do so and when. We have noted that the incidence of many carcinomas increases exponentially with age (Fig. 2.2), probably due
to the accumulation of a number of random mutations. Some people will be lucky
and not acquire the requisite number of mutations at critical sites in the genome,
others will be unlucky. We all know of someone who has died of lung cancer at 40
years of age, while another smoker will live on, in apparently similar circumstances,
to 80 and beyond. We can attribute it to luck, but of course, there may be underlying
genetic factors (nature) such as the ability to repair damaged DNA.

The first association between occupation and cancer was made by a British surgeon,
Percival Pott, at the end of the eighteenth century. He found that cancer of the scrotum
occurred in chimney sweeps in whom, to quote his words, 'the disease . . . seems to
derive from a lodgement of soot in the ruggae (folds) of the scrotum'. Since that time
the search for such occupational hazards has unearthed more substances known to
cause cancer in humans than any other type of study. After the demonstration in 1915
that coal tars painted repeatedly on rabbits' ears produced cancers, came the discovery
that the active constituent was an aromatic hydrocarbon called benzo(a)pyrene (Fig.
2.5). Like other polycyclic hydrocarbons, this compound is metabolized by the
cytochrome P450-dependent mono-oxygenase system to an *ultimate* carcinogen – the
metabolite that reacts with DNA. First, the 7,8-position double bond is opened enzymatically and the epoxide is formed; this 7,8-epoxide is converted to 7,8-diol, which
can undergo a second epoxidation at the 9,10-position to form the ultimate carcinogen

Table 2.3. *Established carcinogenic agents for humans*

Agent	Site of cancer	Occupation
Occupational exposure		
Aromatic amines	Bladder	Dye and rubber workers
Arsenic	Skin	Copper and cobalt smelters,
	Lung	pesticide manufacturers
	Liver	
Asbestos	Lung	Asbestos miners, asbestos
	Pleura	insulation handlers
Ionizing radiation	Lung	Uranium miners
	Bone	Luminizers
Polycyclic hydrocarbons	Skin	People exposed to tars and oils
	Lung	(roofers, asphalters)
UV light	Skin	Outdoor workers

Agent	Site of cancer	Reason for exposure
Medical exposure		
Alkylating agents	Bladder	Cancer chemotherapy
	Bone marrow	
Ionizing radiation	Site of handling, or exposure	Isotope handling, thyroid irradiation
Oestrogens		
Unopposed	Endometrium	Post-menopausal hormone replacement therapy
Diethylstilboestrol	Vagina (off-spring)	Prevention of miscarriage
Thorotrast	Liver (angiosarcoma)	X-ray contrast medium

Agent	Site of cancer
Exposure through life-style	
Aflatoxin	Liver
Alcoholic drinks	Upper gastrointestinal tract and liver
Betel chewing	Mouth
Dietary factors	
e.g. fat, excessive meat consumption, nitrates, cooking habits	Colorectum, stomach, breast, endometrium
Parasites	
Schistosoma spp.	Bladder, bowel, liver
Clonorchis sinensis	Bile duct
Tobacco smoking	Oral cavity, respiratory tract, bladder
UV light	Skin
Oncogenic viruses	Many (see text)

which can bind to DNA. What happens to DNA which has been modified by the formation of nucleic acid *adducts* with large bulky hydrocarbon molecules? Hopefully an excision repair mechanism will ensure that the DNA sequence of bases is faithfully restored, but if there is absent or faulty repair there could be mutations at the DNA sequence level. Apart from xeroderma pigmentosum, ataxia telangiectasia, Fanconi's anaemia and Bloom's syndrome are other cancer-prone conditions thought to involve

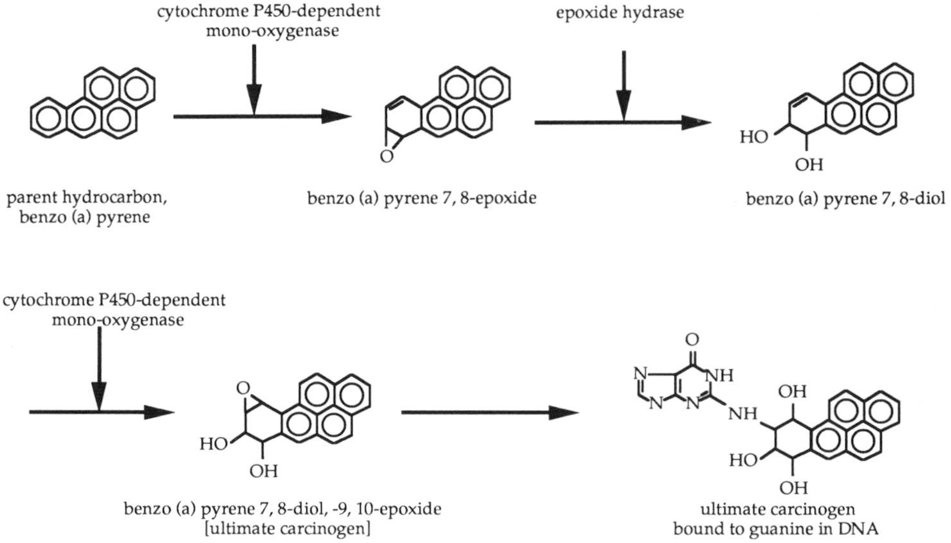

Fig. 2.5 The metabolism of benzo(*a*)pyrene resulting in the formation of a DNA-binding metabolite.

defects in either DNA repair or genomic stability. Bloom's syndrome is associated with a particularly high incidence of malignant tumours, with the mean age at cancer diagnosis being only 25 years. Here defects in the BLM protein, which is thought to be an ATP-dependent helicase (any enzyme which facilitates separation of the two DNA strands), may be responsible for chromosome non-disjunction after DNA synthesis.

Occupational, medicinal and social hazards

Aromatic amines, particularly 2-naphthylamine, were discovered to be bladder carcinogens through their use in the manufacture of aniline dyes. Ionizing radiation is a well known carcinogenic agent, and before the advent of proper safety regulations, was a frequent cause of cancer, particularly on the hands of radiologists. Uranium miners suffered an excess of lung cancers due to inhalation of radon gas, while workers who painted the luminous dials on watch faces tended to develop bone sarcomas because of the habit of shaping the paint brush in the mouth to obtain a fine point, and thus ingesting minute quantities of radium – a bone-seeking element. Survivors of the atomic bombs at Hiroshima and Nagasaki, observers at nuclear test explosions, and people living in the vicinity of the Chernobyl nuclear accident have all shown increased cancer incidence; with respect to the latter, after 10 years there is reported to be a 100-fold increase in childhood thyroid cancers in the Ukraine and Belarus. There is also some evidence of clustering of leukaemia victims in the close vicinity of atomic ordnance factories and nuclear waste reprocessing plants.

Some mineral fibres are associated with carcinogenesis, the best known being the thin (0.25 µm diameter) crocidolite fibres of blue asbestos, implicated in lung carcinomas and mesotheliomas. The exact mechanism by which asbestos fibres increase the incidence of cancer is unclear, but the fact that combined cigarette smoking and asbestos exposure dramatically increase cancer risk suggests that the fibre may simply be acting as an irritant, increasing cell turnover, and thereby increasing the likelihood of damaged (mutated DNA) being copied into subsequent generations of cell progeny.

There are several highly publicized cases where medical intervention for treatment or diagnostic purposes has lead to a rise in cancer incidence. Like many of the occupational hazards, these have been recognized and the causative practises abandoned; nevertheless we can learn much from them. Thorotrast was widely used from the 1930s to the 1950s as a contrast medium in diagnostic radiology, particularly angiography; however, thorotrast is a colloidal suspension of thorium dioxide, a natural emitter of alpha radiation. It was taken up by the body's macrophages, such as those lining the vascular sinusoids of the liver, and as we now know, caused the development of angiosarcomas (malignant tumours of vascular endothelial cells). Increasingly, exposure to very low doses of radiation is being appreciated with a putative link between childhood exposure to routine chest X-rays to monitor tuberculosis and women developing breast cancer. A further well known example was the occurrence of vaginal adenocarcinoma in women in their late teens or early twenties when they had been exposed to diethylstilboestrol *in utero*. This synthetic oestrogenic agent was used in the 1950s in the treatment of threatened miscarriage, primarily in the USA.

We have already noted the significant role played by diet in the causation of many tumours. A further source of carcinogen may be drinking water, contaminated with nitrates from the run-off from agricultural land where nitrate fertilizers have been used. Nitrates and nitrites are also used as food additives and can be readily converted into nitrosamines (established carcinogens in rodents), by intestinal bacteria. Aflatoxins are mycotoxins produced by the fungus *Aspergillus flavus*, and aflatoxin B_1 is one of the most potent carcinogens known in experimental systems, with its epoxide derivative able to bind to DNA (Fig. 2.6). The fungus grows on stored food in the tropics where there is a high incidence of hepatocellular carcinoma, but the

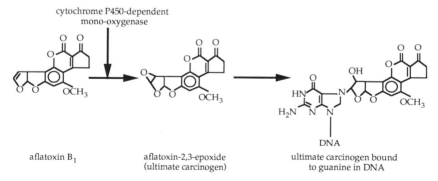

Fig. 2.6 The structure of the mycotoxin aflatoxin B_1 and formation of the major DNA-binding metabolite.

situation is complicated by the high incidence of hepatitis B virus infection, another factor definitely associated with liver cancer.

Exposure to *radiation*, electromagnetic or particulate, can be damaging to DNA, right down at the energy levels of UV light. The incidence of skin cancers, particularly malignant melanoma and basal cell carcinoma, is increasing world-wide. This is most notable in hot countries with fair skinned populations such as in Australia, but also in Europe where the fashion for the past two generations has been to sport a suntan. Naturally pigmented skin is protected from the damage caused by UV light but sun burning results in reduced ability of DNA repair and thus an increased cancer risk. High energy radiation is not generally met with daily, except perhaps low doses of cosmic radiation or background radiation from ores and radon gas in some geographical locations.

Parasites can also precipate the development of cancer. For example, liver flukes such as *Schistosoma* spp. and *Clonorchis sinensis* are associated with bladder cancer and cholangiocarcinoma respectively, and previous exposure to a malaria parasite (*Plasmodium* spp.) seems to be associated with Burkitt's lymphoma and the Epstein Barr virus (EBV). At certain stages in their life cycle *Schistosoma* spp. inhabit the mesenteric veins and *Clonorchis sinensis* the bile ducts, where they induce inflammatory and delayed hypersensitivity reactions in the tissues; when tumours are found they are often associated with these parasites in various stages of development. The aetiology of the relationship of *Plasmodium* spp. and EBV is unknown, but prior infection with the protozoan parasite is suspected to render the lymphoid system of the host amenable to infection by the virus.

The relationship of *viruses* to carcinogenesis is becoming of profound importance as virus life cycles inherently affect host cell DNA. Cancer-causing viruses are called *oncogenic viruses*. The first report that tumours could be induced in naïve animals by treatment with a cell-free filtrate from a virus infected source was by Ellerman and Bang, in 1908, with chicken erythroblastosis (erythroid leukaemia), followed in 1910 by Peyton Rous with the transference of an agent able to cause sarcomas in chickens. Such demonstrations showed that it was possible to transmit tumours from one animal to another, in the manner of an infectious disease, which led to the discovery of the transmissible agent – a virus, as the pores of the filter were too small to permit the passage of bacteria or whole tumour cells. Though only about 17–20% of human cancer is thought to be associated with viruses (Table 2.4), the study of oncogenic retroviruses in animals has had a fundamental effect on our understanding of neoplasia and has led to the discovery of *oncogenes*. Oncogenic viruses are classified according to whether they contain DNA or RNA in their genome; DNA tumour viruses are the major cause of human virally-induced cancers.

DNA oncogenic viruses

The mechanisms by which DNA viruses initiate the neoplastic process are fundamentally different from those of the RNA tumour viruses. Basically, DNA tumour viruses encode proteins which interact with critical cellular growth-regulatory molecules,

Table 2.4. *Human cancers associated with virus infection*

Cancer	Virus	Type
Burkitt's lymphoma	Epstein-Barr virus	DNA
Nasopharyngeal cancer	Epstein-Barr virus	DNA
Hepatocellular carcinoma	Hepatitis B virus	DNA
Cervical carcinoma	Human papillomaviruses	DNA
Leukaemia	HTLV-I and HTLV-II	RNA
Lymphoma and Kaposi's sarcoma	HIV-1 and HIV-2	RNA

Abbreviations: HTLV, human T cell leukaemia/lymphotropic virus; HIV, human immunodeficiency virus.

sabotaging their function. EBV is common, causing such diseases as glandular fever, but in certain geographical locations which are also favoured by malaria carrying mosquitoes, EBV is associated with carcinogenesis. In the Far East, EBV infection is associated with nasopharyngeal carcinoma while in Africa it is associated with lymphoma. Rare cases of Burkitt's (African) lymphoma occur without EBV infection, but in both African and non-African types there are characteristic translocations involving the c-*myc* gene (see Chapter 3, section 3.1) on chromosome 8 and one of the immunoglobulin genes on chromosome 14, 2 or 22. In the case of EBV infection there is good circumstantial evidence that the presence of the viral genome may have initiated the translocation. HBV is associated with low standards of hygiene in daily life and liver infection is rife in many parts of the Third World. Fragments of the viral genome can often be found incorporated into the genome of the tumour cells, suggesting that hepatocellular carcinoma (HCC) is associated with HBV infection, perhaps through the virus causing insertional mutagenesis (see Fig 2.8) The HBV X-protein (pX) coded for by the *X*-gene could also be involved in the development of HCC, for like many other proteins encoded by DNA viruses, pX has transactivating activity on a number of cellular genes. This action of pX may involve protein–protein interactions between pX and cellular transcription factors such as AP-1 (commonly a heterodimer of Fos and Jun) or CREB (cyclic AMP response element and binding protein). HPV DNA is found in DNA of the cells of many tumours of the cervix, so here too the circumstantial evidence for oncogenic activity is very strong. There are at least 60 distinct types of HPV, but preinvasive lesions (cervical intraepithelial neoplasia, see Chapter 4, section 4.3) and invasive cancer are commonly associated with certain types, notably types 16, 18, 31, 33 and 35. Protein products of the so-called early (E) genes maybe responsible for the ability of HPV to cause neoplastic transformation; the E6/E7 genes of HPV may produce proteins which complex with tumour suppressor gene products such as pRb and p53 (see Chapter 3, section 3.3 and Fig. 3.18).

The *adenoviruses* are peculiar in that they readily infect humans, but appear not to be linked to an increased incidence of cancer, whereas they readily induce tumours in laboratory animals. The adenovirus genome persists in animal cells, and the carcinogenic effect could also be due to the ability of the products of the *E1A* and *E1B* genes to sequester p53 and pRb. In humans, adenovirus infection may lead to rapid cell death.

RNA oncogenic viruses

Only one family of RNA viruses, the retroviruses, cause tumours. These are small single-stranded animal viruses. Soon after infection the RNA genome is copied into double-stranded DNA by an RNA dependent DNA polymerase – *reverse transcriptase* – carried by the virus particle, thus creating a DNA *provirus*. RNA tumour viruses are, at present, not thought to be a major cause of human cancers, though there are strong associations between the human immunodeficiency viruses (HIV-1 and HIV-2) and AIDS-related malignancies such as Kaposi's sarcoma, and between the human T cell leukaemia/lymphotropic viruses (HTLV-I and HTLV-II) and T cell leukaemia/lymphoma. How these retroviruses induce neoplasia is not entirely clear, but it may be a combination of an impairment of the immune system to kill tumour cells together with a stimulation of cell proliferation in uninfected or infected immune competent, or other cells; such cells would be 'targets' for further neoplastic changes. In the case of HTLV-I and adult T cell leukaemia, a protein known as the tax protein transactivates a number of cellular cytokine genes in infected cells (see below). Liver cancer associated with HBV infection may be caused by a similar sort of mechanism; infected hepatocytes are killed by cell-mediated immune reactions leading to regenerative hyperplasia, and such cells are at greater risk of undergoing neoplastic change. Although the role of immune surveillance has been largely discounted to explain the increased incidence of many cancers in an ageing population, there seems little doubt that immuno-suppression is a significant risk factor for the development of virus-associated human cancers.

The RNA viruses that cause malignancy in animals have done so much for our understanding of the molecular biology of neoplasia. In each RNA genome of a replication-competent retrovirus there are at least three gene sequences – *gag, pol* and *env*. The *pol* gene encodes the reverse transcriptase, *gag* encodes the internal proteins and *env* encodes the envelope proteins. These genes are flanked by unique sequences, U5 and U3, at the 5′ and 3′ ends, and short repeat (R) RNA sequences (Fig. 2.7A, B). U5 is bound by the primer binding site and is the first portion of the retroviral genome to be transcribed by the reverse transcriptase, and therefore becomes the 3′ long terminal repeat (LTR) of the integrated provirus. In short, the reverse transcriptase creates, from a single stranded RNA genomic precursor, a double-stranded DNA provirus ready for integration into the host cell DNA. Retroviruses are very efficient at integrating their entire genome into the host cell's DNA, and this integration is stable and permanent, particularly since the effects are generally not cytopathic.

There are a number of retroviral mechanisms of cellular transformation including *insertional mutagenesis*, *transactivation* and *oncogene transduction*, and these are discussed below.

The *slow transforming* viruses (e.g. mouse mammary tumour virus – MMTV; avian leukosis [lymphoma] virus) do not readily *transform* (convert into a neoplastic state)

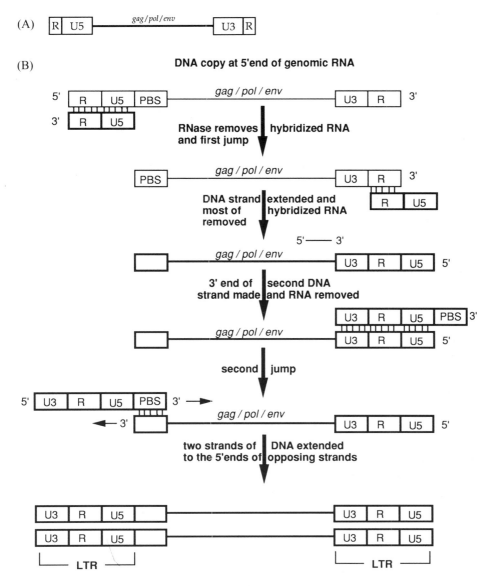

Fig. 2.7 (A) Structure of a typical slow-transforming retroviral genome. (B) Utilizing reverse transcriptase, this single stranded RNA genomic precursor is converted into a double-stranded DNA provirus ready for integration into chromosomal DNA. The provirus now has symmetrical long terminal repeats (LTRs) which contain the promoting and enhancing sequences.

cells, but cause tumours only after long latent periods. For successful tumour formation these viruses insert the double-stranded DNA copy – the provirus – into the host genome in the vicinity of a proto-oncogene, perhaps into elements involved in transcriptional control of the proto-oncogene (Fig. 2.8). This can lead to overexpression of the proto-oncogene, perhaps under the control of a virus promoter, present in the LTR region of the integrated viral genome, resulting in inappropriate

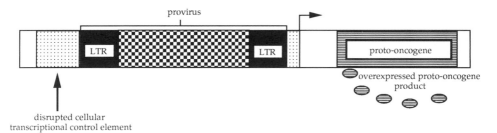

Fig. 2.8 Insertional mutagenesis involves integration of the provirus, usually upstream from a proto-oncogene, but disrupting its transcriptional control leading to over-expression of the encoded protein.

production of the particular protein. Studies on lymphomas induced in birds by avian leukosis virus infection after a long latency period, suggest that for tumour production the provirus has to integrate in the vicinity of the c-*myc* gene, usually with the 3′ LTR upstream of the proto-oncogene. Likewise, mouse mammary tumour virus proviral DNA can integrate randomly into host cell DNA, but mouse breast carcinoma cells have a consistent provirus integration site on chromosome 15, near, but never interrupting, a 30 kilobase sequence. This DNA segment has now been identified as the proto-oncogene *int-1*, whose expression is normally confined to neural tube morphogenesis and spermiogenesis. *Int-1* may code a growth factor, and the gene has considerable homology to *wingless*, a gene family coding for proteins with a role in *Drosophila* development, including segment polarity.

Proviruses are, therefore, acting as mutagens – disrupting host gene expression at the site of their insertion, and this process has become known as insertional mutagenesis. The likelihood that an infected cell will undergo a critical site-dependent proviral integration and transformation is probably very rare, explaining perhaps why such tumours tend to be monoclonal (derived from a single cell, see Chapter 4, section 4.8).

The human T cell leukaemia virus (HTLV-I) is replication-competent, carries no oncogene, integrates at random, but can induce a monoclonal leukaemia after a long latent period. The transforming capability of HTLV-I resides in the unique 3′ genomic structure called the X region, which encodes for at least three proteins, seemingly the most important being the Tax protein (Fig. 2.9). This viral-encoded protein not only increases the rate of proviral transcription, but transactivates host cell enhancers and promoters. These elements include the enhancers and promoters for the IL-2 receptor gene and the granulocyte macrophage-colony stimulating factor (GM-CSF) gene, and overproduction of the proteins encoded by these genes will cause expansion of the target cell population, with perhaps further mutation-like events needed for successful transformation.

So far, we have described the actions of retroviruses which contain the genes needed for their own replication, and whose tumourigenic effects take a long time to be manifest. *Fast-transforming* viruses, however, induce tumours in infected animals in a matter of days or weeks. These viruses include all the sarcoma viruses of both birds

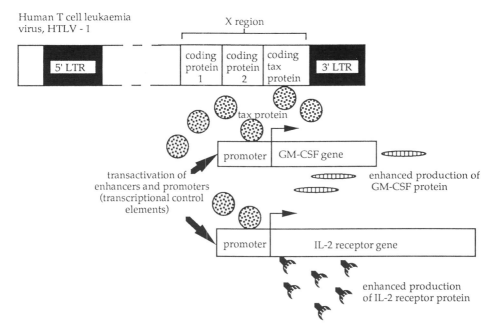

Fig. 2.9 Proto-oncogene activation by a DNA provirus as illustrated by the ability of the human T cell leukaemia virus (HTLV-I) encoded Tax protein to stimulate interleukin -2 (IL-2) receptor and granulocyte/macrophage colony stimulating factor (GM-CSF) gene expression in infected lymphocytes – transactivation.

and rodents, and many of the leukaemia causing viruses. Analysis of the viral genomes reveal that such viruses have acquired new genes, usually at the expense of genetic information coding for their own replicative genes. These new, substituted genes were found to be responsible for the rapid transforming abilities of the viruses and were therefore termed *oncogenes* or *onc* genes, and the mechanism has become known as oncogene transduction. At least 50 or more different viral oncogenes (v-*oncs*) have been identified in this way, each given a three letter code denoting the tumour and/ or the species in which the gene was first discovered:

v-*myc*	Chicken myelocytoma (chronic myeloid leukaemia)
v-*sis*	Simian (monkey) sarcoma
v-*myb*	Chicken myeloblastosis (acute myeloid leukaemia)
v-*erbB*	Chicken erythroblastosis (erthyroid leukaemia)

The first acutely transforming oncogenic retrovirus to be described was the Rous sarcoma virus, which is in fact unusual in that it is the only member of this group to be replication competent (Fig. 2.10). This is because the transduced *src* (sarcoma-producing) oncogene is 3' to the structural genes. This diverse group of viruses also commonly produces polyclonal tumours, presumably a reflection of the high efficiency of transformation in the infected cells. One of the most important discoveries in cancer research was that these retroviral transforming genes had cellular

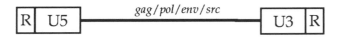

Fig. 2.10 Structure of the Rous chicken sarcoma retroviral genome which unlike other acutely transforming retroviruses retains all its structural genes as well as having an oncogene (*src*).

ancestors, a fact that has shaped our present day ideas of how the neoplastic state is initiated and even maintained. Nucleic acid hybridization studies demonstrated that the v-*onc* sequences showed significant homology to sequences found in the DNA of totally normal cells. It is now believed that the v-*onc*s are, in fact, homologues of normal cellular genes that have been picked up by the viruses during the course of evolution. The cellular counterpart may be called a c-*onc* gene, but this term suggests that the gene is an oncogene, whereas the more appropriate term *proto-oncogene* implies that the gene has only 'potential' oncogenic activity. How the retroviral genomes have picked up cellular sequences is unclear, though it could be that after integration into the host DNA 5′ to a particular proto-oncogene, transcription of the viral genome is altered (Fig. 2.11). This may involve a loss of the 3′ portion of the provirus, or inefficient 3′ LTR polyadenylation signals, and/or the loss of the 5′ portion of the proto-oncogene, leaving a structural gene in frame with the proto-oncogene, permitting

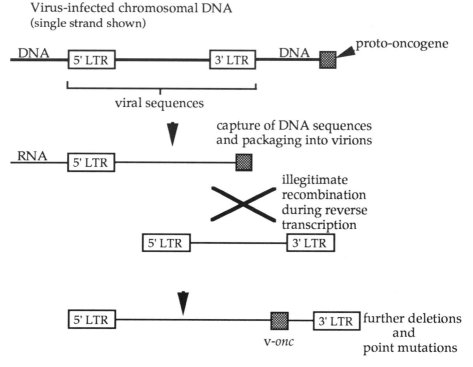

Fig. 2.11 Possible scheme for the evolutionary capture of a cellular proto-oncogene, its packaging into a virion, and, on infection of another cell, recombination with a wild-type viral genome producing a provirus with a transforming v-*onc* – oncogene transduction. LTR, long terminal repeat.

'read-through' transcription and the incorporation of the proto-oncogene. This transcript can be packaged into a virion along with a wild-type retroviral genome, and, after infection of another cell, these two RNA species could undergo reverse transcriptase mediated recombination between their 3′ ends allowing integration of the oncogene-containing genome into chromosomal DNA.

2.6 Further reading

Alderson, M. (1986). *Occupational Cancer*. London: Butterworths.

Doll, R. & Peto, R. (1981). *The Causes of Cancer*. Oxford: Oxford University Press.

Fine, H. A. & Haseltine, W. A. (1993). RNA tumour viruses. In *Cancer Medicine*, 3rd edn. ed. J. F. Holland, E. Frei, R. C. Bast, D. L. Kufe, D. L. Morton & R. R. Weichselbaum, pp. 265–82. Philadelphia: Lea & Febiger.

Gallo, R.C. (1995). Human retroviruses in the second decade: a personal perspective. *Nature Medicine*, **1** (8); 753–9.

3

The genetic basis of cancer

3.1 Identifying the genes

Introduction

Proto-oncogenes are normal cellular genes encoding cytoplasmic and nuclear proteins, responsible for the cell's normal proliferation and differentiation programmes. These genes encode a variety of proteins involved in mitogenesis and differentiation which are organized into a cascade of reactions (Fig. 3.1).

There are examples of proto-oncogene products associated with each of these stages (see below). The oncogenic activity of the v-*onc* genes seems to be due to either quantitative changes in the levels of expression or differences between the viral and cellular homologues leading to the production of a protein with oncogenic activity. More important probably, in the case of human tumours, proto-oncogenes can be involved in tumorigenesis through point mutation, gene amplification or chromosomal translocation. Studies on tumour tissue have identified at least a further 20 c-*onc* genes that appear to have no association with retroviral oncogenes; these include *hst* (<u>h</u>uman <u>st</u>omach cancer) and *bcl-2* (<u>B</u> <u>c</u>ell <u>l</u>ymphoma).

This information has been gathered from three major approaches: (i) DNA transfection, (ii) mapping of insertional mutagenesis in virally induced tumours and (iii) analysis of chromosomal translocations.

Gene transfer

This is achieved by the technique of DNA *transfection*, in which DNA isolated from tumour cells is introduced into relatively normal cells. The recipient cells used are often the mouse fibroblast line, NIH/3T3. Normally these cells grow as a monolayer in a petri dish and stop growing when they make contact with each other, referred to as *contact inhibition*. Loss of contact inhibition, with the result that cells pile up on top of one another to form a focus, is a cardinal property of transformed cells *in vitro*. Cells which stably incorporate non-murine DNA containing the critical sequences encoding the transforming gene(s) will form these foci (Fig. 3.2). To identify the

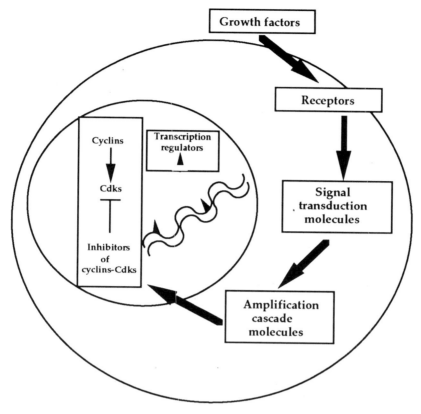

Fig. 3.1 Categories of molecule that regulate cell growth, many of which are encoded by proto-oncogenes.

actual gene responsible for the cells' transformed phenotype, transfection of DNA from the transformed foci is carried out a second and third time, this whittles down the amount of non-murine DNA carried over. This type of analysis found that the *ras* family of proto-oncogenes was abnormally activated in about 20% of human tumours tested by this means; *ras* genes being originally identified from retroviruses which caused rat sarcomas.

Insertional mutagenesis

As discussed in Chapter 2, long latency viruses like the avian leukaemia viruses (ALVs) lack v-*onc* sequences, but a DNA copy of their genome (the provirus) can become integrated within chromosomal DNA. The mode of this integration generates long terminal repeat (LTR) structures in which the U5 region is duplicated at the 3' end and U3 at the 5' end (see Fig. 2.7). As a consequence, one LTR can be used to promote the production of virus progeny, and since the regulatory elements for viral transcription are now found also at the 3' end they can serve as promoters or enhancers for adjacent cellular genes. Analysis of B cell tumours induced by ALVs in chickens

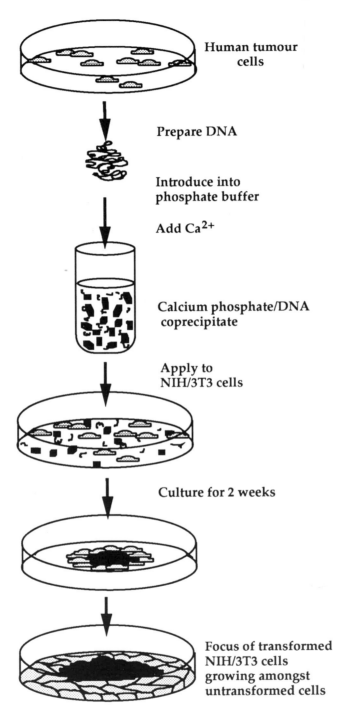

Human tumour
cells

Prepare DNA

Introduce into
phosphate buffer

Add Ca^{2+}

Calcium phosphate/DNA
coprecipitate

Apply to
NIH/3T3 cells

Culture for 2 weeks

Focus of transformed
NIH/3T3 cells
growing amongst
untransformed cells

Fig. 3.2 The prototypical transfection experiment for demonstrating a cellular oncogene.

Table 3.1 *Examples of consistent chromosome abnormalities in human tumours*

Tumour	Chromosomal abnormality	Comment
Chronic myeloid (granulocytic) leukaemia (CML)	Reciprocal exchange of the ends of chromosomes 9 and 22	Fusion of c-*abl* and *bcr* genes; 210 kDa fusion protein acts as a tyrosine kinase constitutively
Burkitt's lymphoma	Reciprocal exchange of the end of chromosome 8 with either the end of chromosome 14, 2 or 22	c-*myc* gene becomes controlled by regulatory sequences of Ig genes
Follicular lymphoma	t(14; 18) chromosome translocation	Over-expression of *bcl-2* gene protects against the apoptotic tendency of germinal centre cells

reveals that the LTR can function as a promoter for transcription of the cellular *myc* gene. Many other proto-oncogenes have been found to be abnormally expressed through promoter insertion, and in many cases the integrated provirus is no longer intact, i.e. one of the LTRs as well as some of the viral replicative coding sequences are lost.

Chromosomal abnormalities

Chromosomal abnormalities in tumours were recognized at the end of the nineteenth century, and we now realize that distinct translocations lead to the activation of proto-oncogenes or the creation of tumour-specific fusion proteins. In both categories the encoded proteins are often transcription factors, and this disruption of transcriptional control highlights the importance of this process in the development of cancer. Chromosomal abnormalities are sometimes specific for a particular tumour type, and their identification in cytological preparations of metaphase chromosomes from tumour cells can lead to the recognition of an incriminating proto-oncogene (Table 3.1).

It is not known why such consistent structural rearrangements occur; certain changes may happen preferentially, but it is more likely that they occur at random and that selection acts to eliminate the vast majority which do not provide the cell with a proliferative advantage. Chronic myeloid leukaemia (CML) is a well differentiated haemopoietic stem cell malignancy that inevitably progresses to acute leukaemia, i.e. the tumour cells become more primitive and more aggressive. This invariably involves further chromosomal alterations. The affected cells from the majority of patients with CML contain a reciprocal translocation, t(9:22), which gives rise to a small 22q- chromosome called the Philadelphia (Ph') chromosome (Fig. 3.3). As a result of this, the c-*abl* proto-oncogene (known from retroviruses), on the long arm of chromosome 9 is juxtaposed to a gene in the <u>b</u>reakpoint <u>c</u>luster

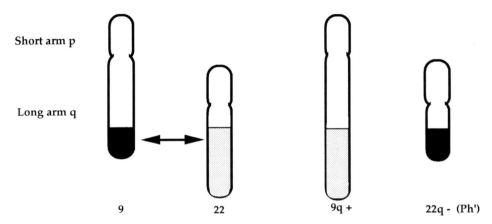

Fig. 3.3 In chronic myeloid leukemia the chromosomal translocation joins the *bcr* gene on chromosome 22 to the *abl* gene from chromosome 9 thereby generating the Philadelphia chromosome.

region (hence *bcr*) of chromosome 22. The *bcr-abl* gene product (p210) has constitutive phosphorylating activity, thus promoting cell proliferation through an unchecked positive influence on kinase-dependent, growth regulatory, signal transduction pathways. Expression of p210 might also suppress apoptosis in the face of cell-damaging agents such as irradiation.

The chimaeric RNA of such a gene fusion is providing an important target for polymerase chain reaction (PCR)-based detection of residual tumour cells after treatment. PCR is a technique for the *in vitro* amplification of specific DNA sequences by the simultaneous primer extension of complementary strands. The method hinges on the ability of DNA polymerases to carry out the synthesis of a complementary strand of DNA in the 5′ to 3′ direction using a single stranded template (Fig. 3.4), although starting from a double stranded region. The PCR employs two primers, each complementary to opposite strands of the region of DNA of interest, which has been denatured by heating. The primers are orientated so that their 3′ ends point toward one another along the intervening sequence: this results in the *de novo* synthesis of the region of DNA flanked by the two primers.

The PCR reaction can be divided into three stages (Fig. 3.5):

(i)   Denaturation of template DNA (rendered single stranded) by heating to ~94 °C
(ii) Annealing of the two primers (single stranded DNA about 20 bp long) to the complementary sequences in the template DNA, usually at ~50 °C
(iii) In the presence of a DNA polymerase, the incorporation of nucleotides into new DNA strands that are initiated from the primer sequences. Repetition of this cycle results in a selective exponential increase in the concentration of the target sequence.

In the early descriptions of PCR, the DNA polymerase was heat labile and had to be replenished after each denaturation step. However, a relatively heat-resistant

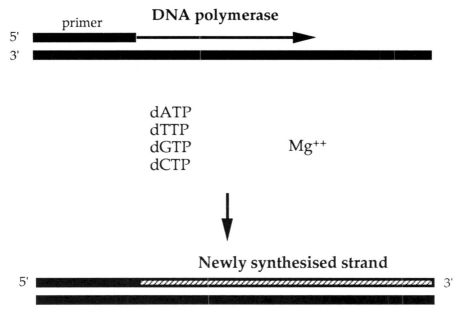

Fig. 3.4 Primer extension: DNA polymerase extends a primer by using a complementary DNA strand as a template.

DNA polymerase (*Taq* polymerase) is now used, which survives the denaturation process and does not have to be replenished each cycle. This enzyme is derived from a bacterium, *Bacillus thermoaquaticus*, that normally exists in hot springs.

The PCR technique is an invaluable technique for the analysis of gene expression, since mRNA reverse transcribed into complementary DNA (cDNA), may then be subjected to conventional PCR amplification – this process is called reverse transcriptase PCR (RT–PCR). In the case of hybrid *bcr-abl* mRNA, whose detection would signal the presence of residual tumour cells in CML after treatment, RNA can be extracted from white blood cells and subjected to RT-PCR. To detect the hybrid mRNA, a set of primers complementary to an *abl* exon and a *bcr* exon are used, so only the hybrid and not the normal transcripts of *bcr* and *abl* will be exponentially amplified. The PCR products are subjected to electrophoresis through an agarose gel, and detection could then involve conventional ethidium bromide staining of the gel, or, if greater sensitivity of detection is needed, the DNA can be transferred to a nylon membrane and hybridized to a radiolabelled oligonucleotide probe (Southern blotting, see below).

A quite different translocation occurs in Burkitt's lymphoma, a malignancy of B lymphocytes. Here 90% of patients have a (8;14) translocation, exchanging the c-*myc* gene on chromosome 8 with that of the immunoglobulin heavy chain on chromosome 14 (Fig 3.6); in the remaining patients the c-*myc* gene exchanges with, or comes in close contact with the kappa (κ) or lambda (λ) light chain genes on chromosomes 2 and 22 respectively. In all cases, of course, this results in the c-*myc* gene being physi-

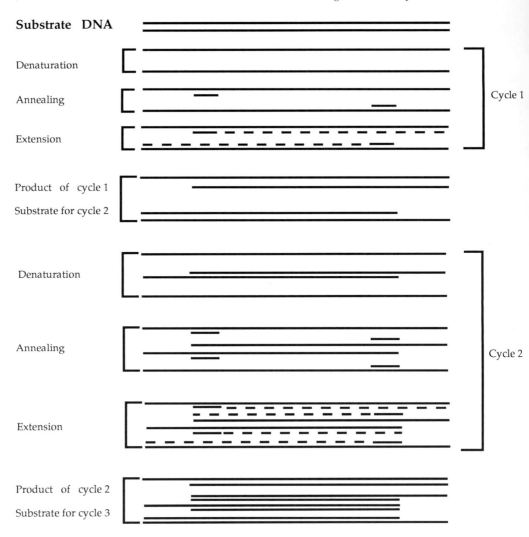

Fig. 3.5 Schematic representation of the polymerase chain reaction (see text for details).

cally adjacent to regulatory sequences for genes that are highly transcribed in mature B lymphocytes, i.e. the immunoglobulin genes. Constitutive overexpression of c-*myc* follows, thus presenting the cell with a persistent, positive signal for continuous cell cycling.

The *bcl-2* gene is located on chromosome 18, and is not generally expressed in lymphoid follicular centre cells which undergo apoptosis (see Chapter 5, section 5.3) unless they are rescued and converted into long-term memory cells by antigen driven selection. Translocation of the *bcl-2* gene to a transcriptionally active site may be expected to increase *bcl-2* expression and protect cells, which under normal circumstances would undergo apoptotic cell death.

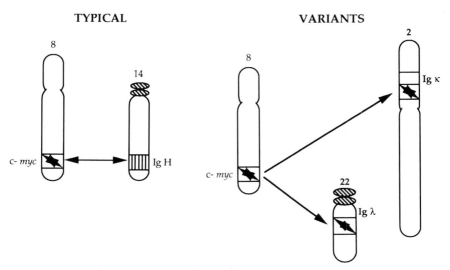

TYPICAL **VARIANTS**

Fig. 3.6 Schematic representations of the common and rarer chromosome translocations in Burkitt's lymphoma.

3.2 Oncogenes

Introduction

It is now generally believed that most human neoplasia results from abnormalities in proto-oncogene expression, genes whose normal function is to control cell proliferation and/or differentiation; thus the genes become *oncogenes* (cancer-causing). They may function as oncogenes because either their protein product is abnormal (e.g. through a point mutation in the gene), or there is a quantitative defect (too much, too little) in transcription of the gene. Two fundamentally different genetic mechanisms appear to be operative during tumour development:

- Enhanced or aberrant expression of proto-oncogenes.
- Loss or inactivation of tumour suppressor genes.

Oncogenes classically act in a dominant fashion – that is alteration of *one* allele is sufficient to cause transformation. They can be regarded, on the one hand, as a *foot on the accelerator* in the drive towards cell proliferation. Anti-oncogenes, better known as *tumour suppressor genes,* are, on the other hand, *a foot on the brake*, in that their protein products appear to inhibit cell proliferation. These genes generally appear to act in a recessive fashion, in that loss of suppressor function requires inactivation of *both* alleles, usually by chromosomal deletion, point mutation or both. Most of our knowledge of tumour suppressor genes comes from studies of familial cancers, where there is an inherited disposition to develop certain types of tumour (see below).

A convenient way of arranging proto-oncogenes is in a cascade of signal transduction based on their supposed functions (Fig 3.7); oncogene products are involved in all the known major stages. What is fascinating is that the studies analyzing animal

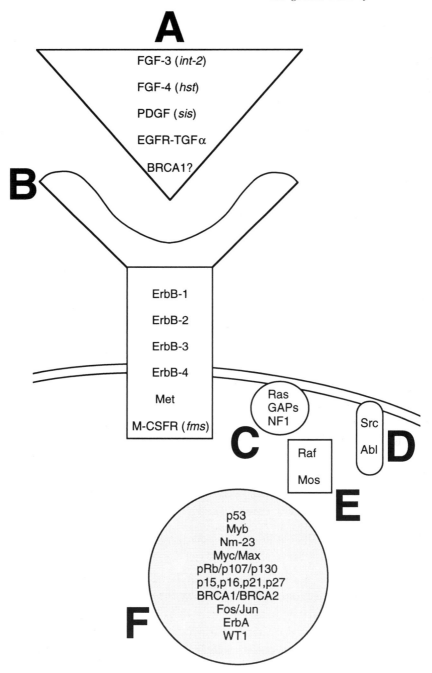

Fig. 3.7 Schematic diagram of the cellular compartments where some of the major proto-oncogene and tumour suppressor gene protein products act. A, As growth factors; B, as growth factor receptors; C, as membrane-associated guanine nucleotide-binding proteins and their regulatory molecules; D, as membrane-associated tyrosine kinases; E, as cytoplasmic serine/threonine kinases; and F, as nuclear factors, predominantly transcription factors.

tumours deliberately induced by mutagenic agents or viruses have found mutations in certain genes (proto-oncogenes). The same kinds of genes are also mutated or abnormally expressed in human sporadic tumours. This is part of the revolution in cancer research that has been taking place over the last 10–15 years.

Oncogenes with products related to growth factors

If oncogenes can produce a continuous supply of growth factors that can act in an autocrine way (see Chapter 5, section 5.2), then neoplastic growth might result. Platelet derived growth factor (PDGF) is found in high concentrations in platelets, and is normally released after wounding, to stimulate the healing process. The v-*sis* gene of simian sarcoma virus encodes a protein product, p28^{sis}, closely related to the B chain of PDGF. The p28^{sis} is, in fact, a homodimer of B chains, and probably acts intracellularly to stimulate continuous cell proliferation in infected cells – NIH/3T3 cells can be transformed by the viral oncogene but not by exogenously added PDGF. Over-expression of PDGF is not common in human tumours, but the observation was nevertheless exciting since it demonstrated a central tenet of tumours – a capacity for continuous cell proliferation. Genes which make up the fibroblast growth factor (FGF) gene family can also act as oncogenes; the *hst* gene was originally found in the amplified DNA of a human stomach tumour, while the *int-2* gene was originally discovered in mice where it was activated by insertional mutagenesis following integration of mouse mammary tumour virus (MMTV). In humans the *hst* (FGF-4) and *int-2* (FGF-3) genes are close to one another on chromosome 11, and are commonly co-amplified in many human tumours, particularly breast carcinomas. The gene encoding transforming growth factor α (TGFα) may be a potential oncogene. TGFα acts *via* the epidermal growth factor receptor (EGFR), and an autocrine loop involving TGFα and EGFR is operative in many tumours. TGFα expression is certainly increased in many human tumours, and the growth of such cells in culture can be impaired by monoclonal antibodies to TGFα. Over-expression clearly confers a growth advantage on some transformed cells, and could be vital for cells transformed by other oncogenes.

Oncogenes with products related to growth factor receptors

There are many proto-oncogenes, e.g. c-*erbB-1*, c-*erbB-2*, c-*erbB-3*, c-*fms* and c-*erbA* that encode the receptors of growth factors or hormones. Mutated to oncogenes by fast-transforming viruses, insertional mutagenesis or chemical mutagens, the net result is the same – the genes code for faulty receptors which behave as though a stimulating ligand was bound, even when it is not, thus stimulating the cell inappropriately. The first indication that altered receptors could be important for transformation came from the discovery that the viral oncogene v-*erbB* of avian erythroblastosis virus (AEV) encoded a protein corresponding to a truncated (shortened) epidermal growth factor receptor (EGFR). This protein lacked most of the extracellular ligand binding domain (see Fig. 5.13) with the result that it could then seemingly generate intracellular signals in the absence of binding ligand. Thus the gene encoding the normal EGFR became

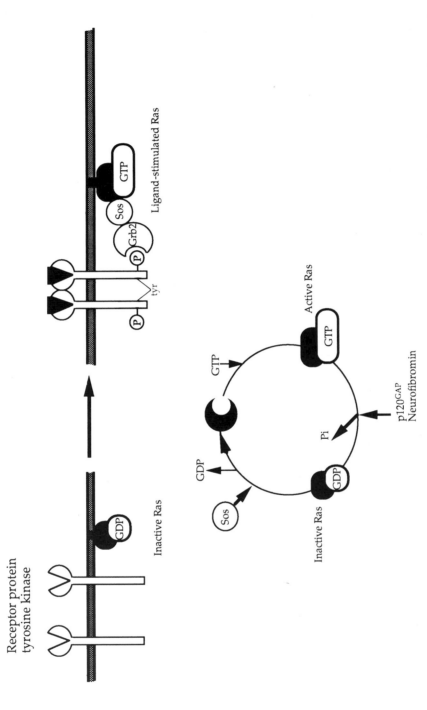

Fig. 3.8 Proposed model for the activation of Ras by the binding of ligand to receptors, resulting in their dimerization and receptor tyrosine (tyr) phosphoryl-ation (P). The autophosphorylation of tyrosine residues results in binding of Grb2:Sos complex (growth factor receptor bound protein 2: son of sevenless), and Sos, one of a family of guanosine nucleotide exchange factors, promotes the release of GDP from Ras and the binding of GTP.

known as c-*erbB-1*. The EGFR-related receptor proto-oncogene c-*erbB-2* (in the rat called *neu*) can produce a transforming protein through conversion of a valine to a glutamic acid residue in the transmembrane domain of the receptor molecule. This was first noted in a rat neuroblastoma induced by transplacental chemical carcinogenesis using nitrosourea. Over-expression of c-*erbB-2*, principally through gene amplification, may be associated with more aggressive tumour behaviour, particularly in breast cancer. Analysis of retroviral infected transformed cells has yielded other examples of incriminating mutant receptors, including the v-*fms* oncogene of feline sarcoma virus encoding a mutant receptor for macrophage-colony stimulating factor (M-CSF) and the v-*erbA* oncogene of AEV encoding a mutant nuclear receptor for thyroid hormone. Of course it is important to note that over-expression of a normal receptor, particularly in situations where its ligand is available, may also contribute to the malignant phenotype. Over-expression of EGFR, with or without gene amplification, is seen in many human tumours, and is a well known feature of the vulval carcinoma cell line A431, and could be expected to give the tumour cells a proliferative advantage (see Fig. 5.17).

Oncogenes with products related to guanine nucleotide-binding proteins

The Ras superfamily comprises at least 50 closely related proteins that share the ability to bind and hydrolyse guanosine triphosphate (GTP) to guanosine diphosphate (GDP). These GTPases regulate a diverse array of cellular functions including cell proliferation and differentiation, and the Ras superfamily proteins belong to a broader family of GTPases including the heterotrimeric ($\alpha\beta\gamma$) G proteins. The *ras* (rat sarcoma) proto-oncogene products are proteins of 21 kDa ($p21^{ras}$) attached to the plasma membrane. In the inactive state they bind GDP, but after activation of plasma membrane receptors following binding of growth factors, they are able to bind GTP and then slowly catalyse its hydrolysis to GDP (Fig. 3.8). $p21^{ras}$ is active in the GTP-bound form and has a growth-promoting effect. The *ras* oncogenes were discovered in two retroviruses known as the Harvey and Kirsten murine sarcoma viruses, which caused rat sarcomas; the cellular *ras* genes were mapped to different chromosomes and became known as c-H-*ras* and c-K-*ras,* another *ras* gene, c-N-*ras,* was detected in neuroblastoma DNA by transfection. The viral $p21^{ras}$ proteins are able to bind to GTP, but the rate at which hydrolysis to GDP occurs (i.e. GTPase activity) is less than with the normal cellular $p21^{ras}$ proteins. Nucleotide sequence analysis showed that in each case this was due to a single nucleotide change at either codon 12 or 13 or 59–61 leading to the substitution of different amino acid residues. The same event occurred in the neuroblastoma N-*ras* gene. Single point mutations seem to be totally responsible for the changes in biological activity of Ras proteins, leading to the accumulation of $p21^{ras}$ in the active GTP-bound form.

The activity of Ras proteins is vital in signalling by both non-receptor protein tyrosine kinases (PTKs), e.g. Src, and receptor protein tyrosine kinases (PTKs), involved in both cell proliferation and differentiation. Ras-GTP controls a mitogen activated protein (MAP) kinase cascade, and it appears that its major function is as a plasma

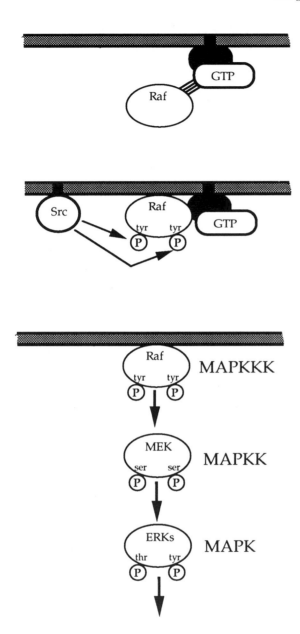

Activation of transcription

Fig. 3.9 In its activated GTP-bound form, Ras brings Raf to the inner surface of the plasma membrane, where it is activated by tyrosine (tyr) phosphorylation (P) through the action of Src. Raf functions as a mitogen activated protein kinase kinase kinase (MAPKKK), which sets in train a cascade of phosphorylation reactions ultimately leading to the phosphorylation of transcription factors.

membrane targeting signal for the serine-threonine kinase, Raf (Fig. 3.9). This kinase was first characterized as the product of the v-*raf* retroviral oncogene, and differs from the product of the normal cellular proto-oncogene (c-*raf*), by having deletions at the amino terminus. It now appears that the non-receptor PTK, Src, activates Raf by tyrosine phosphorylation. Activated Raf functions as a MAP kinase kinase kinase (MAPKKK) which phosphorylates a downstream dual specificity MAPKK known as MEK (MAPK/ERK kinase). In turn, threonine and tyrosine phosphorylation activates MAPKs, also known as ERKs (extracellular regulated kinases) which phosphorylate transcription factors involved in controlling gene expression.

Like other oncogenes, mutant *ras* genes are dominantly transforming, and are the most frequently detectable alteration in some human tumours, notably pancreatic cancer. Overall, mutations in one of the *ras* genes are found in ~40% of human cancers. How such relatively small changes in amino acid sequence affect activity is not entirely clear, but it seems likely that the mutation alters the intrinsic GTPase activity of p21^{ras} and the association between p21^{ras} and GTPase activating proteins (Ras GAPs). GAPs stimulate the intrinsic GTPase activity of p21^{ras} so that it enters the inactive GDP-bound state. Two mammalian GAPs have been identified, a ubiquitous protein known as p120^{GAP} which increases the GTP hydrolysis on Ras by up to 20,000 fold, and a GAP-related protein (p280^{NF1} neurofibromin) encoded by the *NF1* gene. Defective *NF1* is responsible for the human disorder, type 1 neurofibromatosis (or von Recklinghausen neurofibromatosis), and the normal gene encodes a protein with considerable homology to the catalytic domain of p120^{GAP}. The disease shows autosomal dominant inheritance and affects 1 in 3500 individuals of all races. Tissues from the neural crest are affected, and diagnostic features include benign tumours (neurofibromas) and flat pigmented lesions (café au lait spots). Patients with defective *NF1* are at increased risk of developing certain malignancies, especially malignant peripheral nerve sheath tumours, e.g. malignant schwannomas. It appears that both p120^{GAP} and p280^{NF1} are negative regulators of p21^{ras}, and that loss of p280^{NF1}, at least in Schwann cells, is sufficient to keep p21^{ras} in the activated state. The cell-type restriction of NF1 disease could be due to the fact that in other cell types p120^{GAP} is sufficient for negative regulation of p21^{ras}. It seems most likely that neurofibromin (p280^{NF1}) is a tumour suppressor gene product, and that patients with germ line mutations have loss or mutation of one *NF1* allele, and therefore produce less neurofibromin than normal. This situation would be analogous to other inherited predispositions to cancer where individuals have single mutant alleles of tumour suppressor genes (*p53* in Li-Fraumeni syndrome; *Rb* in juvenile retinoblastoma), see below. Malignancy could result from loss or mutation of the remaining *NF1* allele.

Oncogenes with products related to membrane-associated tyrosine kinases

There is a range of proteins that have the characteristic enzymatic property of phosphorylating proteins at tyrosine residues. Typically these PTKs are involved in the process of signal transduction. The best characterized of the non-receptor PTKs is the product of the cellular *src* gene, which produces a phosphoprotein of 60 kDa (pp60^{c-src})

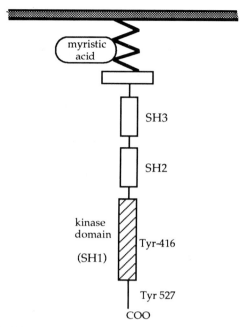

Fig. 3.10 Structure of the membrane-associated tyrosine (tyr) kinase, pp60$^{c\text{-}src}$.

generally associated with the inner surface of the plasma membrane (Fig. 3.10). *Src* is part of a multi-gene family, and all PTK members have regions of homology; the kinase domain is Src homology 1 (SH1) domain, and the region between residues 137 and 241 is well conserved between members, hence the SH2 domain. A further domain of approximately 60 amino acids is known as the Src homology 3 (SH3) domain. The gene derives its name from the fact that the gene responsible for the transforming activity of the Rous sarcoma virus (v-*src*) is derived from the cellular gene. The oncogenic activity of the Rous sarcoma virus (RSV) in chickens was first demonstrated by Peyton Rous back in 1910, when he found that a filter-passing agent from a tumour extract could transmit the tumour to other fowl. The RSV is unusual amongst fast-transforming viruses in that it retains all its replicative genes in addition to the oncogene, v-*src* (see Fig. 2.10). The mutant v-Src protein has amino acid deletions making it slightly smaller than the c-*src* gene product, but the molecular weight is still approximately 60 kDa, and it becomes readily phosphorylated at serine and threonine residues in transformed cells, hence it is known as pp60$^{v\text{-}src}$. Little is known about the cellular targets phosphorylated by the *src* gene product, but some seem to be associated with cell adhesion to the extracellular matrix and others to the attachment of actin microfilaments to the plasma membrane; cells containing pp60$^{v\text{-}src}$ show reduced adhesion to the extracellular matrix and tend to round up – properties common in tumour cells. Naturally, the Src protein is well positioned to mediate dramatic cytoskeletal rearrangements. Cells transformed by pp60$^{v\text{-}src}$ also show increased levels of tyrosine phosphorylated p74$^{c\text{-}raf}$ and a five-fold increase in p74$^{c\text{-}raf}$ associated serine/threonine kinase activity, and this is involved in activating transcription factors (see Fig. 3.9). Src may also be involved in controlling cell cycle progression by other means; a protein, Sam68 (<u>S</u>rc <u>a</u>ssociated in <u>m</u>itosis, 68 kDa) is tyrosine phosphorylated during mitosis. Src activity is normally repressed through the interaction of its SH2 domain and a phosphorylated tyrosine residue (Tyr 527), but the dephosphorylation of Tyr 527 during mitosis allows it to bind to targets such as Sam68 through the Src SH2 and SH3 domains; Sam68 is thought to be involved in RNA trafficking.

The c-*abl* proto-oncogene encodes a protein of between 145 and 150 kDa, which like the product of the *src* gene, is located on the inner surface of the plasma membrane. The c-*abl* proto-oncogene product also has tyrosine kinase activity and is expressed constitutively in CML when the c-*abl* gene is transferred from chromosome 9 to chromosome 22 (the Philadelphia chromosome), see Fig. 3.3.

Oncogenes with products related to cytoplasmic serine/threonine kinases

There are several cytoplasmic gene products which seem to be involved in the signal transduction pathways, and are implicated in transformation. Two of these genes, c-*mos* and c-*raf* encode protein kinases which phosphorylate serine and threonine residues on proteins leading to the activation of transcription factors (see Fig. 3.9). The significance of alterations in these genes in human tumours is poorly understood, though the v-*mos* product is associated with <u>mo</u>use <u>s</u>arcomas in mice infected with the murine sarcoma virus. In the frog *Xenopus*, the c-*mos* product appears responsible for holding the oocyte in metaphase during meiosis.

Oncogenes with products related to nucleus-associated molecules

Several oncogene products are localized to the nucleus. The *myc* oncogene was one of the first nuclear oncogenes to be defined, and was found to be the transforming gene of the <u>my</u>elo<u>c</u>ytomatosis viruses, retroviruses that cause myeloid leukaemias and other neoplasms in infected chickens. Its fascination has been its involvement, not only in tumours caused by retroviruses, but also in tumours associated with translocations (e.g. Burkitt's lymphoma, see Fig. 3.6) and where insertional mutagenesis (avian leukaemia virus) has led to increased c-*myc* expression and tumour formation. In fact, there is a series of *myc* genes, including N-*myc* and L-*myc*, first detected in neuroblastomas and small cell lung carcinomas respectively, both of which were discovered through gene amplification. The *myc* genes all encode proteins of approximately 62 kDa, which contain regions rich in basic amino acids suggesting a DNA binding capacity, which are more abundant in proliferating cells. The Myc protein generally forms heterodimers with an 18 kDa protein – Max, and Myc-Max heterodimers act as DNA-binding transcription factors recognizing CAC(G/A)TG sequences, thus activating transcription from these sites. Another DNA-binding protein is encoded by the c-*myb* proto-oncogene, again it was first identified as the transforming gene of avian <u>my</u>elo<u>b</u>lastosis virus (v-*myb*), which causes myeloblastic leukaemia in chickens. Like other viral oncogene products, the viral Myb protein differs from its normal cellular counterpart, with extensive stretches of amino acids deleted at both the N- and C-terminals.

Other nuclear oncogenes are also closely linked to the regulation of gene expression (transcription). Gene transcription is controlled by proteins (transcriptional factors) with DNA-binding motifs which bind to specific nucleotide sequences, 'promoters' and 'enhancers', close to the initiation codon of each gene. The *fos* gene product is a phosphoprotein of 55 kDa (pp55$^{c\text{-}fos}$) whose expression is enhanced in many cells within minutes of application of proliferative and differentiating stimuli. The *fos* gene product is a transcription factor. In retroviruses containing *fos* (e.g. FBT mouse osteos-arcoma virus) the gene can be altered allowing for a greater stability of *fos* mRNA. Relatively recently it has been shown that the c-*fos* gene product can form a complex with the c-*jun* proto-oncogene product to form a transcription factor known as AP-1. Very specific binding can occur between the two proteins due to their so-called 'leu-cine zipper' regions – regions containing five leucine residues at regular spaced inter-vals. Given the importance of gene expression for proliferation and differentiation, it is hardly surprising that alterations in nuclear proto-oncogenes encoding transcription factors are implicated in tumorigenesis.

3.3   Tumour suppressor genes

Discovery

In considering the somatic mutation hypothesis for explaining how cancer arises, two large classes of genes need to be considered. So far we have discussed oncogenes, originally discovered through the study of critical genes in the acutely transforming retroviruses, but we also need to examine a second class called anti-oncogenes or more correctly tumour suppressor genes. These genes were identified through the study of hereditary cancers, though the term 'hereditary cancer' is a misnomer in that what is inherited is a *predisposition* to cancer. The existence of tumour suppressor genes had long been suspected from the occurrence of non-random chromosome loss from particular tumours, suggesting that loss of specific gene products was required for tumorigenesis to occur.

For many of the common as well as some of the rarer human cancers there appears to be at least one inherited form; i.e. all cancers exist in both a hereditary and non-hereditary (sporadic) form. Tumour suppressor genes were discovered in retinoblastoma, a rare malignant tumour derived from retinal cells, which occurs almost exclusively in chil-dren. In 1971, Knudson postulated that this rare childhood tumour (100 cases per annum in the UK) was triggered by two successive lesions in the cell genome. In proposing this, he examined the two forms of the disease – familial and sporadic. Tumour suppressor genes produce cancer in a recessive mode, one normal allele seems to be adequate to protect against a particular cancer. In the strict Mendelian sense, recessive alleles are expressed in the homozygous, but not in the heterozygous state – what is expressed in the homozygous state is a lack of tumour suppression caused by the mutation or loss of both alleles. Sporadic cases of retinoblastoma, found usually in older children, are rarer

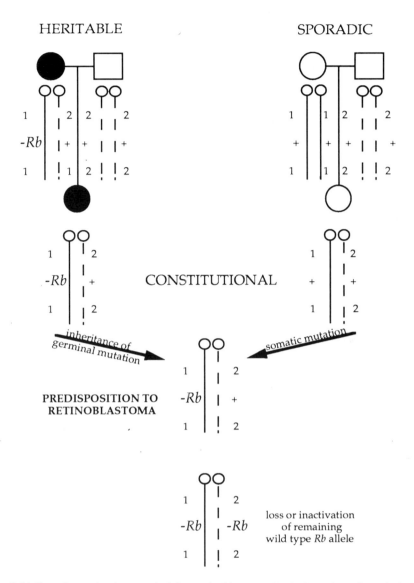

Fig. 3.11 Genetic mechanisms underlying retinoblastoma. In the hereditary form (left) the child inherits a chromosome 13 from her affected mother which carries a recessive defect at the *Rb* locus (designated −*Rb*), and so is genotypically +/− at this locus in all her cells. A retinoblastoma (or other tumour, see Table 3.2) would develop through loss or mutation of the remaining dominant wild-type *Rb* allele in an appropriate cell, e.g. retinoblast. In the sporadic form (right), both copies of the *Rb* gene must be lost or inactivated through somatic mutation in the same cell for a tumour to develop.

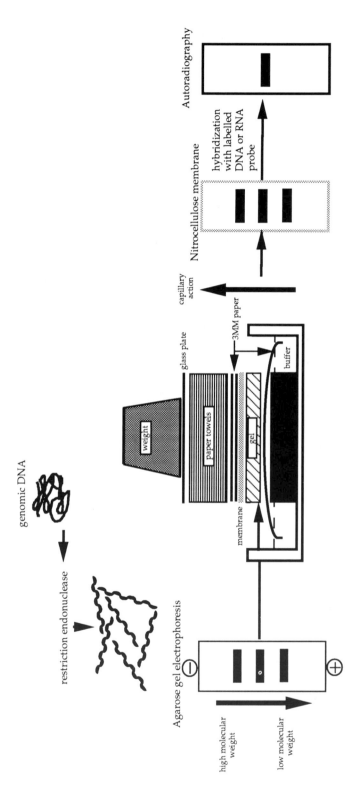

Fig. 3.12 Genomic Southern blotting for the detection of specific DNA sequences. DNA digested by a restriction endonuclease(s) is separated according to size; DNA is negatively charged so the smallest fragments will migrate furthest towards the anode. DNA rendered single-stranded by alkali, is then blotted onto a nitrocellulose sheet by capillary action. The DNA fragments, still arrayed by size, can now be probed for specific nucleotide sequences using a ^{32}P-radiolabelled nucleic acid probe. The probe will hybridize to complementary sequences in the DNA, and can be localized by exposing the sheet to X-ray film.

than familial cases, and are thought to involve sequential loss or mutation of both the *Rb* gene alleles (Fig. 3.11). Thus, the genotype changes from normal (+/+) to heterozygote (+/−) to abnormal homozygote (−/−), which develops cancer in a recessive manner – two somatic mutations. This is clearly a very rare event. However, in the familial cancers, one of these mutations is in the germ line, thus all cells, including retinoblasts, are heterozygous at the *Rb* locus. A likelihood of mutation or loss of the remaining wild-type *Rb* allele is much more likely than two somatic mutations at the same locus, and indeed, compared to the sporadic form, familial retinoblastoma is seen in younger children and is often bilateral.

The retinoblastoma susceptibility gene, *Rb*, encodes a 105 kDa nucleoprotein (p105^{Rb} or pRb) which in its under-phosphorylated state binds to the transcription factor E2F (a heterodimeric protein composed of an E2F [adenovirus early gene 2 factor] and a DP [differentiation protein] family member). E2F plays an important role in the control of the transition from G$_1$ to S. Hyperphosphorylation of pRb at the end of G$_1$ may allow release of these transcription factors, and certainly prevents interaction of pRb with newly synthesized E2F proteins, leading to cell cycle progression. Though originally named because of its importance in retinoblastoma, abnormalities of the *Rb* gene are thought to be important in the development of several other neoplasms, notably sarcomas. This is well illustrated by the fact that patients with bilateral (familial) but not unilateral retinoblastoma have a high incidence of the development of independent second-site tumours, particularly osteosarcomas. Thus, there is evidence of a genetic association (lack of the same suppressor gene(s) function) between apparently disparate tumour types. Further evidence of a central role of pRb in cell cycle control comes from the information that, like p53, another growth-suppressing protein found in the nucleus, pRb is inactivated (sequestered) by the transforming proteins of DNA tumour viruses such as SV40 and human papillomavirus. It appears that both pRb and p53 need to be inactivated before full viral transformation can occur.

Detection of tumour suppressor genes by loss of heterozygosity

The steps that lead to homozygosity of a mutant suppressor allele usually involve the flanking chromosomal regions as well. Thus, it is possible to trace the presence or absence of a mutant gene by following a marker which is situated close by on the same chromosome. Many of these markers are highly polymorphic since they contain a restriction endonuclease site which differs between individuals; the recognition site for a restriction endonuclease may be lost by alteration of just one base pair. This creates a *restriction fragment length polymorphism* (RFLP), which can be readily detected by Southern blotting with a radiolabelled DNA probe. The term Southern blotting was coined from the original description by Ed Southern of being able to transfer size-fractionated DNA from an agarose gel onto a solid support (nylon or nitrocellulose membrane), followed by hybridization with a labelled probe (Fig. 3.12). Since the amount of radiolabelled probe that hybridizes to a Southern blot is proportional to the number of gene copies present in the target DNA, the technique can be used quantitat-ively to detect gene amplification, e.g. c-*erbB-2* in many breast cancers.

Genomic DNA is much too large to migrate through an agarose gel, and must be first cleaved into smaller manageable fragments using an appropriate 'restriction endonuclease'. These enzymes have evolved to protect bacteria from invasion by fore-ign DNA molecules, e.g. viruses. There are over 180 of these enzymes, and all recog-nize specific nucleotide sequences; most recognize either four base- or six base-pair recognition sites, and these sequences are often palindromes, i.e. the 5′ to 3′ sequence in the upper strand is identical to the 5′ to 3′ sequence in the lower strand (Fig. 3.13). So-called 'six-base cutters' like EcoR1 are more widely used than four-base cutters since the recognition site will occur less frequently in a stretch of DNA, thus the fragments will be longer and more likely to contain useful information.

RFLPs occurring through variations in the non-coding DNA sequences are extremely frequent, though the variations in the size of fragments detected by an appropriate probe need to be quite large (50–100 base pairs) if they are to be clearly separable on a gel – allowing for the absence of one to be detectable – this is known as an *informative pattern*.

DNA cut with restriction enzymes migrates according to size by electrophoresis in an agarose gel, the small fragments migrating furthest. The DNA fragments in the gel are then denatured into single strands and transferred by the technique of Southern blotting to nylon membranes where they are hybridized to the appropriate radiolabel-led probe. Examination of the autoradiographs shows that normal somatic cells from an individual who is heterozygous for a particular marker will yield two bands, but if tumour tissue from the same individual has a deletion of the marker on one of the pair of chromosomes, this will result in a single band (Fig. 3.14). This situation is referred to as a *loss of heterozygosity* (LOH), and the repeated observation of LOH of a specific chromosomal marker in cells from a particular tumour type suggests the presence of a closely mapping tumour suppressor gene, the loss of which is involved in tumour pathogenesis. LOH of course, still leaves the tumour hemizygous for the

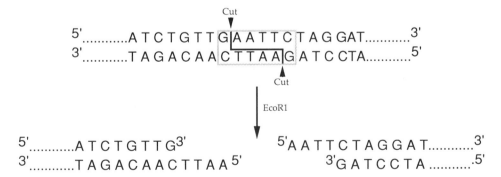

Fig. 3.13 Digestion of DNA with the restriction endonuclease EcoR1 which recognizes a six base-pair sequence GAATTC, which, because of the staggered cut makes 'sticky' ends.

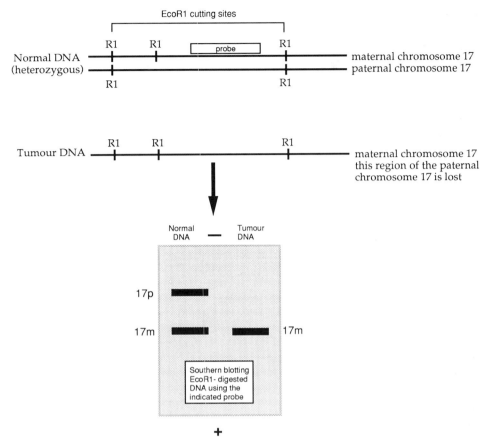

Fig. 3.14 The use of restriction fragment length polymorphisms and Southern blotting to detect loss of heterozygosity in tumour tissue. In this example, normal cells are heterozygous for an EcoR1 recognition site. After digestion, electrophoresis, and Southern blotting, the DNA is probed with the probe to the region as indicated, revealing a heterozygous banding pattern (reflecting the presence of both polymorphisms, one on each chromosome). However, if one of the chromosomes from tumour tissue from this individual shows loss of this pattern, then this suggests the presence of a closely mapping tumour suppressor gene which has been lost.

detected segment, nevertheless if this region contains a non-functional allele because of either a pre-existing inherited mutation or an acquired somatic mutation then this incriminates the particular locus in tumour formation. Thus, LOH usually unmasks a more subtle recessive mutation in the retained copy of a tumour suppressor gene. Mapping of homozygous deletions within regions showing a high frequency of LOH has also incriminated the loss of certain alleles in particular tumours. Using a large repertoire of polymorphic DNA markers, specific tumours have been surveyed systematically looking for repeated instances of LOH, and following this relatively simple approach a number of tumour suppressor genes have been well categorized (Table 3.2).

Table 3.2 *Tumour suppressor genes whose loss or mutation is implicated in human cancer*

Gene	Chromosome	Possible function of protein product	Common tumours
APC	5q	Forms complex with α- and β-catenin and tubulin	Colorectum (familial and sporadic)
WT1	11p	Transcriptional and post-transcriptional regulator	Wilms' tumour
Rb	13q	Regulates availability of E2F family of transcription factors	Retinoblastoma, osteosarcoma, small cell lung carcinoma
p53	17p	Transcription factor for *WAF-1/Cip1*	Breast, lung, colon, brain, pancreas (Li-Fraumeni syndrome)
p16	9p	Inhibitor of cyclin-Cdk complexes	Pancreas, gliomas
NF1	17q	Negative regulator of Ras	Malignant Schwannoma
DPC4	18q	Involved in TGFβ-induced growth suppression	Pancreas
DCC	18q	Cell adhesion molecule	Colon
BRCA1	17q	Secreted growth factor (granin family member)	Breast and ovary, also prostate and colon
BRCA2	13q	Unknown	Breast (female and male), prostate and others
nm23	17q	Nucleoside diphosphate kinase	Breast, many others

APC *(Adenomatous polyposis coli)*

Tumour suppressor genes seem to be very important in large bowel carcinogenesis. In the hereditary condition, familial adenomatous polyposis (FAP), the affected individuals develop hundreds or even thousands of small benign tumours (adenomas) in their colorectal mucosa. If not treated by prophylactic colectomy, FAP patients invariably develop colorectal adenocarcinoma. Point mutations in a candidate tumour suppressor gene *APC* in the germ line appear to confer susceptibility to colonic cancer, and result in a shortened *APC* gene product, probably due to the insertion of a stop codon. While the inherited allele is mutated, the normal allele seems to be lost in the transition to carcinoma. This acquired loss of heterozygosity for chromosome 5q can be detected by RFLP. Adherent junctions are organized around cell–cell adhesion molecules known as cadherins (Fig. 3.15), and these complex with membrane proteins such as α- and β-catenins and p120, the latter being a target for Src kinase. In addition to the membrane-associated cadherin–catenin complex, the α- and β-catenins form a complex with the tumour suppressor protein APC (a 300 kDa protein of 2843 amino acids) in the cytoplasm. The cadherin–catenin complex is a candidate receptor for the contact inhibition signal that helps regulate proliferation, while the APC-catenin complex may be part of the transduction pathway for this signal. This hypothesis would fit the observed mutant APC phenotype – a moderate deregulation of the colonic

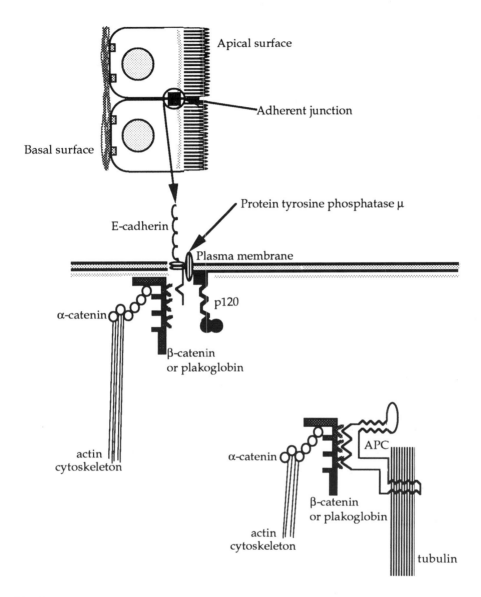

Fig. 3.15 Epithelial cells have adherent junctions (zonula adherens) at their apices in which E-cadherin mediates cell–cell adhesion. On the cytoplasmic face is a multi-protein complex of catenins, and α- and β-catenins also form a cytosolic complex with the adenomatous polyposis coli (APC) protein, which also binds tubulin.

epithelial hierarchy. In addition to APC mutations, the observation of frequent deletion and LOH on chromosome 3p in many tumours, suggests that disturbance of β-catenin could also be involved in neoplastic development.

WT1 *(Wilms' tumour)*

Double allelic loss of a tumour suppressor gene is also thought to be responsible for the childhood renal tumour, Wilms' tumour, both in familial and sporadic forms. Like familial retinoblastoma, the chromosome from one parent is thought to already carry a specific deletion or mutation of a tumour suppressor gene, but this time on the short arm of chromosome 11; one further mutation being needed in the familial form for reduction to homozygosity to be acquired. WT1 may bind to both DNA and RNA, and therefore may be involved in both transcriptional and post-transcriptional (controlling constitutive and alternative splicing, translation) regulation.

p53

The *p53* gene encodes a protein product of 53 kDa and was identified by David Lane in 1979, when it was found to form a complex with the transforming large T antigen of SV40 virus. *p53* was initially placed in the oncogene camp since it could collaborate with cotransfected *ras* in the transformation of NIH/3T3 cells. Subsequently it became clear that this initial work had been with mutant *p53* cDNA clones, and wild-type *p53* cDNAs were strongly suppressive of the transformed phenotype. It is now clear that *functional* deletion of both wild-type *p53* alleles is necessary to cause malignant trans-formation, but *p53* does not necessarily conform to the principles used to define other tumour suppressor genes: one mutant *p53* gene can act as a dominantly transforming oncogene. Normal p53 protein is thought to oligomerize into a multi-subunit complex which acts as a brake on cell proliferation through being a transcriptional regulator, but defective subunits of an oligomerizing protein (e.g. mutant p53 protein molecules) seem to combine with wild-type monomers and inactivate the complex as a whole. The p53 protein promotes transcription of the *Cip1/WAF-1* gene (Cdk-interacting protein/wild-type p53 activated fragment), whose protein product, p21^{Cip1}, is a universal inhibitor of cyclin-dependent kinases (Cdks) and so might be expected to check cell cycle progression at many points in the cell cycle (Fig. 3.16). The protein, p21^{Cip1} also binds to DNA polymerase δ auxiliary protein (also known as proliferating cell nuclear antigen, PCNA, see Chapter 5, section 5.1), blocking its function in DNA replication but not in DNA repair.

Cell proliferation is achieved through an orderly progression around the cell cycle (see Chapter 5, section 5.1), and this in turn is controlled by protein complexes of cyclins and Cdks. The cyclin is thought to be a regulatory molecule, while the Cdk functions as the catalytic subunit, phosphorylating fundamental elements such as the Rb protein, which is necessary for the transition into DNA synthesis (Fig. 3.19). Five major classes of cyclins (termed A through to E) have been described, whose expression is cell cycle-dependent (Fig. 3.17B); likewise, multiple Cdks have been

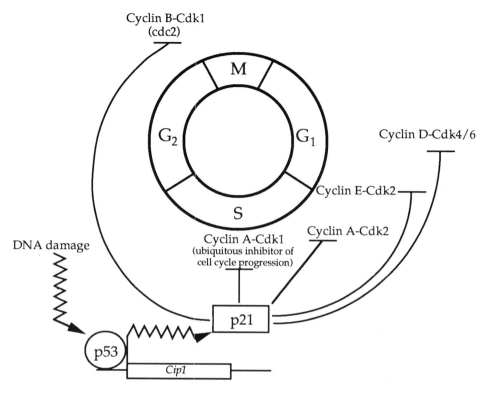

Fig. 3.16 p21, encoded by *Cip1*, is a universal inhibitor of cyclin-dependent kinases, inhibiting cell cycle progression at many points. DNA damage leads to the accumulation of transcriptionally active p53 that induces expression of p21 mRNA and protein.

identified whose abundance varies depending on the cell cycle phase. Cyclin D-Cdk4 complexes seem to govern G_1 progression, cyclin E-Cdk2 controls the G_1 to S transition, progression through S is regulated by cyclin A-Cdk2 and cyclin B-Cdk1 (also known as Cdc2) controls entry into mitosis. There is growing evidence for the involvement of mutations in cyclin and Cdk genes in tumorigenesis, thus the genes can also be considered as proto-oncogenes.

The protein, p21^{Cip1}, is only one of an emerging set of proteins that act as negative regulators of cyclin-Cdk complexes, others named from their apparent molecular weight include p15^{Ink4B}, p16^{Ink4A} and p27^{Kip1}; the genes that encode these Cdk-inhibitory molecules have been designated the *CKI* genes. These genes including *Kip1* (<u>k</u>inase <u>i</u>nhibitor <u>p</u>rotein 1) and *Ink4* (<u>in</u>hibitor of Cd<u>k4</u>) are commonly upregulated by TGFβ, correlating with cell cycle arrest. Alternatively, the adenovirus E1A protein can rescue cells from TGFβ-induced arrest by binding to p27^{Kip1} and disabling its function. Point mutations in *p16* are found in 40% of pancreatic adenocarcinomas, while, unusually for a tumour suppressor gene, many pancreatic tumours and glioblastomas have a homozygous deletion of *p16*. Normally, cell cycle progression can be induced by destroying these inhibitors through attaching them to ubiquitin, thus marking them for degradation. In turn, cyclin-Cdk complexes can also be turned off by destroying the

(A)

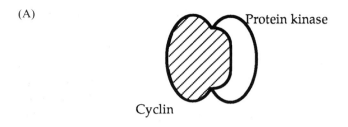

(B)

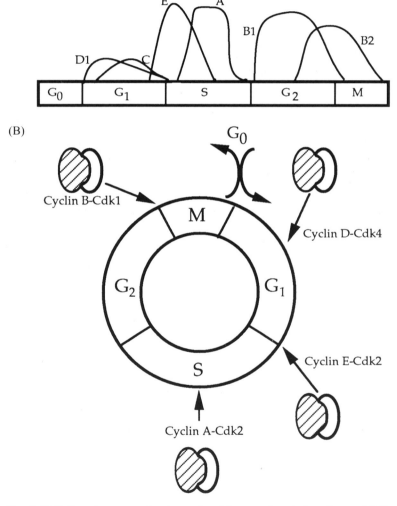

Fig. 3.17 Cell cycle progression is regulated by complexes of cyclins and Cdks. (A) The cyclin is the regulatory molecule and the Cdk is the catalytic subunit. (B) The expression of the cyclins is cell cycle-dependent, and the activity of each cyclin-Cdk complex is regulated by a set of inhibitory proteins (p15, p16, p21, p27) and ubiquitin-mediated proteolysis.

cyclin through ubiquitin-mediated proteolysis. Thus ubiquitin may be a major player in cell cycle control.

Although p21^{Cip1} appears to be the most pleiotropic mediator of p53-dependent cell cycle arrest, other genes are transcriptionally activated by p53 and may also have a role in arresting cell cycle progression. The growth arrest and DNA damage gene, *Gadd45*, appears to be such a candidate, and the protein may block DNA replication and enhance nucleotide excision of damaged DNA. Like *Gadd45*, the *Mdm2* gene has p53 responsive elements. The Mdm2 protein (human homologue of murine double-minute 2) is a 90 kDa zinc-finger protein (p90) that binds directly to p53 and abolishes p53's transcriptional activity. The Mdm2 protein may also bind to pRb, so a single proto-oncogene which is amplified in a variety of tumours, can bypass the usual p53 and pRb checks on cell cycle progression.

p53 *and* pRb *are major cell cycle regulators*

Mdm2 proteins not only repress the transcriptional activity of the p53 protein, and bind to pRb, affecting pRb's ability to sequester proteins such as the E2F transcription factors which stimulate transcription of genes implicated in the induction of DNA synthesis, but they may also directly activate E2F/DP1 activity. Though initially the two suppressor proteins, p53 and pRb, were considered as separate entities, it now appears that p53 and pRb may act in the same pathway to arrest the cell cycle. A number of viral proteins as well as the cellular protein Mdm2 bind to and inactivate p53 and/or pRb (Fig. 3.18). The transforming protein of the SV40 virus, the large T antigen, may mimic the action of mutant p53, sequestering wild-type p53 in inactive complexes which are prohibited from reaching the cell nucleus. The E6 transforming protein of the human papillomavirus (HPV) and the E1B oncoprotein of adenovirus also bind to p53 and inactivate its transcriptional activity. Similarly, under-phosphorylated pRb molecules are functionally inactivated when complexed with

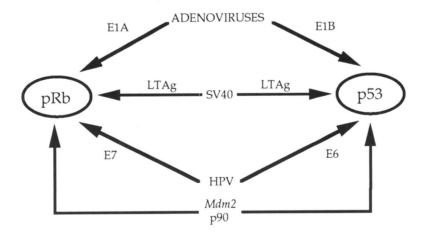

Fig. 3.18 A variety of viral proteins, as well as p90, the product of the *Mdm2* gene, bind the important cell regulatory proteins pRb and p53 and abolish their function.

either the SV40 large T antigen, the HPV E7 protein or the adenovirus E1A protein. This inactivation of pRb by viral transforming proteins is because they bind to the 'Rb pocket', a sequence of 400 amino acids which normally binds the E2F transcription factor. Other so-called pocket proteins are p107 and p130 which are associated with E2F at different stages of the cell cycle. It appears that loss of one of the tumour suppressor gene functions is compensated for by the activity of the other, but high transformation strains of tumour viruses that encode proteins that bind and inactivate both p53 and pRb permit tumour formation through unrestrained E2F induction of DNA synthesis. A working model for a potential link between p53 and pRb in normal cell cycle regulation is presented in Fig. 3.19. p53 influences the activity of cyclin-Cdks that phosphorylate pRb, *via* p21^{Cip1} production. High levels of p21^{Cip1} could inhibit cyclin-Cdk2 thereby maintaining pRb in the under-phosphorylated state, in this state pRb complexes tightly with E2F transcription factors and blocks the transcription of genes required for cell cycle progression. If indeed pRb does function downstream from p53, it would explain how viral proteins such as E7, which sequester under-phosphorylated pRb, can override a p53-induced cell cycle arrest. Highly phosphorylated pRb cannot bind E2F transcription factors and E2F response sites are present in a number of genes implicated in the induction of DNA synthesis. In turn, cyclin E-Cdk2 and all the other cyclin-Cdks may be switched off by proteins encoded by the *CKI* gene family, which themselves are activated by the plasma membrane binding of inhibitory growth factors such as TGFβ.

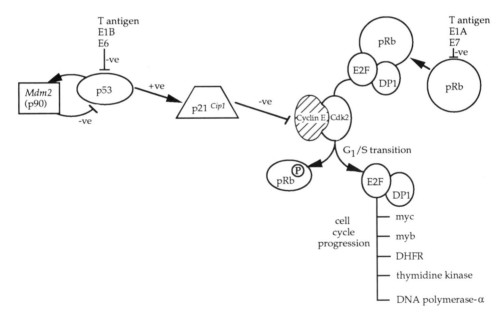

Fig. 3.19 Tumour suppressor proteins p53 and pRb can act in concert to block cell cycle progression. Phosphorylation of pRb allows the transcription factor complex E2F-DP1 to promote the transcription of a variety of genes involved in DNA synthesis. p21, transcriptionally regulated by p53, can inactivate cyclin-Cdk2 and thus inhibit pRb phosphorylation. DHFR, dihydrofolate reductase.

The function of p53 has been likened to that of a 'molecular policeman' or 'guardian of the genome' – when DNA is damaged, p53 accumulates dramatically (up to 60-fold) and switches off replication to allow time for DNA repair. If repair fails, p53 may trigger apoptosis (see Chapter 5, section 5.3). Cells in which p53 is mutated, or bound to viral proteins, cannot carry out this protective arrest, and are more likely to accumulate genetic mutations and are, thus, more prone to malignant transformation. Like other defective tumour suppressor genes, mutant *p53* alleles can be passed through the germ line enhancing the predisposition of affected individuals to the development of a number of tumours. Li-Fraumeni syndrome patients have *p53* germ line mutations which have a 'high penetrance', that is 90% of affected individuals will develop cancer. Tumours which develop include soft tissue sarcomas, astrocytomas and breast carcinomas, but if point mutations in *p53* create dominant negative alleles that disrupt normal cell regulation, how can such changes be tolerated during embryological development? The answer is that it is probably a question of dosage; various mutant alleles encode a variety of amino acid substitutions, some of which are minimally dysfunctional while others create strongly penetrant, dominant negative activity. Abnormalities of *p53* are the commonest genetic abnormality in human cancer, maybe being involved in up to 70% of tumours; antibodies are commercially available to immunocytochemically detect mutant p53 which is much more stable in the cell than the short-lived normal p53 protein.

DCC (*Deleted in colorectal cancer*)

Observations of frequent allele loss involving chromosome 18q lead to the cloning of another tumour suppressor gene, termed *DCC*. *DCC* is expressed ubiquitously in normal adult tissues, and encodes a transmembrane protein very similar to the neural cell adhesion molecules (N-CAM). These molecules are involved in cell-cell and cell-extracellular matrix interactions, and loss or derangement of such molecules can be expected to lead to altered adhesion and to the diminution of the growth-restraining signals associated with such adhesion. Allelic losses (LOH) affecting 18q are detected in 70% of primary colorectal adenocarcinomas, and together with the reduced or lost expression of *DCC* mRNA in more than half of these cases, suggest the retained *DCC* allele is frequently mutated.

DPC4

The vast majority of pancreatic carcinomas show allelic loss at chromosome 18q, but sometimes this does not involve *DCC*; a gene designated *DPC4* (deleted in pancreatic carcinoma locus 4) is commonly homozygously deleted or one allele is missing and the other mutated. The *DPC4* gene has sequence similarity to the *Drosophila* gene *mad* (mothers against *dpp*), and in *Drosophila* homozygous *mad* mutants have a similar phenotype to those with mutations in the decapentaplegic (*dpp*) gene, a gene which encodes a member of the TGFβ superfamily. Thus *DPC4* appears to be involved in some aspect of the TGFβ pathway of growth inhibition.

nm23-H1 *and* nm23-H2

Two homologous genes, *nm23-H1* and *nm23-H2*, encode the A and B polypeptide subunits of a nucleoside diphosphate (NDP) kinase, often referred to as Nm23/NDP kinase. Although the *nm23* gene was originally considered to be a tumour suppressor gene because a reduced expression of the encoded enzyme was found to correlate with a high metastatic potential in some tumours (notably breast carcinomas), its higher than normal expression in other tumours is positively correlated with proliferation and progression – this questions the wisdom of placement of the gene exclusively in the suppressor camp.

BRCA1 *and* BRCA2, *genes for breast and ovarian cancer susceptibility*

The recognition of an inherited predisposition to cancer can be almost impossible in an individual case since the heritable cancer may look just like its non-heritable counterpart. In the rare *inherited cancer syndromes*, which account for only about 1% of cancer incidence, it is often the association of characteristic phenotypic abnormalities with a particular cancer which identifies that cancer as being of a heritable type. For example, if colorectal cancer arises within the setting of multiple intestinal adenomatous lesions, this is a strong indication that this is a case of familial adenomatous polyposis. Similarly, in the case of multiple endocrine neoplasia type 2 (MEN type 2), medullary carcinoma of the thyroid or phaeochromocytoma of the adrenal medulla may arise within a setting of C cell, adrenal medullary and even parathyroid hyperplasias.

A genetic predisposition is also indicated if the cancer is rare (e.g. retinoblastoma), and several cases occur in one family or multiple primaries occur in one individual. However, if the cancer is common, like breast cancer, the significance of several cases in one family is more difficult to assess with regard to a genetic predisposition, and, in addition, no distinguishing phenotype marks any heritable form. However, there is now unequivocal evidence that about 5–10% of breast cancer cases are due to an inherited predisposition, and the incriminating gene, known as *BRCA1*, was localized to chromosome 17q by *genetic linkage analysis* in families with many cases of early onset breast cancer. Sporadic breast cancer is most commonly diagnosed in the 55–65 year old age group, but the familial type presents much earlier, often in women in their thirties and even late twenties. Linkage analysis is based on the ability to find DNA markers of known chromosomal location that are consistently co-inherited with the disease state (taken to represent the presence of the disease gene) in affected families. If the DNA marker and the gene responsible for the disease are close together on the same chromosome, they will tend to be inherited together and are said to be 'linked' (Fig. 3.20). However, if the marker and the disease gene are quite far apart, then the chance that they will part in some offspring due to crossing-over at meiosis will be increased. The probability that the observed inheritance pattern of the marker and the disease occurs because they are physically linked (at a specified distance) on the same chromosome is calculated, and expressed as a ratio relative to the probability

(A)　　　　　　　　　　　　　　　　　　　(B)

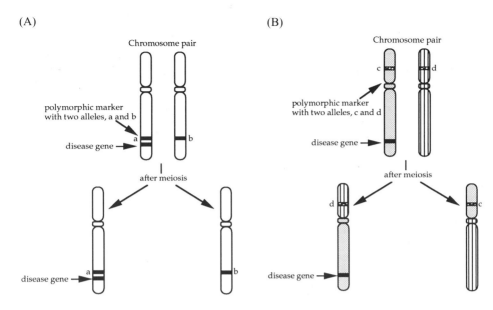

Fig. 3.20 The principle of genetic linkage analysis, a technique which has been used to localize the *BRCA1* gene to a specific region on the long arm of chromosome 17. (A) If the disease gene and marker locus are close together on the same chromosome, they will be inherited together, and are thus 'linked'. (B) If the disease gene and the marker are far apart on the same chromosome, they will not show linkage and will tend to segregate independently of each other.

that the same result would have occurred by chance (the marker and the disease gene are unlinked). This ratio expresses the odds for (or against) linkage and since the logarithm of the ratio is used it is known as the 'LOD' score (logarithm of the odds). A LOD score of >3 is considered proof of positive linkage (odds of 1000:1 in favour of linkage). Using a series of highly polymorphic markers, *BRCA1* has been narrowed down to a region on 17q flanked by markers *D17S776* and *D17S78*.

It appears that in almost all families with familial breast and ovarian cancer, and in about half those families with breast cancer alone, the *BRCA1* gene is mutated. The protein encoded by *BRCA1* is large, 190 kDa, and it may function as a transcription factor since it contains a zinc finger, and some mutations remove the last pair of cysteine residues. Alternatively, BRCA1 protein has some sequence homology with the granin protein family, whose members possibly function as precursors of biologically active peptides as well as being involved in the packaging of peptides into secretory vesicles. The BRCA1 protein has been reported to be present in such vesicles, and most *BRCA1* mutations produce truncated proteins which lack growth-suppressive properties. Thus, BRCA1 could be a secreted growth factor, a novel property for a tumour suppressor gene product. Indeed, since *BRCA1* mRNA expression is enhanced in mice during pregnancy, BRCA1 may mediate protection by inhibiting proliferation of breast epithelial cells during pregnancy and lactation. In breast and ovarian cancer families, loss of heterozygosity studies consistently show 17q loss in the cancers, leaving mutant *BRCA1* on the remaining chromosome 17. These observations support the 'two-hit' hypothesis, strengthening the belief that *BRCA1* is a tumour suppressor gene. One surprising finding is the lack of somatic *BRCA1* mutations in sporadic breast and ovarian cancers, the conventional wisdom being that genes involved in susceptibility to cancer also undergo mutation in sporadic cancers. In a substantial proportion of breast cancer families, the disease is not linked to *BRCA1*. Another genomic linkage search was initiated, and a new susceptibility gene, *BRCA2*, was located to 13q12–13. Interestingly, *BRCA2* mutations show a strong association with male breast cancer, though only a small proportion of affected males in the families develop the disease (~5% by age 70). LOH on chromosome 13q occurs in many cases of sporadic breast cancer and other tumours, suggesting there is a mutated tumour suppressor gene in this region. *BRCA2* could be this gene, though it is important to exclude the possibility of inactivation of the *Rb* gene.

3.4   Summary of the molecular mechanisms of cancer pathogenesis

Overview

The behaviour of normal cells seems to be regulated by growth promoting proto-oncogenes, counterbalanced by the growth-constraining tumour suppressor genes. Alterations (point mutation, gene amplification, insertional mutagenesis, translocations) that potentiate the activities of proto-oncogenes create the oncogenes that promote growth and the establishment of the malignant phenotype. Conversely, genetic alterations in tumour suppressor genes result in a loss of growth restraint normally imposed by the protein products of these genes. The end product of these two events would seem to be the same – deregulated cell behaviour (proliferation and differentiation). However, accumulating evidence suggests that the development of many malignant tumours requires *both* types of change in the tumour genome.

In vitro systems such as the mouse NIH/3T3 cell line for the identification of oncogenes are rather too simplistic. Here a transfected *ras* oncogene can cause transformation, but the target cells are already abnormal in becoming established in culture. A better test of function of an altered gene is to reinsert it into an organism and to see what effect it has. Modified genes can be inserted into fertilized oocytes and the newly adopted genes will be passed on to the progeny – animals that have been permanently altered in this way are called 'transgenic'. Transgenic mice have made an important contribution to our understanding of neoplasia. An oncogene can be linked to a suitable DNA promoter, and will either be expressed in many tissues or only in a few, according to the tissue specificity of the associated promoter. For example, transgenic mice carrying either the v-H-*ras* oncogene or the c-*myc* oncogene driven by the MMTV promoter/enhancer, will develop mammary tumours in a time-dependent manner (Fig. 3.21). However, the vast majority of mammary gland cells expressing either the *myc* or H-*ras* oncogene do not become malignant, showing that a single oncogene is not sufficient to cause neoplastic transformation. When the MMTV/v-H-*ras* and MMTV/c-*myc* transgenic strains are crossed to yield hybrid mice expressing

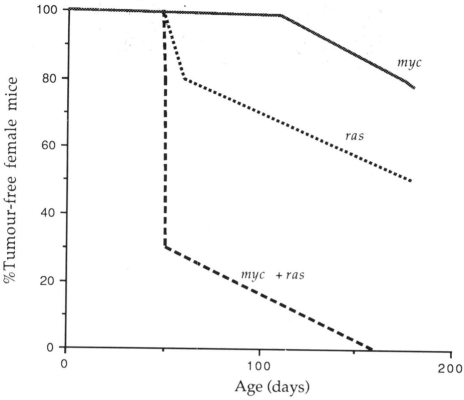

Fig. 3.21 Co-expression of *myc* and *ras* in transgenic mice results in a dramatic and synergistic acceleration of tumour formation. (Redrawn from Sinn *et al.*, 1987, *Cell*, **49**, 465–75.)

both oncogenes, then there is a dramatic and synergistic acceleration of tumour formation (Fig. 3.21). Nevertheless, there is still a lag before any tumours are formed, they still arise stochastically and are still a very rare event amongst all the non-malignant mammary cells. Taken together these observations suggest that even two oncogenes, by themselves, are not sufficient to induce malignant transformation, and further randomly generated changes are necessary for the malignant phenotype to arise.

Colorectal cancer is a major cause of cancer death in the Western world, and the widespread availability of fresh tissue from potentially curative resection specimens has resulted in this tumour type being more thoroughly investigated than probably any other type. Experiments in animals involving chronic administration of carcinogens, such as dimethylhydrazine, have shown that first the colonic epithelium becomes generally hyperplastic, followed weeks or months later by the development of discrete benign tumours (adenomas). Some time later carcinomas arise. In humans too, there is now overwhelming evidence of an adenoma–carcinoma sequence, colorectal carcinoma is usually preceded by the development of an adenoma(s), and the malignant change occurs within this precursor lesion. Familial adenomatous polyposis patients who refuse treatment following the detection of colorectal adenomas invariably develop carcinomas within a few years. Other circumstantial evidence for an

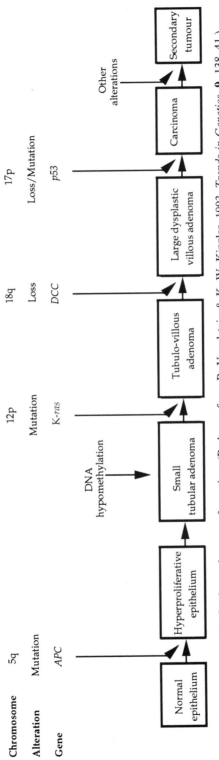

Fig. 3.22 A genetic model of colorectal tumour formation. (Redrawn from B. Vogelstein & K. W. Kinzler, 1993, *Trends in Genetics*, **9**, 138–41.)

adenoma–carcinoma sequence comes from health screening of apparently well people; the average age of people with the diagnosis of a single adenoma is significantly lower than that of people with a single carcinoma. More direct evidence for this sequence came from careful inspection of histological sections of large tumour resection specimens that had adjacent adenomatous tissue. The pioneering studies of Basil Morson in the 1970s unequivocally showed, not only that residual adenomatous tissue could often be found in association with frankly malignant tissue, but also that this adenomatous tissue was commonly thrown into finger-like (villiform) projections and the component cells were very abnormal – dysplastic (see below). The molecular biology of the 1980s and 1990s has provided an explanation for these histopathological observations. The adenoma and carcinoma are really stages in a disease continuum caused by a stepwise accumulation of genetic errors. The colonic adenoma should be regarded as a preinvasive lesion, though in most other tissues benign tumours appear to have little malignant potential – perhaps they are better able to repair further DNA sequence errors?

The colorectal adenoma-carcinoma sequence – a paradigm of multistage carcinogenesis

Following genetic analysis of adenomatous tissue of various histopathological types and carcinoma tissue, a model of the molecular basis of the adenoma–carcinoma sequence has been proposed (Fig. 3.22). Mutations in four or five genes seem to be required for the development of malignancy, fewer changes suffice for benign tumours. A preferred sequence of genetic alterations is illustrated based on their relative occurrence at the various stages of tumour development, but it is the *total* accumulation of changes rather than the precise order in which they occur which seems to be crucial for the evolution of the malignant phenotype. Present knowledge suggests that the mutational inactivation of tumour suppressor genes is more important than the activation of oncogenes. Mutations in the *APC* and *ras* genes are common in both early adenomas and carcinomas, whereas the alterations in *DCC* and *p53* tend to be found mainly in the large, severely dysplastic adenomas and the carcinomas. Here then, is an explanation for Morson's findings, adenomas become large and severely dysplastic because they have accumulated a sub-critical number of genetic alterations – little else is required to tip them over the edge. Hence the residual adenomatous tissue surrounding carcinoma is generally severely dysplastic rather than mildly abnormal. The genetic model of colorectal neoplasia has two further salient features. First, each mutation initially occurs in a single cell, and the presence of such a genetic alteration provides the cell with a growth advantage enabling it to outgrow its neighbours and become the predominant cell type constituting the neoplasm (Fig. 3.23). Thus, a *ras* mutation could be responsible for the conversion of a small, mildly dysplastic tubular adenoma into a large, severely dysplastic, villous adenoma (Fig. 3.24A, B), through clonal expansion of *one* cell in the small adenoma with the mutation. Second, it is likely that somatic mutation of any of the tumour suppressor genes bestows a growth advantage, for if it did not, it might be difficult to amass

NORMAL EPITHELIUM

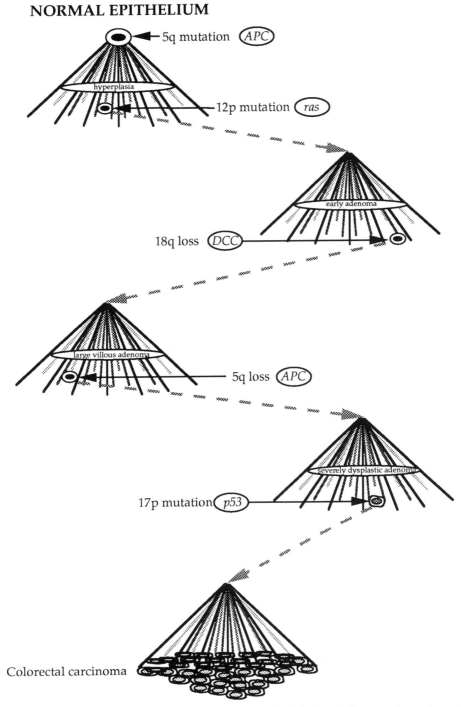

Fig. 3.23 In the evolution of a colorectal carcinoma, it is believed that a variety of genetic events occur, each in turn allows the affected cell to outgrow its neighbours. Successive rounds of mutation and clonal expansion eventually leads to the production of the malignant genotype. The diagram depicts just one of probably thousands of different routes leading to a colorectal carcinoma.

(A)

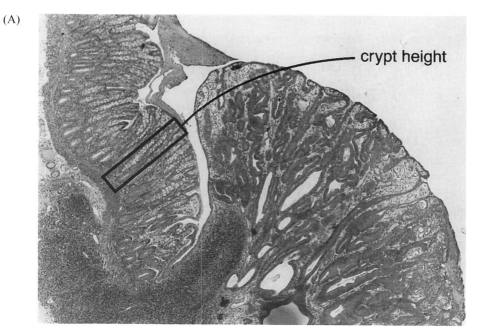

(B)

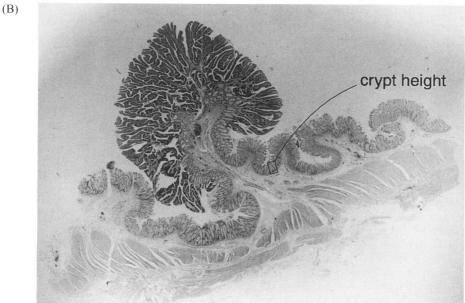

Fig. 3.24 Photomicrographs illustrating (A) a small tubular adenoma which presumably has fewer genetic alterations than (B) a villous adenoma which may only require one further gene mutation in a single cell to produce the malignant tumour. Note the relative enormity of the villous adenoma by comparing the depth of the normal crypts (boxed) in the two micrographs.

enough cells to allow a reasonable chance for the crucial second event – inactivation of the remaining allele. We have already seen that mutation of one *p53* gene results in a protein product that can inactivate the wild-type protein, and the *DCC* gene may also not conform to a recessive model. Mutation of one *DCC* allele may be sufficient to critically reduce the expression of the corresponding protein; indeed a two-fold decrease in expression of some cell adhesion molecules has been found to result in a thirty-fold reduction in cell adhesion. The *DCC* gene encodes a cell adhesion molecule, the reduced expression of which could lead to diminution of the growth-restraining signals associated with such adhesion.

Thus, though tumour suppressor genes have been hypothesized to act recessively (i.e. both maternal and paternal copies of the gene need to be inactivated for the growth suppressive function to be eliminated), studies of colorectal neoplasia, for example, suggest that dominant negative and dosage effects need to be integrated into the conceptualization of suppressor gene action.

3.5   Further reading

Cordon-Cardo, C. (1995). Mutation of cell cycle regulators. Biological and clinical implications for human neoplasia. *American Journal of Pathology,* **147**, 545–60.

Cox, L. S. & Lane, D. P. (1995). Tumour suppressors, kinases, and clamps: how p53 regulates the cell cycle in response to DNA damage. *BioEssays*, **17**, 501–8.

Fearon, E. R. & Vogelstein, B. (1990). A genetic model for colorectal tumorigenesis. *Cell*, **61**, 759–67.

Fearon, E.R. & Vogelstein, B. (1993). Tumor suppressor genes and cancer. In *Cancer Medicine*, 3rd edn., ed. J. F. Holland, E. Frei, R. C. Bast, D. L. Kufe, D. L. Morton & R. R. Weichsel-baum, pp. 77–90. Philadelphia: Lea & Febiger.

Hollywood, D., Sikora, K. & Ponten, J. (1995). Oncogenes. In *Oxford Textbook of Oncology*, vol. 1, ed. M. Peckham, H. M. Pinedo & U. Veronesi, pp. 54–73. Oxford: Oxford Medical Publications.

Klein, G. (1993). RNA tumour viruses. In *Cancer Medicine*, 3rd edn., ed. J. F. Holland, E. Frei, R. C. Bast, D. L. Kufe, D. L. Morton & R. R. Weichselbaum, pp. 65–77. Philadelphia: Lea & Febiger.

Knudson, A. G. (1985). Hereditary cancer, oncogenes, and antioncogenes. *Cancer Research*, **45**, 1437–43.

Quilliam, L. A., Khosravi-Far, R., Huff, S. Y. & Der, C. J. (1995). Guanine nucleotide exchange factors: activators of the Ras superfamily of proteins. *BioEssays*, **17**, 395–404.

Rabbits, T. H. (1994). Chromosomal translocations in human cancer. *Nature*, **372**, 143–9.

Sandberg, A. A. (1990). *The Chromosomes in Human Cancer and Leukaemia*, 2nd edn. New York: Elsevier.

The European Journal of Cancer (1995) Volume 31A. Colorectal Cancer: from Gene to Cure, 1029–386. (Whole issue).

van Rensberg, E. J. & Ponder, B. A. J. (1995). Molecular genetics of familial breast-ovarian cancer. *Journal of Clinical Pathology*, **48**, 789–95.

4

Tumour behaviour

4.1 Introduction

Even in the Western world, many of the patients who develop cancer today will not be alive in five years time. If cancer at any site could be diagnosed while the disease was still localized, the survival rate would be immeasurably improved, simply using the existing modes of treatment. Unfortunately many cancers have already spread before they become symptomatic, and therefore in the absence of spectacular advances in the treatment of metastatic disease, it becomes important still to pay great attention to the prevention and early detection of malignancy. We have already mentioned the epidemiological and experimental studies incriminating chemical and infectious (particularly viral) agents in the aetiology of many human cancers, and these data are used in implementing cancer prevention (e.g. giving up smoking, modifying dietary habits, safer working practices). Another approach to reducing cancer mortality has been directed at the recognition of *preneoplastic conditions* and the early detection of the antecedents of cancer, the *preinvasive states*, sometimes known as *precancerous states*. Nomenclature has been notoriously difficult in this field, but we may define preneoplastic conditions as circumstances which pose an increased risk of eventually developing cancer, whereas preinvasive states are changes which occur, at a cellular level in a tissue, which carry a (variably) increased risk of evolving into a malignant tumour. It is the recognition of these states of higher than normal risk which is so vital, in order to develop programmes for screening, preventative treatment and education.

4.2 Preneoplastic conditions

The agents which bring about such conditions can not generally, with one or two exceptions, be considered as carcinogenic in their own right. The overriding theme seems to be one of hyperplasia as a consequence of long standing inflammatory disease (Table 4.1). Why should hyperplasia increase the risk of cancer development? Perhaps this is best illustrated by studies of experimental carcinogenesis in the rat liver. In the adult rat, hepatocytes are essentially in the G_0 phase of the cell cycle (Chapter 5, section 5.1), and exposure to established hepatocarcinogens does not result

97

Table 4.1. *Preneoplastic conditions*

Organ	Agent/condition	Effect on tissue	Tissue response
Oesophagus	Oesophagitis	Chronic damage	Regenerative hyperplasia Metaplasia (Barrett's oesophagus)
Stomach	Chronic atrophic gastritis	Chronic damage	Regenerative hyperplasia Intestinal metaplasia
Colon	Inflammatory bowel disease particularly ulcerative colitis	Chronic damage	Regenerative hyperplasia
Intestines	Resection	Mucosal damage at anastomotic site	Regenerative hyperplasia
Lung	Tobacco smoke	Chronic irritation	Squamous metaplasia
Liver	Hepatitis B virus	Chronic hepatocyte damage	Cirrhosis
	Chronic alcoholism	Chronic hepatocyte damage	Cirrhosis
Bile duct	*Clonorchis sinensis*	Chronic irritation	Hyperplasia
Urinary bladder	*Schistosoma haematobium*	Chronic irritation	Squamous metaplasia Hyperplasia

in liver tumours. However, if the liver is hyperplastic at the time of exposure to the same carcinogens, then tumours are produced. Thus protocols for inducing liver tumours are designed so that carcinogen exposure occurs either during the period of postnatal liver growth or shortly after partial hepatectomy, when large numbers of potential target cells are in the cell cycle. It is believed that the effects of genotoxic (mutagenic) chemicals are negated if affected cells are allowed time to carry out DNA repair before undergoing normal semi-conservative replication of DNA during the cell cycle. However, if damaged cells are already in the cell cycle, then there is a much greater likelihood that mutated DNA will be faithfully copied and thus be present in all the cellular progeny derived from an initially affected cell.

The degree of risk which hyperplasia poses to an individual patient is impossible to predict, whereas preneoplastic conditions such as defective DNA repair (e.g. *xeroderma pigmentosum*) which are genetically determined, show a clear pattern of Mendelian inheritance and pose a much more predictable risk of cancer development. Throughout the gastrointestinal tract, chronic inflammation can be considered a preneoplastic condition of very variable risk. The hyperplastic mucosa may have supervening dysplasia (see below), a preinvasive state, and therefore a clear distinction between preneoplastic and preinvasive states cannot always be made.

Metaplasia is often found in connection with chronic inflammation and hyperplasia, and may indeed be the parent tissue of many malignant tumours. The reason for this is unclear, it could be simply that the metaplastic epithelium has a higher than normal rate of cell turnover, but alternatively the metaplasia may have already sustained genetic damage (with or without dysplasia). Squamous metaplasia of the respiratory airways and urinary bladder often co-exists with squamous carcinoma, while in the stomach the well differentiated intestinal-type of gastric carcinoma is thought to arise from a particular type of incomplete intestinal metaplasia in which sulphomucin secreting columnar cells are interspersed with intestinal-like goblet cells. Since hepatocellular carcinoma is invariably associated with the abnormal healing response which results in cirrhosis, the classification of cirrhosis as preneoplastic or preinvasive is problematical. Like the experimental studies, it may simply be that the increased hepatocyte turnover in the regenerative nodules represents a more susceptible target population for independent carcinogenic events (e.g. aflatoxin binding), but in the case of HBV infection, viral genome integration may have already destined some cells to become preinvasive.

4.3   Preinvasive states

As opposed to preneoplastic conditions which pose a generally unpredictable increased risk of tumour development, preinvasive states represent cellular changes which are the antecedents of malignant tumour development. Into this category are placed dysplasia, carcinoma *in situ* and some, if not many, benign tumours.

Dysplasia is a common antecedent of invasive carcinoma in many tissues, including oesophagus, colon, stomach and lung. Dysplasia can be graded as mild, moderate or severe, which probably represents a continuum leading to invasive carcinoma; there is a *dysplasia-carcinoma sequence* akin to the adenoma-carcinoma sequence (Figs. 3.22 and 3.23). In affected tissues, dysplasia may be recognised by:

- Increased numbers of mitoses, some of which are abnormal.
- Cellular and nuclear pleomorphism (variation in their shape, size and staining).
- A higher nuclear/cytoplasmic ratio, and increased nuclear DNA (recognized by hyperchromatism, i.e. more darkly stained nuclei).
- Altered differentiation (usually the cells show impaired differentiation), e.g. in the bowel, mucous-producing cells elaborate little or no mucous; in squamous epithelia the surface cells fail to flatten parallel to the surface (loss of polarity).
- Disorganization of the general hierarchical organization of tissues.

Some of these features are schematically illustrated in Fig. 4.1 (A–C), and it is generally believed that the degree of dysplasia reflects the risk of the likelihood of imminent neoplastic transformation. In the uterine cervix, the practice of grading dysplasia into mild, moderate and severe has been abandoned in favour of describing the changes in terms of *cervical intra-epithelial neoplasia* (CIN). This is graded from CIN1 (previously mild dysplasia), through CIN2 (moderate dysplasia) to CIN3 (severe dysplasia or carcinoma *in situ*), a spectrum of a single disease process carrying an increasing risk of the development of invasive squamous carcinoma. Grading is based on the extent to which the stratified squamous epithelium is affected; normally cell proliferation is the province of the basal layer and when cells migrate suprabasally

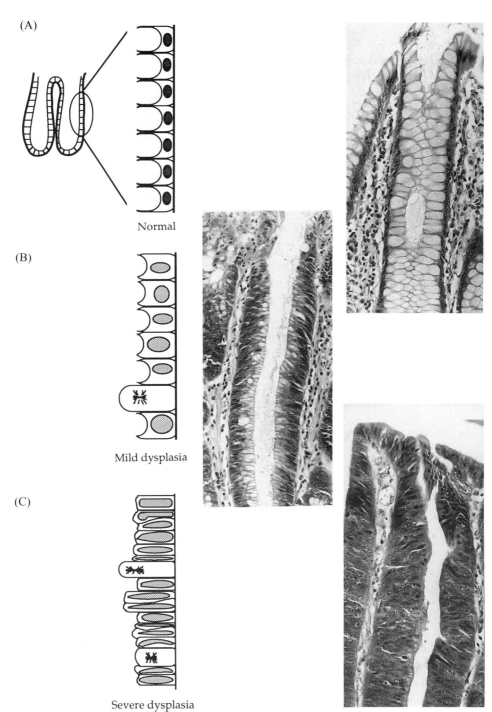

(A)

Normal

(B)

Mild dysplasia

(C)

Severe dysplasia

Fig. 4.1 Schematic and photomicrograph representations of the degrees of dysplasia which can occur in the essentially mucous-secreting colonic epithelium, comparing normal epithelium (A) with moderate (B) and (C) severe dysplasia.

they cease proliferation and orientate themselves parallel to the surface, generally becoming more flattened with small, hyperchromatic nuclei. CIN is recognized by a failure to implement this maturation process partly or wholly: cell proliferation occurs above the basal layer and cells fail to flatten and orientate themselves (loss of polarity) parallel to the surface (Fig. 4.2A–C). CIN1 is recognized histologically by an absence of maturation in the bottom one-third of the epithelium, CIN2 is characterized by a failure of cells to mature appropriately in the lower two-thirds of the epithelium, while in CIN3 undifferentiated cells occupy the full thickness of the epithelium. CIN is, of course, asymptomatic and is detected by examination of cervical smears (see Fig. 1.8).

In the human female breast there are a variety of intraductal and intralobular lesions that are preinvasive, and therefore will progress to infiltrating carcinoma given enough time. Discussion of the full range of such lesions is beyond the scope of this book, suffice it to say that the commonest type of breast carcinoma, ductal carcinoma, probably arises directly from what is termed ductal carcinoma *in situ* (DCIS). In other words the lesion has all the features expected of neoplastic growth (cellular and nuclear pleomorphism, hyperchromatism, frequent mitoses, abnormal mitoses, necrosis and apoptosis), but has not yet invaded (Fig. 4.3). In the skin, Bowen's disease is a classical example of full thickness epidermal dysplasia (carcinoma *in situ*), however, only a very small proportion proceed to invasive squamous carcinoma.

Finally, we need to consider the malignant potential of benign tumours. Studies of colorectal carcinogenesis, on the one hand, certainly suggest that adenomas are preinvasive, and that severe dysplasia is a reliable indicator of imminent malignant transformation. On the other hand, many benign tumours show little dysplasia, and malignant change in them is probably uncommon.

4.4 Benign tumours

Benign tumours are characterized by local growth with compression of the surrounding tissues as they expand, producing a distinguishable edge or capsule. Macroscopically, one of the first observations to be made to determine a tumour's malignancy, or lack of it, is the condition of the tumour's 'pushing' edge, which might have both fibrous and compressed normal tissue components in a solid organ (Fig. 4.4). Non-malignant tumours are easily removed surgically because of this boundary, often they can be 'shelled out' like peas from a pod. Benign tumours do not spread to distant sites and any symptoms they might cause are often due to local factors such as pressure on a nerve or perhaps occlusion of a blood vessel, often because of expansion of the neoplastic growth against a rigid barrier (e.g. gliomas in the skull). Benign tumours arising from surface epithelia, because they do not invade inwards, tend to bulge outwards from the surface to form *exophytic* tumours (Fig. 4.5); exophytic tumours arising from mucosal surfaces in the gut often form pedunculated (stalked) adenomas commonly called *polyps* (see Fig. 3.24), though it should be remembered that not all so-called polypoid masses are adenomas (e.g. inflammatory polyps) and some adenomas can be flat (*sessile*).

(A)

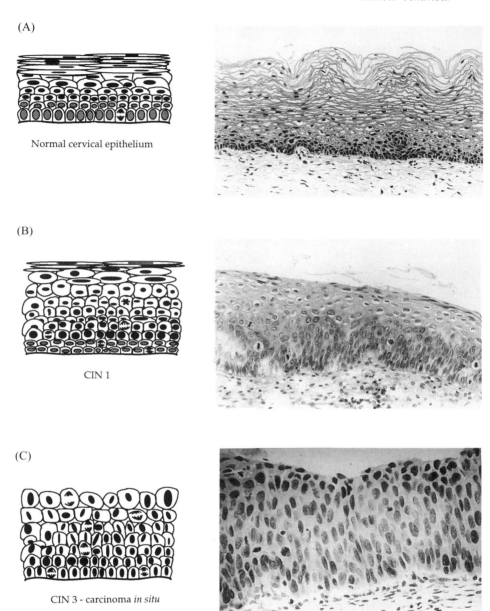

Normal cervical epithelium

(B)

CIN 1

(C)

CIN 3 - carcinoma *in situ*

Fig. 4.2 Schematic and photomicrograph representations of the stratified squamous epithelium lining the uterine ectocervix comparing the normal stratified squamous epithelium (A) with CIN1 (B) and (C) CIN3 (carcinoma *in situ*).

Typically, benign tumours are slow growing, reflected in the comparatively low number of mitotic figures visible histologically, and the cells of the tumour closely resemble each other and the tissue from which they arise. Benign tumours rarely have areas of necrosis and their blood supply keeps up with the tumour growth,

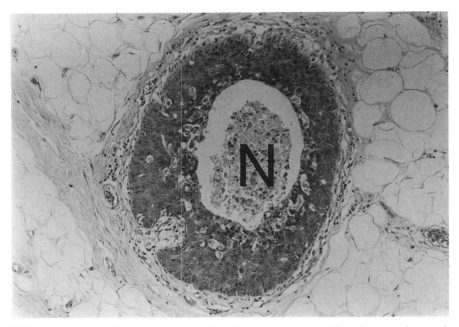

Fig. 4.3 Photomicrograph illustrating a breast ductal carcinoma *in situ*. Note the central necrosis (N) – hence comedo carcinoma.

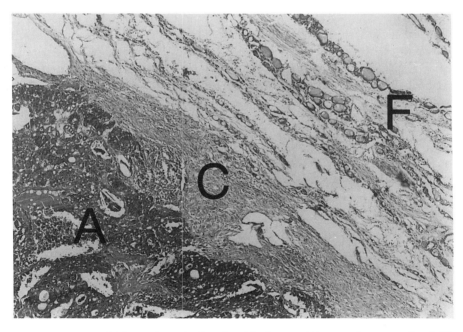

Fig. 4.4 Photomicrograph illustrating a benign thyroid adenoma (A), note the encapsulated (C) boundary between the adenomatous tissue and normal thyroid follicles (F).

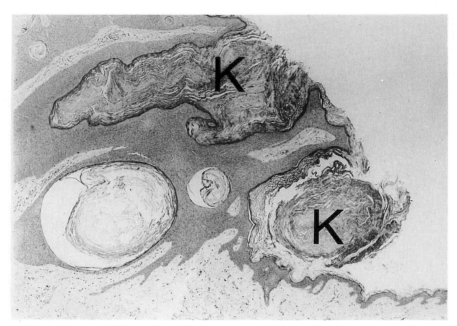

Fig. 4.5 Photomicrograph illustrating a benign tumour of the epidermis, a basal cell papilloma in which there is little mitotic activity and few cellular abnormalities apart from a grossly thickened epidermis, thrown into folds and thus trapping keratinized squames (K) in whorls.

whereas the growth of malignant tumours often outstrips their neo-vascularization and areas of ischaemia occur that result in necrosis. In benign tumours the nuclear/cytoplasmic ratio of the cells (N/C ratio) tends to be low (the nuclei appear relatively small), while the N/C ratio is often high in malignant tumours because the nuclei can be aneuploid and commonly there is a reduced commitment towards a differentiated phenotype, e.g. storage of a secretory product. Table 4.2 summarizes the major histological differences between benign and malignant tumours.

Table 4.2 *Histological differences between benign and malignant tumours*

	Benign	Malignant
Tumour margin	Often 'pushing'	Often infiltrative
Local invasion	Never	Yes
Metastases	Never	Frequent
Resemblance to normal	Good	Variable
Growth rate	Slow	Relatively rapid
Chromosome complement	Diploid	Aneuploidy common
Mitotic activity	Low	High
Abnormal mitoses	Never	Frequent
Cell death	Rare	Frequent (necrosis and apoptosis)
Cell and nuclear pleomorphism	No	Common

4.5 Malignant tumours

Malignant tumours derive their name, 'cancer' (L. crab), because they *invade* surrounding tissue – cords of invasive tumour cells being likened to the claws of a crab protruding from the animal's body. The other unique property or behaviour of malignant, as opposed to benign tumours is their propensity for spread to sites discontinuous with the original tumour mass, a process known as *metastasis*.

Invasion differs from the expansion of benign tumours, in that malignant cells, either singularly or as cords or sheets of cells, infiltrate the neighbouring normal tissue instead of being retained within a well-defined boundary. In epithelial tissues the basement membrane is ruptured, and tumour cells invade the submucosa (Fig. 4.6A, B). For the successful spread of tumour cells, a number of barriers must be breached including:

- basement membranes;
- stromal matrix;
- cell-cell contacts.

The components of the basement membrane include type IV collagen, laminin and other specific glycoproteins, as well as specific proteoglycans, and all these must be degraded for invasion to begin. Likewise the stromal matrix is a considerable barrier to cell movement, and is composed of a diverse array of macromolecules including interstitial collagens, elastin, fibronectin and other glycoproteins and proteoglycans. Invading tumour cells must therefore produce a constellation of degradative enzymes including type IV collagenase, interstitial collagenases and plasminogen activators (these convert the inactive zymogen, plasminogen to plasmin – a broad spectrum protease).

In the early stages of tumour growth it is likely that decreased adhesion of the tumour cells both to one another, to the basement membrane and to matrix proteins will all aid local spread. There are several major groups of cell adhesion molecules (CAMs) involved in cell–cell and cell–matrix adhesion including the *integrins*, *cadherins* and *immunoglobulin superfamily* (Ig-SF) (Fig. 4.7).

The integrins are heterodimers consisting of noncovalently associated α and β subunits that mediate both cell–cell and cell–matrix adhesion. Cadherins are calcium-dependent transmembrane adhesion molecules, and are probably the most important group in the formation of cell–cell associations. The immunoglobulin superfamily encompasses a wide variety of molecules, most of which are involved in cell–cell recognition and includes molecules that function in cellular immunity (i.e. MHC antigens, CD4, CD8 and the T cell receptor), neural development (neural cell adhesion molecule, N-CAM) and signal transduction (the platelet derived growth factor receptor, see Chapter 5, section 5.2). CEA (carcinoembryonic antigen) is an oncofoetal glycoprotein belonging to the Ig-SF and the *DCC* gene encodes a molecule in the Ig-SF with strong homology to N-CAM. It is impossible to make a sweeping generalization about CAMs and tumour progression, but it is likely that initially, tumour cells possess decreased adhesive interactions with surrounding cells and extracellular

(A)

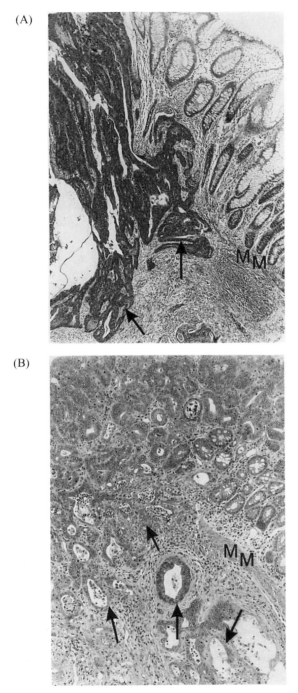

(B)

Fig. 4.6 Photomicrographs illustrating invasive tumours of glandular colonic epithelium, hence colonic adenocarcinomas in (A) human and (B) rat. Note the presence of invasive malignant glands (arrows) in the submucosa beneath the muscularis mucosa (MM).

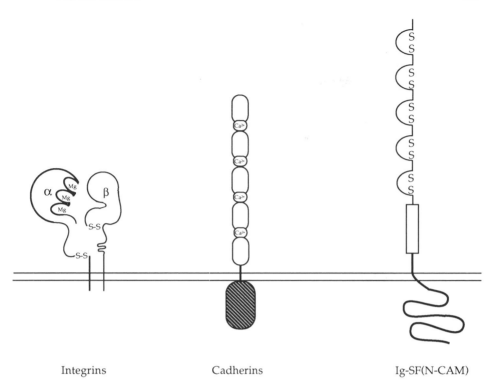

Integrins   Cadherins   Ig-SF(N-CAM)

Fig. 4.7 Schematic diagram of three of the principal cell adhesion molecules involved in cell–cell and cell–matrix interactions.

matrix so that they become detached from the primary tumour; as they invade, CAMs enabling efficient cell–matrix interactions may be over-expressed allowing rapid movement in adjacent tissue and migration into vascular channels. Arrest in the circulation may require firm cell–cell contacts to be re-established, and then to be broken as tumour cells separate from the endothelium. Further migration may then require efficient cell–matrix interactions again. The expression of integrins on tumour cells exemplifies the complexity of the relationship between CAMs and malignancy. Malignant melanomas appear to have a consistent up-regulation of integrins during tumour progression, whereas many carcinomas have fewer integrins than their corresponding normal epithelial cells, and this lack of interaction with the surrounding matrix maybe why such tumours are poorly differentiated (Fig. 4.8). Cadherins, however, connect cells together by so-called homophilic interactions (e.g. E-cadherin binds selectively to E-cadherin), and appear to be consistently under-expressed in invasive epithelial tumours (Fig. 4.9).

Thus, the modulation of CAMs is likely to be critical for the two most significant features of malignant cell behaviour – invasion and metastasis (see below). Transmembrane CAMs can diffuse in the plane of the plasma membrane, so they can accumulate at sites of cell contact, to initiate cell–cell adhesion, as well as being integral parts of intercellular junctions (adherent junctions and desmosomes) which are more

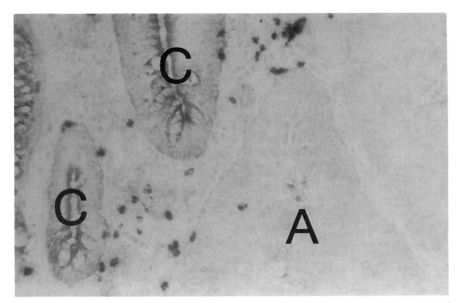

Fig. 4.8 Photomicrograph illustrating the down-regulation of integrin expression in a group of poorly differentiated colonic adenocarcinoma cells (A) as illustrated by reduced immunoreactivity with an antibody raised against the α3 integrin subunit. Note prominent expression in the normal crypt cells (C). (Courtesy of Dr. Massimo Pignatelli.)

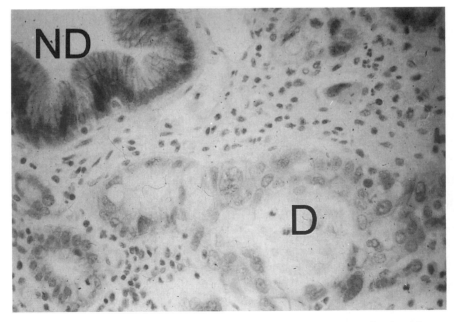

Fig. 4.9 Photomicrograph illustrating the down-regulation of E-cadherin expression in an invasive ductal carcinoma of the pancreas (D) as illustrated by reduced immunoreactivity with an antibody raised against E-cadherin. Note prominent expression in the normal ductal cells (ND). (Courtesy of Dr. Massimo Pignatelli.)

permanent cell adhesion fixtures connecting the cytoskeletal filaments of neighbouring cells. Intercellular junctions are not a feature of embryonic or healing tissues where cell mobility is important, and such structures need to be disrupted for epithelial tumour cells to become detached from one another. In fact, significant alteration in any component of the cadherin–catenin complex (see Fig. 3.15) can result in adherens junction disassembly, and thus non-adhesive and invasive cells.

The pattern of local invasion of a tumour can be haphazard, but may follow a path of least resistance – between muscle bundles, along tubes or ducts, beneath the connective tissue of nerves (perineural invasion, Fig. 4.10) or along lymphatic vessels (lymphatic permeation, Fig. 4.11).

4.6 Metastasis

Introduction

The degree of local spread will generally increase the likelihood of tumour *metastasis*, the process by which a tumour implant becomes established at a site which is discontinuous with the primary tumour. This behaviour is unequivocal evidence of malignancy, the new tumour implant being known as a *tumour metastasis* or *secondary tumour*. The term 'metastasis' frequently refers to the formation of secondary tumours after dissemination through lymphatic or vascular channels, but the shedding of tumour cells into the body cavities (e.g. ovarian cancer cells) and their subsequent

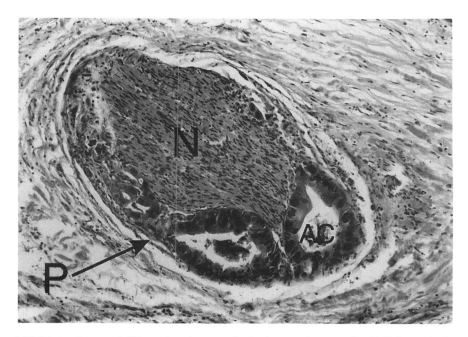

Fig. 4.10 Photomicrograph illustrating the spread of adenocarcinoma cells (AC) beneath the perineurium (P) of a nerve bundle (N).

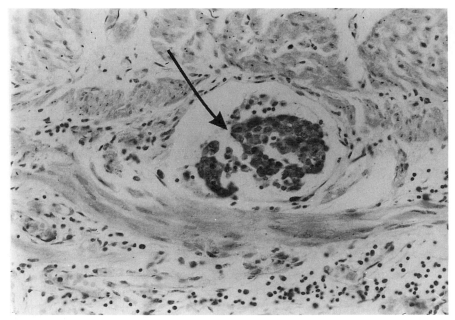

Fig. 4.11 Photomicrograph illustrating the spread of gastric adenocarcinoma cells (arrow) into a lymphatic vessel in the wall of the stomach.

implantation on a new surface (e.g. the serosa of gastrointestinal tract) – transcoelomic spread, is included in the concept. The walls of blood vessels and lymphatics are the first natural obstacles to rapid widespread dissemination of invading tumour cells, and only cells with the necessary degradative enzymes are able to move into the blood or lymph, and then to be carried around the body; the whole process is summarized in Fig. 4.12. The journey through the blood vascular system is extremely hazardous as tumour cells get jostled in a series of high speed collisions with the vessel walls and each other; only a minority of blood-borne cancer cells seem to survive this traumatic experience. Indeed the whole process of metastasis can be viewed as a ladder, and failure to complete any one step will mean no metastasis (Fig. 4.13). Experimental studies have shown that even tumour cells injected intravenously fare badly, with less than 1% surviving for more than 24 hours. Metastases are the **major cause of death** from malignant disease because localized primary tumours in non-vital organs (e.g. skin) are not, in themselves, life-threatening.

The liver is a common site of secondary deposits. When tumour metastases are present the spatial and chemical environment is perturbed, profoundly changing normal liver function. The importance of metastases in the prognosis of cancer cannot be overstated. Primary tumours can be removed by surgery and remaining local involvement can be treated with adjuvant chemotherapy and/or radiotherapy, but it is the persistence of widespread metastatic disease which is difficult to treat that results in mortality.

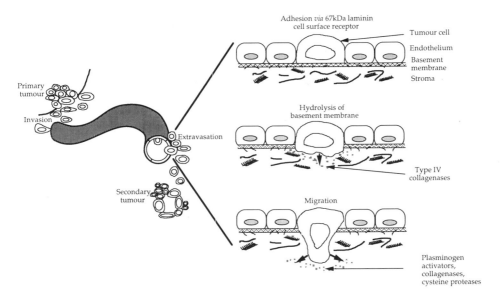

Fig. 4.12 Summary of the metastatic process. To exit the vascular system at a distant site the tumour cells must first cause endothelial retraction followed by adhesion to the underlying basement membrane *via* a 67 kDa laminin cell surface receptor. Basement membrane penetration requires the secretion of a 72 kDa type IV collagenase, and further penetration is aided by the concerted actions of collagenases, plasminogen activators and cysteine proteases.

The major pathways of metastasis

The pattern of metastatic spread is not random and undoubtedly certain tumours 'favour' colonizing particular sites for metastatic growth. This non-random distribution of metastases seems to result from a combination of at least two factors. The distribution of some secondary tumour deposits can be largely explained on mechanistic grounds; tumour cells that are shed into the blood vascular system lodge in the first capillary network they meet downstream. For example, the liver is the commonest site for secondary tumours in patients with primary cancer in the catchment area of the hepatic portal vein, and the lung is the most favoured site in patients with primary tumours draining into the systemic veins. Thus, vascular drainage patterns certainly seem to influence the distribution of secondary deposits from some types of primary tumour. However, the distribution of some tumour secondaries cannot be explained solely on patterns of vascular supply and drainage. In his classical study of breast cancer from almost 1000 autopsies at the end of the nineteenth century, Stephen Paget noted that lymph nodes, liver, lung, bone and brain were commonly involved, whereas the kidney was very rarely involved despite receiving one-quarter of the cardiac output (Paget, S.,1889. The distribution of secondary growths in cancer of the breast. *Lancet* **1**: 571–3). From such data he expounded his *seed and soil* hypothesis, likening cancer cells to 'seeds', which, after being scattered on the 'wind', grow only in sites ('soil')

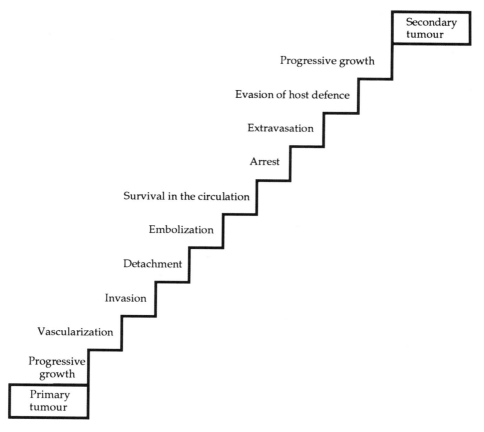

Fig. 4.13 The stairway of metastasis. Each step is a hazardous process and failure at any one step will prevent secondary growth occurring.

that are congenial to their survival and further growth. It is now quite clear that certain sites favour the growth of particular types of secondary tumour, no more so than the adrenal glands where the high frequency of secondary tumours is out of all proportion to the percentage of cardiac output received by these organs. Organ-specific factors which may determine patterns of metastatic growth include:

- local production of paracrine-acting growth factors;
- tissue sensitivity to tumour angiogenic factors;
- tissue specific adhesion properties of the endothelium.

Local production of both inhibitory and stimulatory growth factors may well profoundly influence the ability of recently seeded tumour cells to gain a foothold and colonize a new site, and some growth factors even have opposite effects on different cell types. The growth of tumour foci beyond about a millimetre or so in diameter depends on the formation of new blood vessels to supply these foci – a process known as neovascularization (see below). Growth factors (GFs) such as bFGF and TGFα (see Chapter 5, section 5.2) are produced by tumours and stimulate endothelial proliferation, but the control of angiogenesis may be slightly different in different tissues. A further factor determining patterns of metastasis may be the 'stickiness' of the endothelium, in that endothelia in particular organs have organ specific CAMs which determine which cell–cell interactions occur. There is experimental evidence to support this notion; if tumour cells of one type are incubated with endothelial cells from various organs, then the tumour cells preferentially adhere to the endothelia from organs which are the preferred sites of metastasis *in vivo*. More specifically, there is evidence that V-CAM (vascular cell adhesion molecule), a member of the Ig-SF, functions as an endothelial cell receptor for malignant melanoma and myeloid malignancies expressing the α4β1 integrin. CD44, a cell surface glycoprotein involved in lymphocyte homing, is expressed by many mesenchymal and neuroectodermal tumours. Many mRNA splice variants exist, and they function in adhesion to matrix proteins and hyaluronic acid; transfection of one variant into a non-metastasizing rat pancreatic carcinoma cell line can induce a metastatic phenotype.

The major pathways of metastasis are:

- Across body cavities such as the peritoneal cavity. In this way metastases from an ovarian tumour (Fig. 4.14) might form on the peritoneal surface of the intestine and then spread inwards.
- Embolization *via* the lymphatic system, often 'favoured' by carcinomas; lymph nodes may thus be the first sites of secondaries. Lumps in the axillary

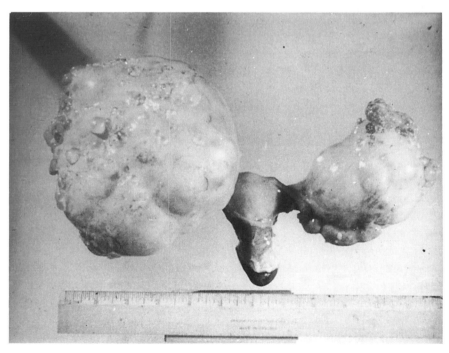

Fig. 4.14 Macroscopic appearance of a cystic ovarian tumour presenting bilaterally; fragments of this tumour readily become detached and can spread across the peritoneal cavity. (Rule in mm.)

and inguinal lymph nodes are easily palpable, and such is the frequency of regional lymph node involvement that they are usually included for radiotherapy whether palpable lesions are discovered or not.

* Embolization *via* the blood system, usually *via* veins rather than arteries. This may be partly because of the relative thickness of the arterial wall, but experimental studies have suggested that the high intra-arterial blood pressure may be a more significant impedance to tumour invasion; reducing the blood pressure has allowed invasion into arteries to occur.

We have already mentioned that metastasis is an inefficient process and that the majority of tumour cells that embolize into the circulation do not give rise to secondary tumours. Do the few cells that survive do so fortuitously, or is there a sub-population of 'metastatically competent' cells in the primary tumour from which the metastases are derived? Experimental studies certainly suggest that there are sub-populations with greater metastatic ability, but even after selecting for these, the process still remains inefficient because of the extremely hazardous journey cells must make in the vascular system, regardless of whether the cells are capable of forming metastases or not. Even if metastases are formed from a sub-population of the primary tumour, generally speaking the microscopic structure of the metastasis conforms quite closely to that of the parent tumour (Fig. 4.15), and this similarity in histological pattern is obviously useful in trying to identify the site of an unknown primary tumour. Information on the genetic basis of the metastatic phenotype is just emerging with the discovery of metastasis-suppressing genes. One of these, *nm23* is found in rodents and humans, and low levels of *nm23* RNA expression are strongly correlated with the metastatic potential of ductal carcinoma of the breast. Thus the *nm23* gene may belong to the expanding family of tumour suppressor genes whose deletion leads to tumour progression (see Chapter 3, section 3.3).

4.7   Tumour heterogeneity

Like normal tissues, tumour cell populations are not homogeneous. This phenotypic heterogeneity is the result of at least two major factors. First, the fact that neovascularization often fails to keep abreast of tumour cell population growth means that hypoxic and anoxic regions are created – hypoxia results in little or no cell proliferation, anoxia results in necrosis (Fig. 4.16A, B). A tumour cannot grow beyond a tiny focus (maximum diameter 200–300 μm) without the induction of new blood vessels (angiogenesis). Growth factors which promote the growth of new capillary sprouts and loops include acidic and basic fibroblast growth factors (aFGF and bFGF), TGFα and vascular endothelial growth factor (VEGF). These can be exported from tumour cells, mobilized from extracellular matrix or released from macrophages attracted to the tumour. These growth factors not only stimulate endothelial cell proliferation, but also promote the endothelial production of matrix-degrading enzymes like plasminogen activator and collagenase.

The second factor contributing to heterogeneity is the ability of tumours to show

(A)

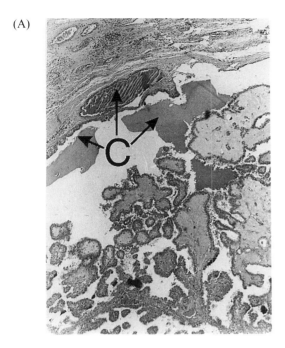

(B)

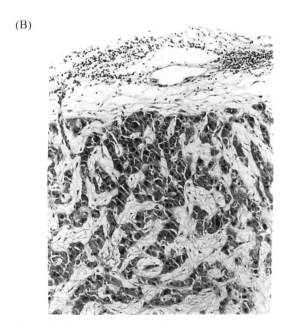

Fig. 4.15 Photomicrographs illustrating the occurrence of secondary tumours in lymph nodes just beneath the capsule. (A) The thyroid papillary carcinoma closely mimics thyroid tissue with lakes of thyroid colloid (C). (B) The hepatocellular carcinoma resembles the normal liver with the large cells arranged in broad bands (trabecular pattern).

(A)

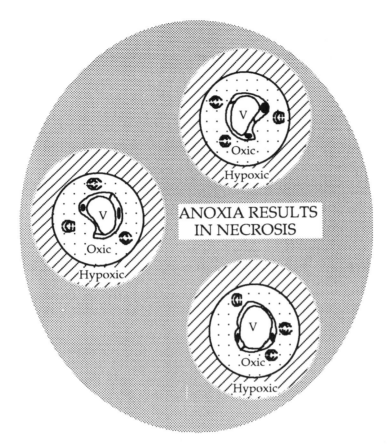

ANOXIA RESULTS
IN NECROSIS

(B)

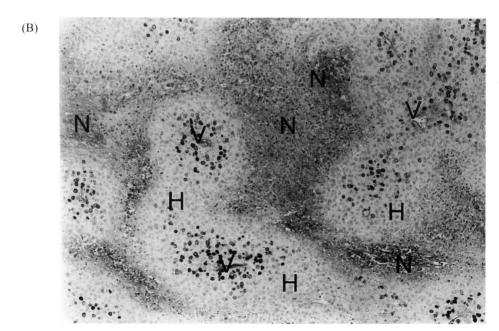

patterns of differentiation (see also Chapter 6, section 6.2) which resemble the maturation sequences (hierarchy) seen in the parent tissue (Fig. 4.17A, B), thus recapitulating the phenotypic diversity of the tissue of origin; it is a common misconception to consider tumours as totally anarchic – they are not. Of course, the differentiation programme of neoplastic cells is not normal, amply illustrated by their ability for local invasion. This heterogeneity creates problems for the cancer researcher who might wish to measure the proliferative rate. If a small number of cells are scanned to estimate the proportion of cells in DNA synthesis (the labelling index, see Chapter 5, section 5.1), then it might well result in the count being biased towards either a well oxygenated area or alternatively a hypoxic region (Fig. 4.16A, B). Short of examining all the cells in the tumour, it is always a problem to decide on how many cells need to be examined to provide a representative sample. Likewise, in the squamous carcinoma (Fig. 4.17A, B), do we estimate the labelling index in the well differentiated area where terminally differentiated and reproductively sterile keratinized squamous cells are in abundance, or do we choose the less well differentiated area where greater proliferation is occurring? A histopathologist would 'grade' the squamous carcinoma according to the 'worst bit', i.e. a poorly differentiated tumour (see Chapter 6, section 6.2).

Many malignant tumour cells contain an irregular number of chromosomes, and are referred to as *aneuploid*, aneuploidy being a state where a cell has a DNA content which is an inexact multiple of the normal (diploid) content. This may be due to a failure of one or more duplicated chromosomes to separate at anaphase, resulting in daughter cells having one or more chromosomes missing or extra. Commonly, aneuploid tumour cells have more than the normal number of chromosomes, but hypodiploid cells do occur, although they are rare. Aneuploidy is associated with increased aggressiveness in tumours, and is responsible for the variations in nuclear size and staining seen in many tumours – this known as *nuclear pleomorphism* (Fig. 4.18A, B). Most of these karyotypic abnormalities seem to occur at random, though we have already noted that certain chromosomal translocations are consistent features of some malignancies (see Fig. 3.3 and 3.6).

Aneuploidy and/or a reduced commitment towards differentiation are responsible for the increased nuclear:cytoplasmic ratio often seen in tumour cells, and aneuploidy is likely to be the cause of the many so-called 'bizarre' mitotic figures so common in aggressive tumours (Fig. 4.19): it is likely that many of these aberrant mitoses result in cell death.

Fig. 4.16 *facing* Tumour heterogeneity due to vascular insufficiency. (A) The model predicts three distinct zones moving downstream from the afferent blood supply – adequately oxygenated, hypoxic, anoxic. (B) Photomicrograph illustrating this zonation in a sheet of anaplastic tumour cells with DNA-synthesizing cells (nuclei labelled by antibody directed against incorporated bromodeoxyuridine and here appearing black, see Chapter 5, section 5.1) close to the blood vessels (V); this region gives way to an area of little or no cell proliferation, presumably due to hypoxia (H) and finally to an area of necrosis (N).

(A)

(B)

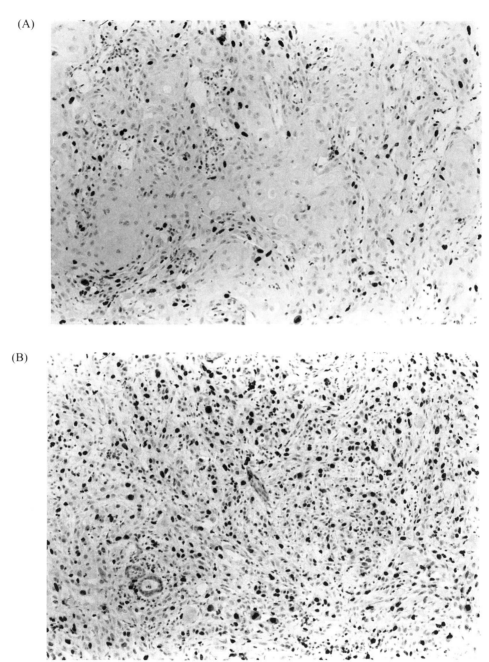

Fig. 4.17 Cells in the cell cycle can be visualized using the MIB1 (Molecular Immunology Borstel) antibody (see Chapter 5, section 5.1). (A) LH side: In the well differentiated areas of this squamous carcinoma the labelled nuclei are on the periphery of the squamous islands. These have keratinized (K) squames at their centre, easily seen in the H&E stained section

(A)

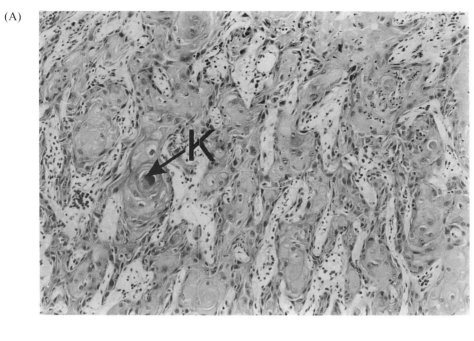

(B)

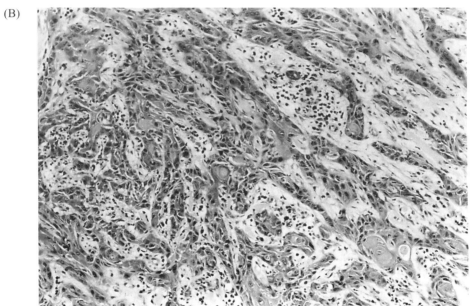

(RH side). (B) LH side: In contrast, there is much more MIB1 labelling in the poorly differentiated areas of the same tumour where large squamous cells are rare, as can be seen in the H&E (haematoxylin and eosin) stained section (RH side).

(A)

(B)

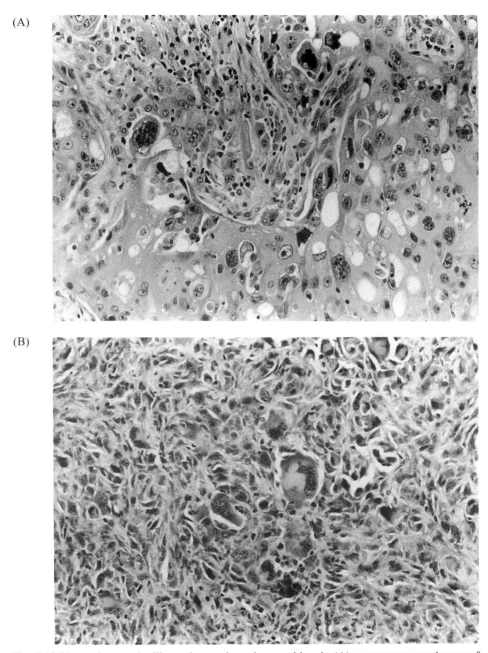

Fig. 4.18 Photomicrographs illustrating nuclear pleomorphism in (A) a squamous carcinoma of the lung and (B) a malignant fibrous histiocytoma.

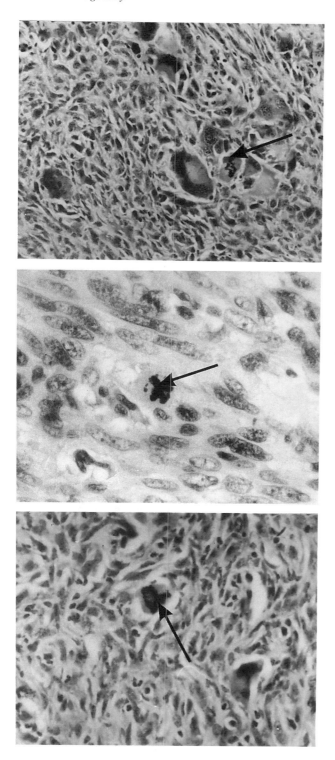

Fig. 4.19 Photomicrographs illustrating so-called 'bizarre' mitotic figures (arrows) which often lead to death of one or both of the daughter cells due to severe chromosomal imbalance.

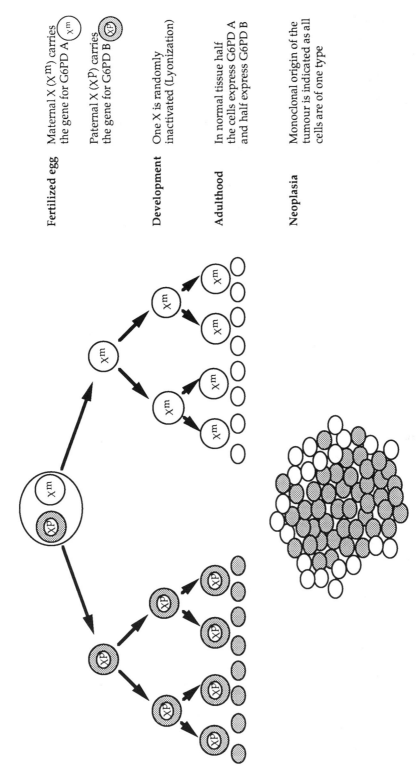

Fertilized egg Maternal X (X^m) carries the gene for G6PD A

Paternal X (X^p) carries the gene for G6PD B

Development One X is randomly inactivated (Lyonization)

Adulthood In normal tissue half the cells express G6PD A and half express G6PD B

Neoplasia Monoclonal origin of the tumour is indicated as all cells are of one type

Fig. 4.20 The monoclonal origin of some tumours can be demonstrated by the presence of just one or other of the G6PD isoenzymes in females heterozygous for this X-linked gene.

Table 4.3 *Methods of clonality determination*

General approach	Methods
X-chromosome inactivation	G6PD isoenzymes
	X-linked RFLPs
Lymphocyte analysis	Immunoglobulin light chain analysis
	Immunoglobulin and TCR gene analysis
Somatic mutation	Cytogenetic analysis
	Detection of chromosome loss by RFLP analysis

Abbreviations: G6PD, glucose-6-phosphate dehydrogenase; RFLP, restriction fragment length polymorphism; TCR, T-cell receptor

4.8 Clonality and stem cells

Evidence for clonality

It is now generally accepted that tumours are *clonally* derived, a clonal population being defined as one composed of cells arising from the mitotic division of a single cell. This belief is consistent with the somatic mutation theory of carcinogenesis which assumes that a tumour arises from the progeny of a single cell that has acquired the appropriate number of somatic mutations (Fig. 3.23). A number of methods have been developed to analyse clonality in tumours (Table 4.3), and all depend upon the demonstration that a cell population is homogeneous with respect to a particular marker.

In females, random inactivation of one X-chromosome occurs in each somatic cell in early embryonic development (Lyonization after Mary Lyon). Therefore females heterozygous for polymorphic X-linked genes are essentially mosaics, roughly half the cells expressing the maternal allele and half expressing the paternal allele. This phenomenon was exploited in the now classical studies of tumours of the uterine musculature, since the enzyme glucose-6-phosphate dehydrogenase (G6PD) occurs in some populations, especially those of African origin in two forms, A and B, which can be easily separated by gel electrophoresis. Normal tissues are a mosaic of both G6PD isoenzymes, whereas tumours arising from a single cell will show a single G6PD isoenzyme phenotype (Fig. 4.20). The majority of tumours analyzed by this technique have been found to be monoclonal in origin, though, of course, this evidence does not rule out the possibility that originally the tumour arose from a group of cells and that only later in its development did the tumour evolve from a single one of these cells.

Molecular probes for X-linked polymorphic genes now make it possible to detect clonal markers by X-linked RFLP analysis in a similar manner to the G6PD isoenzyme studies. Genes which can be used for such analyses include the hypoxanthine phosphoribosyltransferase (HPRT) and phosphoglycerate kinase (PGK) genes, though the heterozygosity rate of these genes is only about 30%, which is clearly a limiting factor. First, normal and tumour DNA are digested with the appropriate restriction endonuclease to distinguish the maternal and paternal copies of the gene through X-linked RFLP (see Fig. 3.14 for approach). Since active and inactive X-chromosome genes are produced by differences in gene methylation, a second endonuclease which only cuts the non-methylated parts of each allele is employed. In a polyclonal population where X-chromosome inactivation occurs randomly, the paternal and maternal alleles are both cleaved to some extent by this enzyme, and therefore the intensity of both fragments is less when quantified by autoradiography. However, in DNA extracted from a tumour of monoclonal origin, either *only* the maternal allele or *only* the paternal allele is methylated. The methylated allele is not cleaved by the second restriction endonuclease, whereas the nonmethylated allele is digested completely and hence is not detected. The fact that only one of the two alleles is methylated is evidence of clonality.

One of the classical methods of determining monoclonality in B-cell neoplasms is the demonstration of a single light chain isotype, either κ or λ on the cell surface of neoplastic lymphoid cells. T and B cells rearrange their antigen receptor genes, and thus, T-cell receptor (TCR) and immunoglobulin genes give rise to DNA markers unique to each individual lymphoid cell and its progeny. In a polyclonal lymphoid population these rearrangements are not detected by Southern blotting as they are well below the sensitivity of the method, but in a monoclonal population all cells have the same rearrangement which is readily detected by Southern blotting. A problem with conventional Southern blotting is its inability to detect relatively small gene rearrangements, but the polymerase chain reaction (PCR) now makes it possible to detect clonal markers resulting from very small rearrangements. Such technology is useful for detecting minimal residual disease in lymphoma and leukaemia.

The Philadelphia chromosome (Fig. 3.3) in CML is a consistent, non-random chromosomal abnormality [t(9,22)], which appears in all the tumour cells, and thus behaves as a clonal marker. Cytogenetics, however, has its limitations in that only cells in mitosis can be studied, and increasingly, loss of chromosomal material is being studied by molecular probes. DNA analysis depends on the ability to distinguish the two chromosomal homologues by the detection of RFLPs. We have already mentioned that the analysis is informative if constitutional DNA displays heterozygosity for a particular RFLP (see Fig. 3.14); loss of heterozygosity in tumour DNA indicates loss of one of these polymorphic regions, and would be present in all tumour cells derived from a single mutated cell.

Stem cells – the carcinogen targets and their existence in tumours

We have seen that there is good evidence to support the belief that most, if not all, tumours are clonally derived. We must then enquire about the nature of the carcinogen target cells. It is argued that in many tissues the only cells present for long enough to accrue the requisite number of molecular abnormalities for malignancy are the *stem cells*. The other target cell for carcinogens could be differentiated cells, but they would have to retain or regain the capacity to divide as well as organize tissue-specific differentiation. This concept is known as *dedifferentiation*, but given the inverse relationship between proliferation and differentiation, there is little evidence to support this mechanism.

Certainly in the epidermis, the classical carcinogenesis experiments in which successful promotion could be achieved at long intervals after initiation support the notion that the first event occurs in a long-lived cell (see Fig. 2.3). In the colonic crypt, for example, it is argued that cells in the amplification compartment are doomed to die after a limited number of divisions, and therefore any cell initiated here could not establish a foothold and would move up the 'cell escalator' and be shed from the luminal surface. This is a rather simplistic view since a cell initiated even in its last transit division could acquire stem cell properties, and then evade the cell escalator through invagination into the lamina propria. Perhaps the most persuasive evidence linking stem cells with early molecular events comes from cases of non-lymphocytic leukaemia and myelodysplasia; here clonal markers (e.g. G6PD isoenzymes, X-linked RFLPs) can be found in various cell lineages indicating the involvement of a pluripotential (also called multipotential) stem cell. We can in fact build a model of stem cell behaviour in a tumour which is essentially a caricature of normal behaviour, with the important distinctions of overproduction of (malignant) stem cells and the impaired ability of their progeny to differentiate normally (Fig. 4.21). In, say, a normal epithelial tissue, there are a given number of stem cells which maintain their number while at the same time giving rise to cells which go through a predetermined number of amplification divisions; these cells then lose the capacity to divide, ultimately maturing and dying shortly afterwards. In a tumour there is a block to this orderly process, probably resulting in the accumulation of stem cells as well as other cycling cells that are not the normal differentiated phenotype. These nevertheless usually have a resemblance to the tissue of origin – this is characteristic of many cancers.

Clonogenic assays

As in normal tissues, stem cells in tumours do not display any special markers, though undoubtedly they do exist, albeit in small numbers. This is supported by *clonogenic assays* which indicate that only a small fraction of the cells within a tumour are clonogenic in *in vitro* assays. In such assays, tumour cells are separated from one another by mechanical and/or by enzymatic digestion, and then plated at low density in an artificial test environment, e.g. a sloppy agar-filled petri dish or test tube (Fig. 4.22). Clonogenic cells are defined as those cells capable of forming a large family of descendants in an artificial test environment. The clonogenic cells are operationally those cells capable of producing a macroscopically visible clone of cells (usually at least 50, representing five to six generations of proliferation, chosen to exclude cells that have a limited growth potential as a result of having embarked upon differentiation, or those that have been sublethally damaged by a therapeutic treatment) in a time period of about two to three weeks. The proportion of cells capable of producing such colonies is known as the *plating efficiency*:

$$\text{Plating efficiency} = \frac{\text{no. of macroscopic colonies}}{\text{no. of cells plated}} \times 100$$

Normal renewal

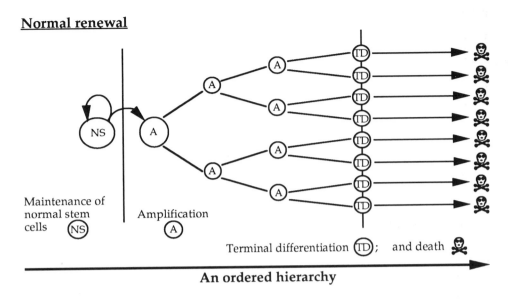

An ordered hierarchy

Neoplasia

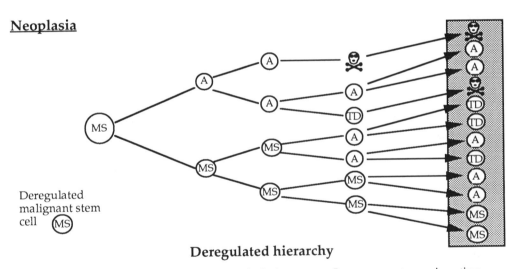

Deregulated hierarchy

Fig. 4.21 The concept of maturation arrest or blocked ontogeny. In a tumour at any given time (shaded box) there will probably be a mixture of malignant stem cells (capable of perpetuating the tumour indefinitely), other replicating cells and some terminally differentiated cells.

The belief that the clonogenic cells from a tumour actually represent the stem cells *in vivo* is supported by the fact that the *in vitro* or *in vivo* efficiency of cytotoxic agents to reduce the plating efficiency of particular tumours is mirrored by their anti-tumour effectiveness *in vivo*. Thus, successful cancer therapy depends on the ability to

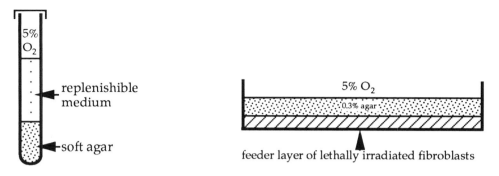

Fig. 4.22 *In vitro* clonogenic assays can be performed in petri dishes or test tubes.

eradicate a small fraction of the tumour cell population – the stem cells. To test the ability of a compound to knock out stem cells *in vitro* or *in vivo* a *cell survival curve* is plotted after treatment (Fig. 4.23 A, B). If 200 tumour cells from an untreated tumour are plated and 20 colonies are scored after a suitable period of incubation, then the plating efficiency would be 10% – this is said to represent the 100% survival value. Other cells from the same tumour can be incubated for, say 24 hours, with varying concentrations of a cytotoxic drug, washed and then plated as before. If prior treatment with 54 ng/ml reduced the plating efficiency to 2 colonies per 200 cells, then the surviving fraction is 0.01/0.1 = 0.1, i.e. 10% (Fig. 4.23A). A cell survival curve is usually plotted on a logarithmic scale of survival because if killing is random (see Chapter 7, section 7.3), then survival will be an exponential function of dose, and this would be a straight line on a semi-log plot. Furthermore, a logarithmic scale is more amenable to gauging subtle effects at very low levels of clonogenic cell survival (Fig. 4.23B).

As in normal tissues, stem cells in tumours can behave as if either unipotential or pluripotential. A squamous carcinoma (Fig. 4.17) which forms keratin 'pearls', on the one hand, is assumed to be derived from a unipotential tumour stem cell, since it mimics the limited behaviour of cells from the basal layer of the epidermis that function to form large families of progeny which differentiate only into keratinized squamous cells. On the other hand, the target stem cells which lead to gonadal teratomas and some haemopoietic tumours are likely to be pluripotential, since resultant tumours are composed of many differentiated cell types. Teratomas in their malignant form often have a mixture of embryonic tissues, but benign teratomas can contain differentiated tissues which ordinarily come from all three germ layers (Fig. 4.24). In many exocrine glands such as breast, salivary glands and pancreas the malignant phenotype is commonly a ductal carcinoma, and it is the ductal epithelium which harbours the stem cells.

4.9   Tissue and clinical effects of tumours

A quite common feature of malignant tumour cells is their ability to promote the growth of surrounding fibrous tissue, a process known as *desmoplasia*. This desmo-

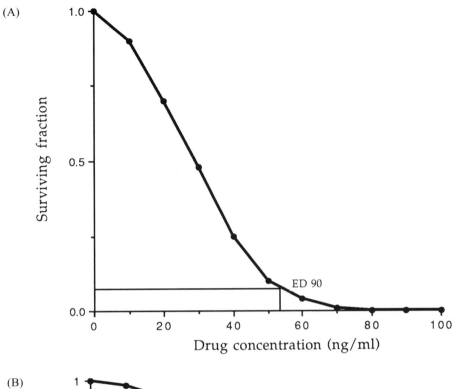

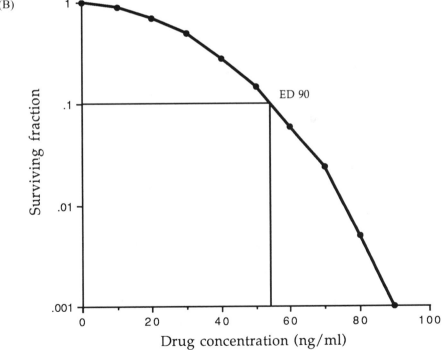

Fig. 4.23 Typical clonogenic cell survival curves for cells incubated with increasing concentrations of a cytotoxic drug prior to plating out on soft agar. (A) Plotted on a linear survival scale and (B) plotted on a semi-logarithmic scale. *ED90* indicates the dose required to kill 90% of the clonogenic cells.

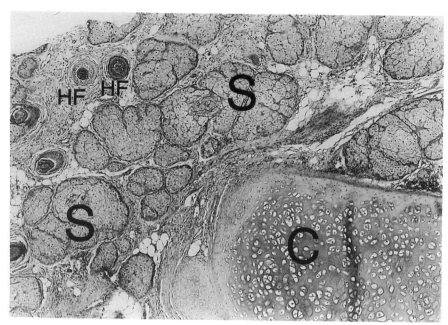

Fig. 4.24 Photomicrograph of a benign teratoma in the ovary illustrating the enormous diversity of differentiated tissues which make up the tumour cell population – suggestive of an origin from a pluripotential stem cell. Tissues include cartilage (C), sebaceous glands (S) and hair follicles (HF).

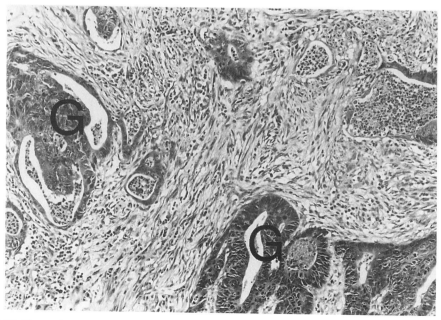

Fig. 4.25 Photomicrograph illustrating an adenocarcinoma which has induced a prominent fibroblastic (desmoplastic) reaction, see the spindle-shaped cells in the tissue surrounding the malignant glands (G).

plastic reaction gives rise to tumours with a firm consistency often referred to as 'scirrhous', which have the feel of an unripe pear when cut. Desmoplasia occurs prominently in basal cell carcinoma (BCC) of the skin where the strong reaction may be instrumental in preventing the metastasis of this otherwise aggressively invasive tumour; it also occurs around many other carcinomas (Fig. 4.25). Since the induction of neovascularization by tumour cell-derived growth factors is a necessary feature of malignant neoplastic growth, it is likely that fibroblast proliferation and collagen synthesis are similarly stimulated, particularly by TGFβ or PDGF. BCC illustrates the fact that malignant tumours of surfaces often cause ulceration, hence 'rodent ulcer' (Fig. 4.26). On external surfaces this increases the risk of infection, while in the gastrointestinal tract occult blood loss can be an important cause of anaemia.

Tumours can also cause local effects through obstruction (e.g. in the gastrointestinal tract) and compression. Even benign tumours can be life-threatening if they occur in a rigid confined site such as the cranium. More widespread effects of tumours can be subdivided into those of a general nature and those specific to particular tumours. Disseminated malignant tumours are commonly associated with features of anorexia,

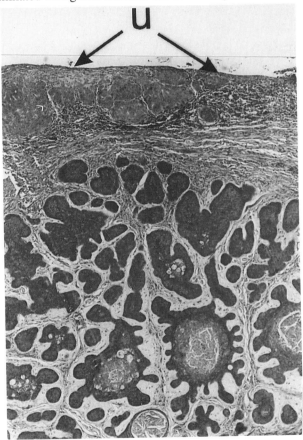

Fig. 4.26 Photomicrograph illustrating a basal cell carcinoma which has caused ulceration (U) of the overlying epidermis.

Table 4.4 *Clinical effects of some tumours*

Tumour	Clinical manifestation	Tumour-derived hormone
Adrenocortical adenoma	Cushing's syndrome	ACTH
Oat cell carcinoma	Cushing's syndrome	ACTH
Parathyroid adenoma	Hypercalcaemia	Parathyroid hormone
Skeletal metastases	Hypercalcaemia	Osteolytic activity of tumour enzymes
Pancreatic insulinoma	Hypoglycaemia	Insulin
Pancreatic gastrinoma	Zollinger–Ellison syndrome	Gastrin
Pancreatic VIPomas	Watery diarrhoea	Vasoactive intestinal peptide
Phaeochromocytoma	Hypertension	Catecholamines
Carcinoid	Acromegaly	Growth hormone

weight loss and muscle weakness. This catabolic clinical state is known as *cachexia*, and is likely to be caused by a combination of endocrine, metabolic and immunological disturbances resulting from tumour-host interactions, and is not simply a result of starvation.

Since well differentiated tumours can retain the functional properties of the parent tissue, their excessive size and relatively autonomous nature (e.g. inoperative negative feedback loops) means that clinical features are common, particularly in endocrine tumours (Table 4.4).

However, some tumours produce products which are unexpected or inappropriate. The best known example of this *ectopic* hormone production occurs in the lung, where the small cell ('oat-cell') variety of lung carcinoma can secrete both ACTH and antidiuretic hormone. Small cell lung carcinomas are also a prime example of the autocrine nature of growth stimulation of many cancer cells (see Chapter 5, section 5.2). Bombesin is released from oat cell tumours which in turn activates bombesin receptors, leading to enhanced growth. The autocrine nature of malignant growth explains the relative autonomous behaviour of malignant cells in culture, and other examples include the stimulation of some sarcomas and gliomas by PDGF, and the stimulation of many carcinomas by TGFα binding to EGFR.

4.10 Further reading

Albelda, S. M. (1993). Role of integrins and other cell adhesion molecules in tumor progression and metastasis. *Laboratory Investigation*, **68**, 4–17.

Carter, R. L. (1984). *Precancerous States*. London: Oxford University Press.

Folkman, J. (1995). Angiogenesis in cancer, vascular, rheumatoid and other diseases. *Nature Medicine*, **1**, 27–31.

Liotta, L. A., Stetler-Stevenson, W. G. & Steeg, P. S. (1993). Invasion and metastases. In *Cancer Medicine*, 3rd edn., ed. J. F. Holland, E. Frei, R. C. Bast, D. L. Kufe, D. L. Morton & R. R. Weichselbaum, pp. 138–53. Philadelphia: Lea & Febiger.

Sell, S. & Pierce, G. B. (1994). Maturation arrest of stem cell differentiation is a common pathway for the cellular origin of teratocarcinomas and epithelial cancers. *Laboratory Investigation*, **70**, 6–22.

Steel, G. G. (1993). Clonogenic cells and the concept of cell survival. In *Basic Clinical Radiobiology*, ed. G. G. Steel, pp. 28–39. London: Edward Arnold.

5

Cell proliferation and cell death

5.1 The cell cycle and how to measure it

Introduction

Although measurements of tumour cell proliferation tell us almost nothing about the growth rate of the tumour, a lot of effort, and no little expense, is being directed at measuring cell proliferation in human tumours. The reasons are twofold. First, the proliferative index may be a prognostic indicator. Second, high levels of proliferation may identify patients who would benefit from particularly aggressive therapy (see below). Until relatively recently this measurement amounted to no more than the mitotic count or mitotic index (see below), or perhaps the labelling index (LI) measured after bromodeoxyuridine injection. However, monoclonal antibodies to proliferation-associated antigens are becoming increasingly available commercially, particularly attractive being the ones that react with formalin-fixed, paraffin wax-embedded tissue sections. This has allowed retrospective studies on archival tissue where patient survival data have already been gathered, and thus the proliferation 'marker' can be quickly evaluated for its usefulness as a prognostic indicator. In some human tumours high levels of proliferation are associated with poorer survival, though the discriminating power of any marker is usually only evident when tumours are arbitrarily divided into say, those with an LI above 10% and those with an LI below 10%. Unfortunately, in the scientific climate of 'publish or perish', the production of each new marker spawns a new round of measuring proliferation in the same tumours which were measured with last year's (or last month's) antibody. Such studies have been likened to 're-inventing the wheel', a criticism probably not too far wide of the mark. Cell proliferation in tumours can also be measured by flow cytometry, and the method can be applied to fresh, frozen and paraffin wax-embedded tissue. The advantage that the technique can analyse thousands of cells very quickly has to be weighed against the fact that included in this analysis are many non-tumour cells, in particular large numbers of inflammatory cells that are commonly present in tumours.

There can be little doubt that cell proliferation is a fundamental process in both health and disease, and that oncologists must be able to measure correctly the 'normal' status if subtle perturbation of the system is to be detected. For example, many internal and external stratified squamous epithelia have pronounced circadian variations in proliferative indices; such oscillations could mask or accentuate perceived induced changes caused by genotoxic carcinogens or promoters. Likewise, the proliferative cells in the various gastrointestinal mucosae are tightly compartmentalized (see Fig. 5.3), and early preneoplastic changes in colonic crypts include fairly small extensions of the proliferative zone into the upper reaches of the crypt. There are many methods available for detecting proliferative cells, but it is important to appreciate the potential pitfalls which may be encountered in accurately quantifying the results.

The cell cycle

Cell population kinetics encompasses a body of methods for quantifying certain *state* parameters and certain *rate* parameters by which a proliferating mass of cells may be characterized. This assessment of proliferative status involves estimates of population size or cell number, the flux(es), which is the rate by which cells enter or leave various compartments or populations, and the time spent within a compartment or the time taken to accomplish some proliferation-related function.

Before addressing these techniques, it is necessary to take a brief look at the cell cycle. It was originally thought that a cell duplicated its DNA in mitosis, then the concept of the cell cycle was formulated in the early 1950s. It was found that broad bean root cells incorporated ^{32}P into their nuclei in a discrete period in their life history, and only a few hours later did the label appear in mitotic cells: hence the existence of a 'G$_2$' period was demonstrated. There are in fact several functional states which proliferating cells can occupy besides mitosis (Fig. 5.1). After completing mitosis (M) the daughter cells enter the Gap 1 (G$_1$) phase in which they spend a period of time, this will vary according to the type of tissue. They then enter the S or synthetic phase where the cell's genetic material is doubled during DNA synthesis. After this there is a second gap phase (G$_2$) before cells divide again. The time between two mitoses is often called the cell cycle time and this varies widely depending on the duration of the G$_1$ phase. Current thinking places a crucial control point, at which cells commit themselves to a further mitosis, firmly in the early G$_1$ phase. This control point is illustrated diagramatically in Fig. 5.1, and has been variously called a 'restriction point' or 'transition point'. There are three potential avenues open to a cell reaching this point in the cell cycle: (i) to recycle; (ii) to 'decycle', and enter a proliferatively quiescent phase, commonly called the G$_0$ phase, from which the cell can be ejected back into the cell cycle if conditions are appropriate or (iii) the cell can decycle and progress upon a course that leads to terminal differentiation, reproductive sterility and eventual death.

In real, normal and tumour cell populations, cells do not all traverse the cell cycle at the same rate, as suggested by the single line describing the cell cycle in Fig. 5.1. Also it is very rare to find all the cells in the cell cycle at any time, although portions of an epithelial cell population may consist solely of proliferating cells. In the mid-crypt region of the rat jejunal crypt all cells are cycling, but, when viewed as a whole, the mucosa is a mixture of proliferating and non-proliferating terminally differentiated

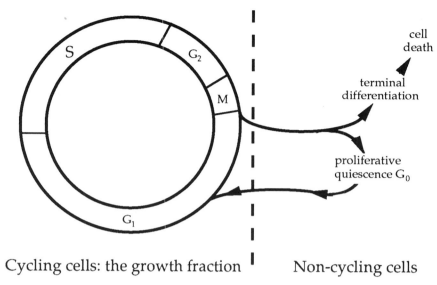

Cycling cells: the growth fraction | Non-cycling cells

Fig. 5.1 Schematic diagram of the cell cycle. G_1 is the most variant phase in the cell cycle and can be almost non-existent in exponentially growing cultured cells, but can be 5–6 days in basal cells in stratified squamous epithelia. Cells commonly complete S phase in 6–8 h, G_2 in 1–4 h and M in 1–2 h. Glandular epithelia (e.g. hepatocytes, renal tubular cells, prostatic acinar cells) are in G_0, these cells are not actively preparing for the next round of cell division, but can be triggered back into the cell cycle.

(end state) cells (see Fig. 5.2A). Likewise, most basal cells in stratified squamous epithelia are cycling (Fig. 5.2B), while suprabasal cells are non-cycling end state cells. Conventionally, those cells born into the proliferative category are designated P cells, and those born into the non-proliferative (quiescent) category are known as Q cells. The ratio of proliferating to non-proliferating cells is defined, in index form, as the *growth fraction* (GF) as:

$$GF = N_P/N_P + N_Q \tag{1}$$

where N_P and N_Q are the numbers of cells in the P and Q compartments respectively. As we shall see, it is possible to estimate the GF in a cell population. In tumours it is not easy on kinetic grounds to distinguish G_0 from terminally differentiated cells, though morphologically it is easy to recognize the latter in well differentiated tumours (see Fig. 4.17A). Many cells in hypoxic regions of tumours (see Fig. 4.16) may be in G_0 and thus relatively resistant to many anti-cancer drugs and irradiation (see Chapter 7, sections 7.2 and 7.3). However, these cells may move from the Q to the P compartment after the destruction of proliferating cells to cause repopulation of the tumour – a phenomenon known as *recruitment*.

Normal tissues are generally classified into one of three types. *Renewing* populations (where cell production is matched by cell loss ensuring no net growth) are a mixture of P and Q cells, but other cell populations can be differently organized. In the adult organism, neurones in the central nervous system (CNS) and cardiac

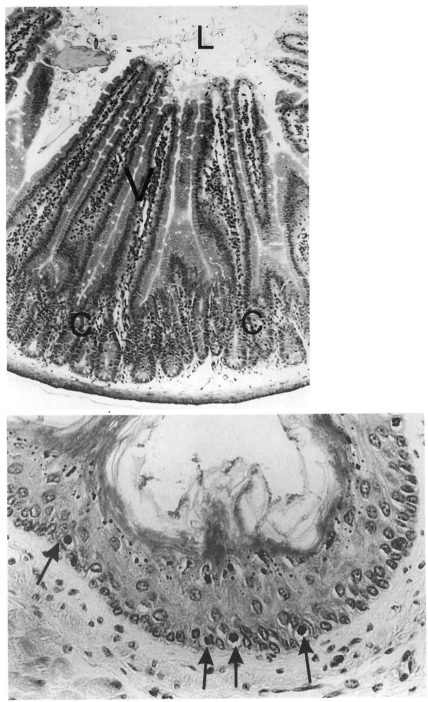

Fig. 5.2 Photomicrographs illustrating the organization of renewing epithelia into proliferating and non-proliferating (terminally differentiated) compartments. In the rat small intestine (A) proliferation is confined to the crypts (C), and the villi (V) which protrude into the lumen (L) are clothed by terminally differentiating cells. In the rat oesophagus (B) proliferation is confined to the basal layer as seen by the presence of vincristine-arrested metaphases (arrows), and the suprabasal cells are terminally differentiating.

myocytes are examples of *static cell* populations; all cells are in the Q compartment, terminally differentiated and unable to re-enter the cell cycle. However, in *conditional renewal* populations most cells are ordinarily resident in the G_0 state, but can be triggered back into the cycling compartment by an appropriate stimulus such as cell loss or increased functional demand. Glandular epithelia such as those of liver, kidney, salivary glands, prostate and thyroid are classic examples of conditional renewal systems, though connective tissue cells such as fibroblasts or skeletal muscle cells can also be placed in this category.

In all renewing populations there is a small number of stem cells, which like their counterparts in tumours have an infinite capacity for self-renewal, but unlike tumours (see Fig. 4.21) they maintain their number, while at the same time producing daughter cells which undergo a limited number of amplification divisions before leaving the cell cycle, terminally differentiating, and eventually dying. In the bone marrow, retroviral lineage marking indicates a common multipotential stem cell, while in rodent thin epidermis it is likely that the stem cells are a sub-population of basal cells, more slowly cycling than the other proliferative cells, and situated in the centre of each epidermal stack. Likewise, in the small intestine where cell migration is essentially unidirectional, the stem cells are thought to be at the beginning of the flux, amongst non-proliferative Paneth cells at the base of the crypt. All gastrointestinal epithelia have a hierarchical organization (Fig. 5.3A, B, C), and this strict division of labour is rapidly lost in dysplastic epithelia, with, amongst other changes, an extension of the proliferative zone to the full thickness of the mucosa.

Cell kinetic methods analyzed on tissue sections

Many of the simplest methods for measuring cell proliferation only give information on the proliferative state of cells, and not the rate at which they are being produced, and these so-called state parameters are described first.

Mitotic count or mitotic index

The mitotic count is often defined as the number of mitoses per 10 high power fields (HPF), whereas the mitotic index (MI) is the proportion of the cell population in mitosis expressed as a percentage. Like any state parameter, the mitotic index depends not only on the rate of transit of cells in mitosis, but also upon how long they remain in the phase, thus an elevation of the mitotic index can be caused simply by an increase in the duration of mitosis. The mitotic count takes no account of cell size: a HPF of a large cell tumour will contain fewer cells than a small cell tumour; thus to compare the mitotic counts of different tumours is frequently meaningless. For this reason, the mitotic index, although more time consuming, is a preferable method of assessing mitotic activity.

Thymidine labelling

There are four bases in DNA, three of them are also found in RNA, so only one, thymine, is unique to DNA. Due to the specificity of the nucleoside thymidine,

(A)

Compartment

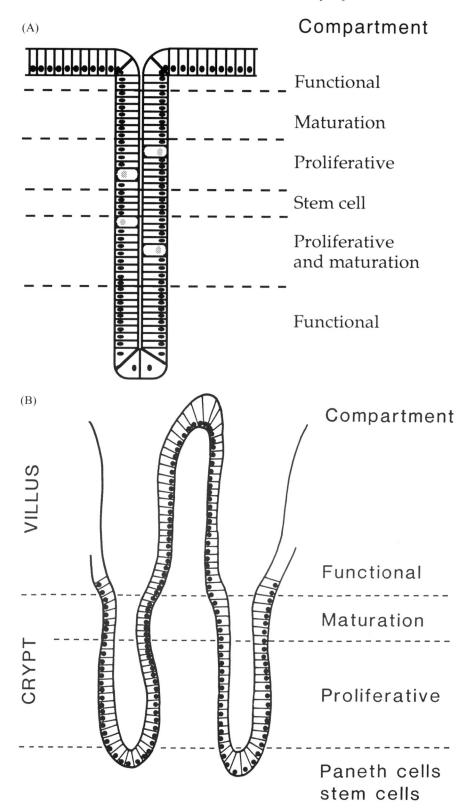

Functional

Maturation

Proliferative

Stem cell

Proliferative
and maturation

Functional

(B)

Compartment

VILLUS

Functional

Maturation

CRYPT

Proliferative

Paneth cells
stem cells

(C)   # Compartment

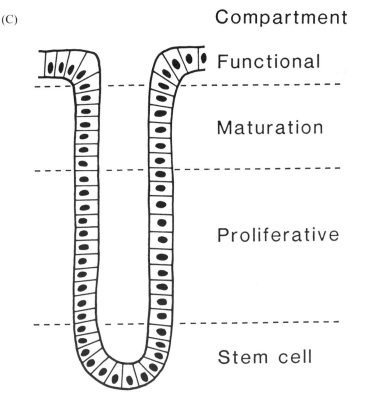

Functional

Maturation

Proliferative

Stem cell

Fig. 5.3 A diagrammatic representation of the kinetic compartments in (A) the gastric gland, (B) the small intestinal crypt and (C) the colonic crypt.

radioactively labelled thymidine (particularly [³H]-thymidine) has been widely used in proliferative studies since the original description of its synthesis in 1957. The flash or pulse thymidine labelling index (TLI%) is a measure of the percentage of cells in the S phase of the cell cycle, and is usually measured at one hour after exposure of the tissue to [³H]-thymidine. Because the S phase is longer than the M phase (Fig. 5.1), TLI is always larger than MI and therefore seemingly more reliable (see below).

The major drawback to the use of [³H]-thymidine in experimental studies is the cost; whole animal labelling is expensive, and added to this is the cost of photographic materials, the employment of a competent autoradiography technician, the utilization of a dedicated Dark Room and the lengthy (2–3 weeks) period over which sections must be exposed to photographic emulsion for the autoradiographic process to take place. For these reasons the use of this former gold-standard of cell proliferation measurements has declined markedly in popularity in recent years, largely superseded by the cheaper and quicker immunohistochemical methods. For proliferation studies in humans the same arguments against the use of [³H]-thymidine apply, and, in addition, there are serious ethical constraints, though the measurement of [¹¹C]-thymidine uptake by positron emission tomography (PET) may be a cheaper and altogether more ethical alternative since the half-life of this radioisotope is measured in hours rather than years.

Knowledge of the TLI, or for that matter the bromodeoxyuridine LI (see below), permits calculation of a very useful parameter called the *potential doubling time* (t_{PD}) through the relationship:

$$t_{PD} = \lambda t_S / LI \tag{2}$$

where λ is a parameter which depends on the position of S in the cell cycle: if S is close to the end of the cycle, $\lambda = \ln 2$, but if S occurs at the beginning of the cycle, $\lambda = 2\ln 2$. If growth is thought to be exponential, as it often is in tumours (see Fig. 5.32), a value of 0.75 for λ is commonly chosen, while the duration of the S phase (t_S) usually comes from an 'educated guess'. The potential doubling time (t_{PD}) is the time it should take for a population to double in size when based *solely* on a consideration of cell production, and is largely used in the context of expanding cell populations such as tumours. Of course, it is commonly recognized that in real life most solid tumours double in size in a time greatly in excess of their t_{PD}, and this is because of *cell loss*. Cell loss becomes an increasingly important determinant of tumour growth rate as tumours enlarge, extending the doubling time, often in the absence of any real decline in cell production rate (see Chapter 5, section 5.4).

Bromodeoxyuridine (BrdUrd) labelling

Though the MI gives an unequivocal measurement concerning cell proliferation, it is generally felt that a measurement of the fraction of cells in S or alternatively the growth fraction is a more accurate figure. This is because the latter is a higher number since the S phase is much longer (about 8×) than the M phase, and therefore a scan of a limited number of cells (e.g. 2000) is more likely to yield a more accurate LI than MI, since mitoses are relatively rare (in comparison to labelled cells) and could be over- or underestimated in a limited count.

Thus with the problems connected with radiolabelled thymidine, alternative S-phase markers have been enthusiastically sought. The first of these to be widely adopted was bromodeoxyuridine (BrdUrd). BrdUrd is a pyrimidine analogue which is readily incorporated into nuclei during the DNA synthetic phase, and there are now various monoclonal antibodies to BrdUrd which can be used on alcohol-based and formalin fixed, paraffin wax-embedded tissue sections. Tissues normally require a period of acid denaturation to render the DNA single-stranded to allow access of the antibody to BrdUrd, and, in addition, those fixed in cross-linking fixatives such as formalin also require proteolytic pretreatment. Microwaving has been reported to obviate the need for these denaturation/digestion steps: – these are all 'antigen retrieval' procedures. Visualization is carried out using a standard indirect immunoperoxidase labelling technique, and the brown diaminobenzidine (DAB) reaction product is easily seen (see Fig. 4.16B). A distinct advantage over autoradiography is that a result can be obtained within a matter of days. With these considerations in mind, BrdUrd labelling is the method of choice for identifying the S-phase fraction, at least in situations where the substrate can be administered; this would apply not only to experimental animals and cell culture systems, but also to certain cancer patient groups where cell kinetic information may be useful in planning therapy.

Alternative labelling methods

Thymidine and BrdUrd labelling both suffer from the disadvantage of the DNA substrate having to be administered prior to detection, so precluding retrospective studies on archival material. This limitation was overcome, at least for human material, by the introduction of the monoclonal antibody Ki-67, which recognized a bimolecular complex of 345 and 395 kDa associated with cycling cells. The human Ki-67 antigen is expressed in all stages of the cell cycle and is thus a measure of the growth fraction, but the original antibody was limited by its recognition of the antigen only in human snap frozen material. The human Ki-67 antigen can now be detected in microwaved archival material (Fig. 5.4) using a newer monoclonal antibody MIB1 (Molecular Immunology Borstel).

The antigen termed proliferating cell nuclear antigen (PCNA) promised to replace Ki-67 because it could be detected immunohistochemically in routinely processed tissue. PCNA is a 36 kDa non-histone nuclear protein required for DNA synthesis and repair, being an auxiliary protein to DNA polymerase delta. Elevated levels of PCNA appear in the nucleus during late G_1, become maximal during S phase, before declining in G_2 and mitosis, and the prototype antibody, PC10, not only labels cycling cells but because of the long half-life of the protein, also cells that have recently left

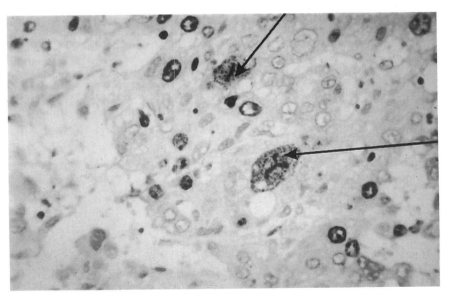

Fig. 5.4 Photomicrograph illustrating MIB1 (Molecular Immunology Borstel) immunolabelling in a human hepatocellular carcinoma; note the labelling of mitoses (arrows) as well as other cells indicating that the Ki-67 protein is expressed throughout the cell cycle.

Table 5.1. *Some of the markers which label cycling cells*

Marker	What it measures	Advantages	Disadvantages
Tritiated thymidine	S-phase fraction	Very specific	Has to be injected Radioactive Expensive
Bromodeoxyuridine	S-phase fraction	Very specific Inexpensive	Has to be administered
Ki-67/MIB series	Growth fraction	No injection	Apparently none
Anti-PCNA	Late G_1-M fraction	No injection	Antigenicity easily destroyed

the cell cycle. However, on the one hand, the antigen can be readily destroyed by prolonged fixation, even after just 48 hours, yet on the other hand, be visualized in 100% of cells by aggressive antigen retrieval procedures. With these caveats in mind, the detection of PCNA should certainly be cautiously interpreted. Table 5.1 summarizes the commercially available markers to identify cycling cells.

Rate parameters: the metaphase arrest technique

Proliferative indices (mitotic and labelling indices) can reflect not only changes in the proliferative rate, but also changes in the phase durations, t_M and t_S respectively. However, the metaphase arrest method provides a firm kinetic parameter, the rate of entry into mitosis (r_M), or the birth rate (K_B), which is not subject to the vagaries of proliferative index measurements. The method can give results over an experimental period as short as 2.5 hours, and involves the study of paraffin wax-embedded sections only. However, the method requires multiple samples over this period, so it is only feasible to apply it to situations where there are many similar tumour-bearing animals (see Chapter 5, section 5.4).

There are many compounds which have metaphase arresting properties, the earliest used was colchicine, and latterly its less toxic derivative, colcemid. More recently the *Vinca* alkaloids vincristine and vinblastine have found widespread usage, and, over a period of two to three hours *in vivo*, generally the agents do not allow anaphase 'escape' or cause premature metaphase degeneration. Arresting agents disrupt the assembly of the mitotic spindle, with the production of the characteristically abnormal mitotic figures which can be easily recognized (Fig. 5.2B).

Basically, the method hinges upon the measurement of the slope of the line which describes the rate of accumulation of arrested metaphases (Fig. 5.5). After a short lag, the metaphase index will increase linearly, and, since each mitosis results in the birth of one new cell, it follows that K_B will equal r_M. Thus, the time taken to double the number of cells already present, t_{PD}, can be derived from the expression:

$$t_{PD} = 1/K_B \tag{3}$$

If, as in many tumours, the population under study is growing exponentially, it will

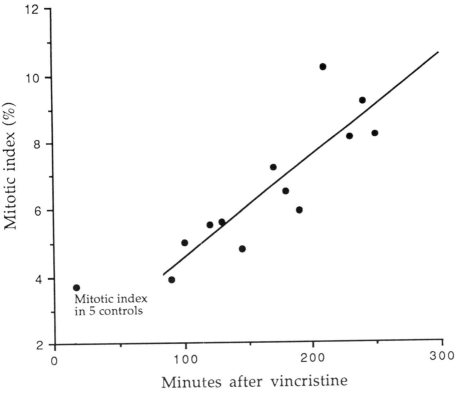

Fig. 5.5 A metaphase arrest line constructed for basal cells in the mouse oesophageal squamous epithelium after injection of vincristine. Note the delay of 75 min before metaphase arrest becomes effective. The slope of the line (fitted by least squares) is about 2%/hour, suggesting a t_{PD} of ~50 h ($t_{PD} = 1/K_B = 1/0.02 = 50$ h) where t_{PD} refers to potential doubling time and K_B is birth rate. In renewing tissues where normally the population is not increasing in size because cell production is matched by cell loss, the term turnover time is often preferred to the potential doubling time.

be necessary to correct for the fact that the absolute rate of cell production is constantly increasing, therefore:

$$t_{PD} = \log_e 2/K_B \tag{4}$$

Which cells to count and how many?

So far we have been largely concerned with visually identifying proliferative cells in tissue sections, be they mitoses, arrested metaphases or labelled S phase and other cycling cells. The problem now facing us is to decide how many cells to score to obtain an accurate index. Unfortunately there is no easy answer, since if the particular labelled cells are relatively scarce a larger sample needs to be scanned than if the labelled cells are more frequent, in order to obtain similar statistical errors of the count – it is common to find sample sizes of between 1000 and 2000 cells chosen, though usually without any statistical basis for the choice. Of course, microscopy is time-consuming, and counting huge numbers of cells might not be worth the extra precision of the count – the trick is to strike the correct balance. One very real problem is tissue heterogeneity in proliferation, in solid tumours we have seen that proliferative cells are often concentrated around blood vessels (Fig. 4.16B) and are relatively scarce as cells differentiate (Fig. 4.17A).

Flow cytometry

In the context of cell proliferation studies, flow cytometry can provide a rapid analysis of the DNA content of thousands of cells and, in tumours at least, significant aneuploid sub-populations (which would otherwise be undetected by other methods) can be readily distinguished. In practice, a single cell suspension is prepared, and for DNA analysis the cells are stained with one of several fluorescent dyes (propidium iodide, acridine orange, ethidium bromide) which stoichiometrically bind to DNA. The cells are then passed in suspension through an exciting laser beam and the resulting fluorescence is collected through a lens and observed by a photomultiplier and converted into a voltage pulse (Fig. 5.6). The pulse height is proportional to the total fluorescence emitted as the cell passes through the beam and is a direct measure of the amount of nuclear DNA – and the data are expressed as a distribution of cellular DNA contents (Fig. 5.7). Since the total DNA content of the cell varies with the stage of the cell cycle, the relative number of cells in each stage of the cell cycle can be estimated, this is usually a computer analysis. Obtaining a monodispersed cell population is probably the most difficult technical task, and there is also the problem of contamination of tumour cell populations by non-tumour cells such as inflammatory cells.

The labelling index can also be estimated by performing a combined BrdUrd-DNA profile; patients can be injected with BrdUrd and the isolated cells incubated with an anti-BrdUrd antibody, these cells are subsequently labelled with an anti-mouse secondary antibody conjugated to a green fluorescent molecule such as fluorescein isothiocyanate (FITC). Cells are then counterstained for DNA content using propidium iodide, a red fluorescent marker. The cells are now passed in suspension through an exciting laser beam and the resulting fluorescence is split by a series of mirrors and lenses, observed by photomultipliers and electronically processed. This simultaneous measurement of the DNA content and BrdUrd uptake in each of thousands of cells is then displayed as a two-dimensional histogram (Fig. 5.8).

Measuring the cell population size

It could be argued that the most meaningful parameter in the context of proliferation is not a state or rate parameter, which, after all, are only 'snapshots' in time, but the net result of any changes in cell proliferation or cell death – the *size* of the population. This could be the cell number, measured either directly in a haemocytometer chamber

(A)   (B)

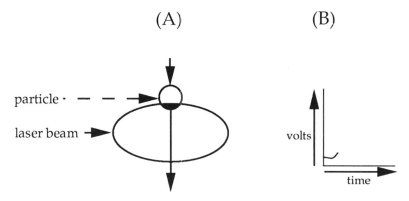

Particle enters laser beam

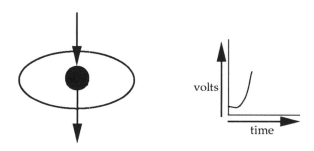

Integrated pulse - particle fluorescence

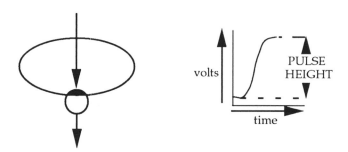

Particle leaves laser beam

Fig. 5.6 The principle of flow cytometry. Stained cells are excited by a laser beam and the resultant fluorescence converted to a voltage.

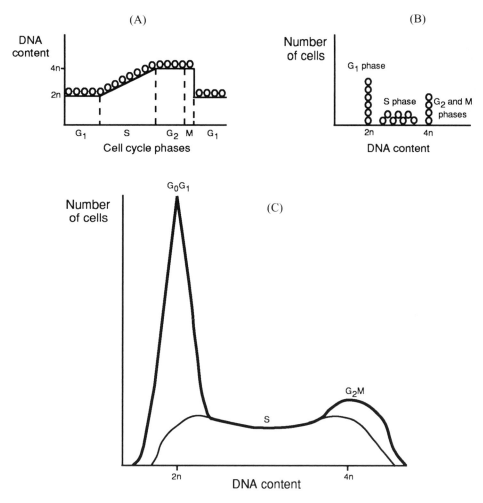

Fig. 5.7 The principle of a DNA histogram as analyzed by flow cytometry. (A) As cells pass through S they double their DNA content, so cells in G_2 have twice the DNA content of G_1 cells. (B) If these cells were sorted from one another on the basis of their DNA content they would segregate in this manner. (C) A typical DNA histogram obtained from a flow cytometer; the exact number of cells in each category is derived from associated computer software.

from a cell culture experiment, or indirectly from a DNA assay applicable to both *in vitro* and *in vivo* systems. There are alternative methods for measuring population size, and for solid tumours it is common to construct a *growth curve* (see Fig. 5.32). This (hopefully) reflects changes in viable tumour cell number, but this is a gross oversimplification since tumours contain many cells which are not tumour cells, furthermore there may well be products of differentiation such as mucin or keratin, and, particularly as tumours get big, they often contain large 'lakes' of necrotic tissue. Despite these shortcomings, it has been possible to gain much information about how

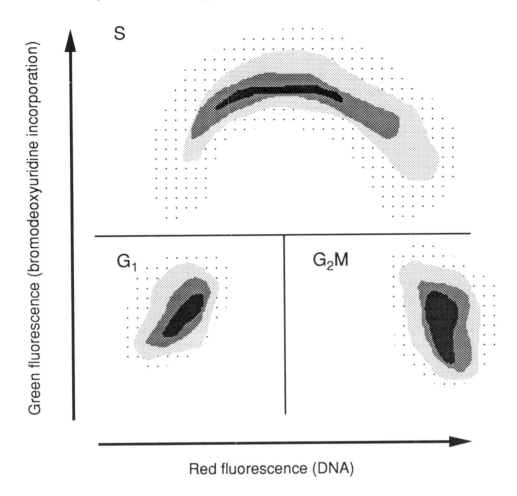

Fig. 5.8 A two-dimensional histogram display of cells in DNA synthesis (green fluorescence) and the simultaneous measurement of DNA content (red fluorescence); note cells in S have a DNA content intermediate between G_1 and G_2M cells.

tumours grow from the analysis of such curves, and this is discussed more fully in Chapter 5 (section 5.4).

5.2   Growth factors and their receptors

Introduction

In the serum of multicellular organisms there is a huge number of polypeptide growth factors that are directly and specifically involved in stimulating cell division and differentiation. They are not the typical cell nutrients that act within cells, but rather they are secreted by cells and water soluble ones interact with specific, membrane-bound glycoprotein receptors that are crucial in the conversion of the first message (the growth factor) into a second or intracellular message. These can act within the cell and initiate a series of biochemical reactions, which eventually result in specific gene expression. Ligand binding can activate one or more of a variety of plasma membrane-associated transducing systems which generate the intracellular signals.

Growth factors are among the most potent of biological substances, being biologically active at concentrations of picograms per ml ($1pg = 10^{-12}g$), while the specificity and magnitude of the response is believed to be mainly due to the type and abundance of membrane-bound receptor rather than the availability of the growth factor. A cell can be basically viewed as a bag, it has an inside and an outside, with the growth factor receptors spanning the plasma membrane like rivets. A cell may alter its receptivity to a peptide growth factor by up-regulation or down-regulation of its surface receptor number, or alternatively the affinity of the receptor for the binding ligand might change, or receptor occupancy may result in a quantitative change in the intracellular signal generated as the secondary event (Fig. 5.9). Receptor down-regulation is commonly seen when a cell is subjected to prolonged exposure to a peptide hormone or growth factor, such as insulin, glucagon and epidermal growth factor (EGF). In the case of EGF (Fig. 5.10), occupied EGF receptors are being continually internalized (endocytosed) and recycled back to the cell surface, with, on average, one-third of the internalized receptors suffering lysosomal degradation on each pass through the cell.

Strategies of chemical signalling

The use of growth factors as a mode of communication between cells allows the producer cells and target cells to be physically separated from one another, though other forms of intercellular communication do exist such as through gap junctions of adjacent cells, and the direct physical contact between cells achieved by the interaction of plasma membrane-bound cell adhesion molecules. Operationally, it is possible to distinguish at least three principal types of growth factor secretion, dependent upon the distance between the secreting cell(s) and the cellular target (Fig. 5.11). In *endocrine* secretion the effector cells are typically in groups surrounded by a rich vascular network, and secrete a hormone directly into blood vessels; the hormone acts on target cells with the necessary receptive machinery, at some distance from the source. Androgens or oestrogens (which are lipophilic and interact with cytoplasmic and nuclear receptors) induce growth in the prostate or endometrium through this means. The immune system too can be regarded as an endocrine system, albeit a mobile one, since the whole range of cellular functions is controlled by an intricate cytokine network (see below).

Paracrine secretion, however, involves growth factors only acting within the immediate vicinity of the effector cells, perhaps within a millimetre or so. This mode of action undoubtedly occurs in the alimentary tract where several families of neuro-endocrine cells produce multiple locally acting peptides, some of which influence growth.

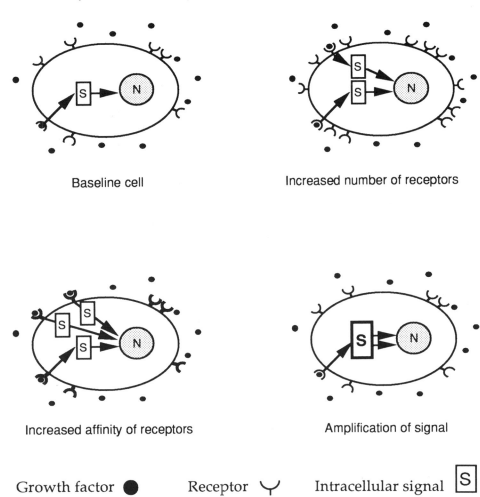

Baseline cell

Increased number of receptors

Increased affinity of receptors

Amplification of signal

Growth factor ●   Receptor ⅄   Intracellular signal $\boxed{S}$

Fig. 5.9 Mechanisms by which a cell can increase its response to a growth factor.

The relative autonomous nature of malignant cells in culture has been appreciated for many years, i.e. they require fewer exogenous growth factors for optimal growth than do their normal counterparts. One explanation was that the malignant cells had the ability to produce their own growth factors, and the same cells had functional receptors for them – a mechanism termed *autocrine* secretion. Such a mechanism could clearly bestow a growth advantage to cancer cells and they would be under less strong external growth control than neighbouring normal cells. Autocrine secretion was first described in rodent cells transformed by sarcoma viruses, where the mixture of secreted polypeptides (originally called 'sarcoma growth factor') contained one growth factor structurally related to (but distinct from) EGF and now called type α transforming growth factor (TGFα), and another distinct growth factor named transforming growth factor beta (TGFβ). Autocrine secretion of TGFα plays an important role in the malignant behaviour of many cell types, and other peptides which function

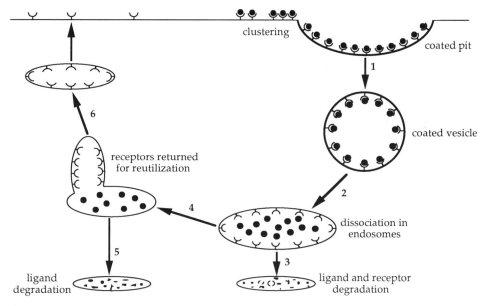

Fig. 5.10 A model of receptor down-regulation, degradation and recycling. Occupied receptors cluster, congregate in coated pits and become internalized within endosomal vesicles. Dissociation within an acidic environment leads to ultimate degradation within lysosomes, though some receptors may be recycled back to the cell surface. (Redrawn from Schlessinger, J., 1988. The epidermal growth factor receptor as a multifunctional allosteric protein. *Biochemistry*, **27**, 3119–23.)

in this way include platelet-derived growth factor (PDGF) produced by osteosarcoma and glioma cells, and bombesin, the tetradecapeptide secreted by human small cell ('oat cell') lung cancers (SCLCs). In these examples it has been possible to inhibit cell growth by antibodies to the peptides, leaving no doubt that antibody therapy can interfere with an essential autocrine pathway intimately associated with aberrant growth of tumour cells.

The signalling pathway activated by an autocrine growth factor can also evoke a negative growth response, i.e. it can act as a 'foot on the brake' rather than a 'foot on the accelerator'. The best known example of such a negative growth factor is TGFβ, a homodimeric peptide, which along with TGFα was responsible for the transforming ability of so-called 'sarcoma growth factor', the mixture of polypeptides secreted into the extracellular medium by mouse 3T3 cells when transformed by Moloney sarcoma virus. The concept of a cell producing its own growth inhibitory substances is not new, there was the *chalone* hypothesis, but it was little more than intellectually appealing until the discovery of TGFβ as the inhibitory molecule produced by, and inhibiting monkey kidney cells. TGFβ is, in fact, a multifunctional agent stimulating the growth of some cells, while being a potent growth inhibitor of others, and even having activities apparently quite separate from proliferation such as promoting collagen synthesis. Thus, like many growth factors, the original name for TGFβ is a misnomer, in that its biological activities extend far beyond the context of its original discovery. In

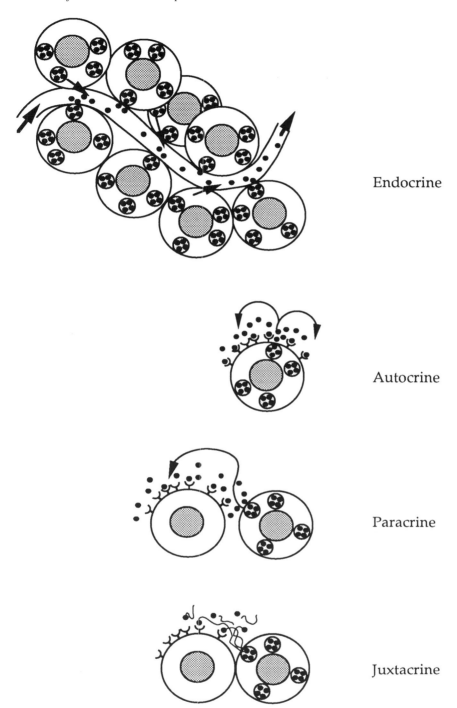

Endocrine

Autocrine

Paracrine

Juxtacrine

Fig. 5.11 Diagrammatic representation of the pathways by which growth factors communicate with their target cells.

summary, the autocrine hypothesis now includes the concept that malignant transformation may be the result, not only of excessive production, secretion and action of
positive autocrine growth factors, but also of the failure of cells to synthesize, secrete
or respond to negative growth factors which they normally release to control their
own growth.

A further type of signalling between cells has been termed *juxtacrine* stimulation.
Many growth factors, including TGFα, are synthesized as membrane-anchored larger
precursor molecules, and it has been suggested that cells expressing the pro-TGFα
molecule can bind to adjacent cells bearing EGF receptors and trigger cell
proliferation.

Growth factors

Table 5.2 summarizes the major growth factor families. EGF was first isolated from
male mouse submaxillary glands by Stanley Cohen in 1962, and like almost every
other growth factor it has a spectrum of biological activities far beyond that from
which its name derives. It is now known to be a major mitogen for many cell lineages
and even has non-related actions such as inhibiting gastric acid secretion. Mouse EGF
is highly homologous with the human polypeptide hormone urogastrone, originally
isolated from the urine of pregnant women and now regarded as the human homologue
of EGF. The members of the EGF family of growth factors are all synthesized as much
larger, membrane-bound, glycosylated precursors, and despite only limited amino acid
sequence homology, the secreted molecules have six conserved cysteine residues forming three disulphide bonds (Fig. 5.12). TGFα, despite only 35% sequence homology
with EGF, has biological activity similar to EGF and binds to the same receptor. As
already mentioned the 160 amino acid cell surface precursor may be biologically
active through interaction with EGF receptors (EGFRs) on the surface of adjacent
cells. As well as being abundant in many tumour cells, TGFα is also widely found in
normal tissues. Amphiregulin was isolated from conditioned medium of MCF-7 breast
carcinoma cells treated with phorbol ester and can be both stimulatory and inhibitory
to cell growth. All these molecules can bind to the same receptor, EGFR, also known
as c-erbB-1, a member of the type 1 family of receptor tyrosine kinases which includes
three more related receptors, c-erbB-2, c-erbB-3 and c-erbB-4.

PDGF is a cationic, disulphide-linked dimeric protein with a molecular weight of
~30 kDa; the PDGF family also includes vascular endothelial growth factor (VEGF).
The subunits of the PDGF dimer are polypeptides designated A or B chains, and
PDGF family members can be either homodimeric (AA or BB) or heterodimeric (AB).
The B chain is 96% homologous with part of the transforming protein product (p28^{sis})
of the simian sarcoma virus which causes sarcomas in baboons. Two distinct PDGF
receptor subunits, designated α and β have been identified. High affinity binding of
PDGF involves dimers of the receptor (either αα, ββ, or αβ), and results in activation
of the tyrosine kinase in the intracellular domain, leading to autophosphorylation of
the cytoplasmic domain of the receptor as well as phosphorylation of other intracellular substrates (see below). Along with platelets, fibroblasts, endothelial cells and

Table 5.2. *Major polypeptide growth factor families*

EGF family	EGF, TGFα
	Amphiregulin
	Heparin-binding EGF
	Pox virus growth factors
	Cripto
	Beta cellulin
Platelet derived growth factor family	PDGF
	VEGF
Insulin-like growth factors	Insulin
	IGF-I
	IGF-II
	NGF
TGF-β family	TGF-β1 to TGF-β5
	Inhibins, Activins
	BMP-1 to BMP-7
Fibroblast growth factor family	FGF-1 to FGF-9
Hepatocyte growth factor	HGF-SF
Trefoil growth factor family	pS2, SP, ITF
Bombesin-like peptides	Bombesin, GRP
Cytokines	Erythropoietin
	Colony-stimulating factors, e.g. G-CSF,
	GM-CSF, M-CSF
	Stem cell factor (c-*kit* ligand)
	IL-1 to IL-12
	Interferon-α, β and γ
	TNFα, TNFβ

Abbreviations: EGF, epidermal growth factor: VEGF, vascular endothelial growth factor; TGF, transforming growth factor; SP, spasmolytic polypeptide; ITF, intestinal trefoil factor; GRP, gastrin releasing peptide; G-CSF, granulocyte colony stimulating factor; GM-CSF, granulocyte-macrophage colony stimulating factor; M-CSF, macrophage colony stimulating factor; IL, interleukin; TNF, tumour necrosis factor; BMP, bone morphogenetic protein.

monocytes, certain tumour cells are sources of PDGF or PDGF-like molecules, and PDGF functions as a mitogen for mesenchymal cells as well as being a powerful chemo-attractant for inflammatory cells. Pericytes (pluripotential stem cells) found in association with the microvasculature in human wound healing situations strongly express the PDGF-β receptor, indicating a role for PDGF in angiogenesis.

Insulin and the insulin-like growth factors (IGFs) have similar structures and biological activities, generally stimulating growth and cellular metabolism. Insulin often acts synergistically with other growth factors while IGF-II has been particularly implicated in foetal development and embryonal neoplasms. IGF-I (formerly called somatomedin C) and IGF-II (formerly called multiplication stimulating activity – MSA) are single chain peptides of 70 and 67 amino acid residues respectively which are highly conserved in different species. Growth hormone stimulates the production of IGF-I, primarily in the liver, though IGF-I mRNA can be found in most tissues.

The TGFβs form a large family of multifunctional peptide growth factors. They are

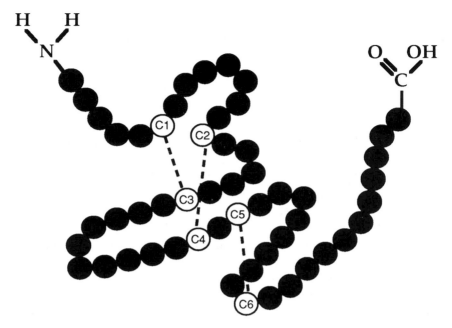

Fig. 5.12 Schematic representation of the 53 amino acid epidermal growth factor molecule. The cysteine bridges are between residues 1 and 3, 2 and 4 and 5 and 6 (numbered from the N-terminal end).

active in the form of disulphide-linked dimers, and both homodimers and heterodimers exist. The originally described form of TGFβ is now designated TGFβ1, and there are a number of closely related peptides (TGFβ2, TGFβ3, TGFβ4, TGFβ5), as well as the more distantly related activins, inhibins and bone morphogenetic proteins (BMPs). The TGFβs are synthesized as large precursor molecules with the mature form of TGFβ at the C-terminus; this is proteolytically cleaved prior to secretion, but both portions remain together upon secretion as a non-covalent complex of the dimeric latency associated protein (LAP) and the processed dimeric 25 kDa TGFβ. This complex is biologically inactive, and release of TGFβ may be facilitated by action of macrophage-secreted proteases on the LAP. TGFβ is generally held to be stimulatory for the growth of cells of mesenchymal origin and inhibitory for epithelial cells, and is also involved in conservation of extracellular matrix molecules. Various members of the TGFβ family have also been implicated in promoting apoptosis, obviously a desirable effect in tumours.

The fibroblast growth factor (FGF) family currently consists of nine structurally related peptide growth factors, designated FGF-1 to FGF-9. Acidic and basic FGFs (FGF-1 and FGF-2) are the prototypic members of this family, both characterized by a high affinity for heparin, and synthesized by a wide variety of normal and malignant cells. FGFs are potent stimulators of endothelial proliferation and therefore probably crucial in tumour angiogenesis as well as during wound healing; basic FGF has shown promise in the healing of ulcers and the growth of skin grafts. Keratinocyte growth factor (KGF; FGF-7) produced by mesenchymal cells, may be one of the mediators of mesenchymal-epithelial interactions since the receptor is found mainly on epidermal keratinocytes, and after wounding, massive increases in KGF mRNA in the underlying dermis precede epidermal proliferation.

Over the last two or three years the search for a humoral regulator of liver growth has increasingly concentrated on the role of hepatocyte growth factor (HGF), also called scatter factor (HGF-SF). HGF is synthesized from a single precursor molecule of 728 amino acids, which is proteolytically processed to form the mature HGF, a heterodimeric molecule composed of a 69 kDa α chain and a 34 kDa β chain. The α chain contains four kringle domains (double loop structures held together by disulphide bonds) reminiscent of various proteases involved in coagulation and fibrinolysis. The β chain has a 37% homology with the β chain of plasmin. HGF is currently considered to be a pleiotropic factor, produced by mesenchymal cells, influencing epithelial cell growth, motility and morphogenesis. HGF was originally termed scatter factor, because the protein from the conditioned medium of human embryonic fibroblasts was able to enhance the local motility (scatter) of a variety of epithelial cells *in vitro*. HGF and scatter factor are identical.

The trefoil peptides are members of a relatively recently discovered group of peptides seemingly of great significance in the field of gastroenterology. The group takes its title from the characteristic trefoil motif, a three loop ('three leafed') structure secured by disulphide bonds based on cysteine residues: the trefoil peptides known to date have either one, two or four trefoil domains. The first molecule characterized was pS2, a single trefoil, whose synthesis could be induced by oestrogens in the MCF-7 human breast cancer cell line. Despite its heritage as a tumour-associated peptide, pS2 mRNA and protein are expressed by the foveolar epithelium throughout the length of the normal human stomach, though its function remains illusive. pS2 is, however, highly homologous with spasmolytic polypeptide (SP), a larger molecule of 108 amino acids, which has two cysteine-rich trefoil domains. This peptide was originally found as a side fraction in the commercial purification of insulin from pig pancreas, and has defined physiological effects on the gut, inhibiting gastric acid secretion and intestinal motility as well as stimulating growth – highly desirable qualities for a putative gut growth factor. Intestinal trefoil factor (ITF), is a recently described single trefoil peptide largely confined to goblet cells. Gastric ulceration and inflammatory bowel disease promote the synthesis of trefoil peptides in regenerating mucosal cells.

Bombesin is a 14 amino acid peptide initially purified from the skin of the frog *Bombina bombina*, and it is homologous to the mammalian peptide, gastrin-releasing peptide (GRP), the largest form of which has 27 amino acids but which has sequence homology with bombesin over the last seven amino acids. Bombesin/GRP has been clearly implicated in the autocrine stimulation of human SCLCs.

A number of regulatory molecules have been identified that particularly influence haematopoiesis, the immune system and inflammation, and these proteins are collectively known as cytokines. Many of these cytokines were called colony stimulating factors (CSFs) because of their ability to stimulate *in vitro* colony formation by progenitor cells in semi-solid media, some have now been assigned appropriate names, e.g. erythropoietin, others have retained their CSF designation, while others have been given an interleukin number. Almost all patients in the later stages of renal failure were anaemic until recombinant human erythropoietin (rhEPO) became available for therapy. EPO is a 165 amino acid residue glycoprotein, and the major stimulus for EPO gene transcription is tissue hypoxia: most EPO is produced by the kidney, and it is likely that the renal source of EPO is a fibroblast-like population of interstitial cells. EPO acts in concert with other growth factors to stimulate the proliferation and maturation of bone marrow erythroid precursor cells, and rhEPO raises the haematocrit and blood haemoglobin concentration in a dose-dependent way. The availability of rhEPO was a major advance in clinical medicine, and it abolishes the need for blood transfusions to correct the anaemia associated with chronic renal failure; it also appears useful in alleviating the anaemia of chronic inflammatory and malignant diseases.

At present the two clinically most important CSFs are granulocyte colony stimulating factor (G-CSF) and granulocyte-macrophage CSF (GM-CSF). Both are glycoproteins, produced by a variety of cell types including macrophages, fibroblasts and endothelial cells, particularly in response to cytokines (tumour necrosis factor α – TNFα; interferon γ – IFNγ) and inflammatory stimuli (endotoxin; lipopolysaccharide – LPS). GM-CSF stimulates the proliferation of granulocyte and macrophage progenitors, and enhances the function of the differentiated cells. Likewise, G-CSF is best known for its stimulatory effects on granulocyte precursor proliferation and survival and function of the terminally differentiated cells. Both CSFs are now widely used in the clinic, particularly for the recovery of haematopoiesis after chemotherapy-induced neutropenias and/or pancytopenias. Neutropenia is a significant dose-limiting toxicity of many cancer chemotherapeutic regimens, therefore CSFs can reduce the risk of infections, reduce the days of hospitalization and decrease the use of antibiotics. Chemotherapy is often accompanied by autologous marrow infusion, and as might be predicted, the clinical benefits of CSFs are less if the bone marrow has been collected after extensive prior chemotherapy, consistent with the hypothesis that a sufficient number of myeloid precursor target cells need to be available for a significant effect.

Stem cell regulation in the bone marrow is a complex process in which there are both positive and negative influences, and it is quite clear that many of the growth factors can act synergistically. For example, some of the interleukins (e.g. IL-1 and IL-3) act on early progenitor cells which primes them to respond more effectively to other more lineage-restricted haematopoietic growth factors, and so combinations such as IL-3 and GM-CSF are proving very effective in alleviating myelosuppression after chemotherapy for cancer. Stem cell factor (SCF or c-*kit* ligand) is another early acting growth factor, which alone, is predominantly a survival factor, but it synergizes strongly with other growth factors, and now recombinant human SCF is finding clinical use in combination with GM-CSF, G-CSF and EPO in promoting the growth of myeloid and erythroid progenitors after cancer chemotherapy.

Many cytokines have been evaluated for their anti-tumour effects; the interferons were the first cytokines to be described and they generally have a cytostatic effect on growth. Tumour necrosis factor is a multifunctional cytokine, which was so named because of its massive lethal effect on animal tumours in response to the treatment of the hosts with Bacillus Calmette-Guerin (BCG) followed by injection with endotoxin. Two related forms of TNF are recognized, TNFα produced largely by monocytes and macrophages, and TNFβ (lymphotoxin) predominantly produced by activated lymphocytes. Both cytokines recognize two cell surface receptors, a high affinity type I receptor and a low affinity type II receptor – the former being associated with receptor-mediated cytotoxicity. TNFs can indirectly cause widespread necrosis through their action on vascular endothelium, so the presence or absence of TNF receptors on specific tumours shows little correlation with the overall cytotoxic effect of the TNFs *in vivo*. Nevertheless, efforts are being made to produce synthetic peptide derivatives of the TNF molecules which are selectively lethal to tumour cells while avoiding the more generally toxic effects.

Growth factor receptors

Receptor structure

Here we are largely concerned with growth factors that are water- rather than lipid-soluble, and because they cannot diffuse across the plasma membrane, they interact with cells by binding to receptors located on the cell surface. Steroids which are the best known examples of lipid soluble hormones can diffuse across the plasma membrane and interact with intracellular receptors.

Cell surface-associated receptors have a similar overall design being composed of an *extracellular* domain responsible for binding the growth factor (ligand), a short hydrophobic *transmembrane* domain, and an *intracellular* domain responsible for initiating the intracellular signal in response to ligand binding (Fig. 5.13). Many, though not all transmembrane receptors belong to a large family of receptor *protein tyrosine kinases* (PTKs), essentially enzymatic proteins with the ability to catalyse the phosphorylation of the amino acid tyrosine in proteins – the phosphorylated forms of many proteins (enzymes) are more active than the non-phosphorylated forms. A classical example of a non-receptor PTK is the protein product pp60$^{c\text{-}src}$ of the proto-oncogene c-*src* (see below), while the EGFR exemplifies the receptors with tyrosine kinase activity.

EGFR, sometimes called c-erbB-1, belongs to the type I family of growth factor receptors which includes three more related receptor molecules c-erbB-2, c-erbB-3 and c-erbB-4. It will be remembered that the viral homologue of the EGFR is v-erbB, the transforming protein encoded by the v-*erbB* oncogene of avian erythroblastosis virus, suggesting the virus has acquired the cellular gene sequences coding for a shortened receptor lacking the EGF-binding domain, which then functions abnormally leading to transformation. The monomeric type I growth factor receptors have two cysteine-rich repeat sequences in the extracellular domain, and Fig. 5.14 illustrates some of the other families of receptor PTKs. Insulin receptors have similar cysteine-rich sequences in a disulphide-linked heterotetrameric structure ($\alpha_2\beta_2$) structure, while FGF and PDGF receptors have immunoglobulin-like repeats in their extracellular domains.

The more detailed structure and regulation of the EGFR will serve as a model of

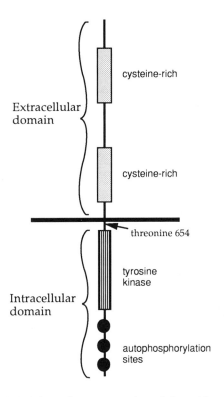

Fig. 5.13 Schematic representation of the epidermal growth factor receptor.

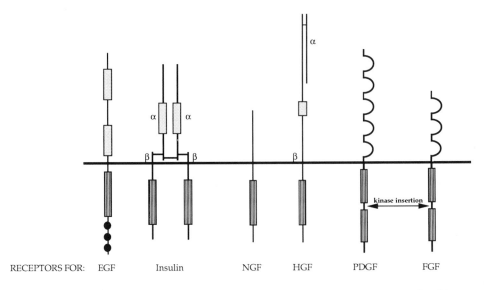

Fig. 5.14 Schematic representation of some of the transmembrane receptor tyrosine kinases. Each receptor family is designated by a prototype ligand. Stippled boxes indicate cysteine-rich domains, and striped boxes indicate tyrosine kinase domains. EGF, epidermal growth factor; NGF, nerve growth factor; HGF, hepatocyte growth factor; PDGF, platelet derived growth factor; FGF, fibroblast growth factor.

growth factor receptors (Fig. 5.13). EGFR is a 170 kDa glycoprotein which spans the plasma membrane once. The 621 amino acid extracellular domain is responsible for ligand (e.g. EGF or TGFα) recognition and binding, and contains two cysteine-rich regions. The hydrophobic transmembrane region is only about 23 amino acids long, and may do little more than anchor the receptor in the plane of the plasma membrane. Separating the transmembrane domain from the cytoplasmic catalytic domain is a juxtamembrane region probably involved in receptor transmodulation, whereby the receptor function is altered by the binding of different ligands to their distinct receptors. Thus, a growth factor such as bombesin, which stimulates the phosphatidyl inositol signalling pathway (see below), can activate protein kinase C (PKC), which in turn phosphorylates serine and threonine residues of the EGFR. Threonine 654 in the juxtamembrane region appears to be a particular target, and its phosphorylation can lead to the loss of the high affinity binding of EGF and/or an inhibition of the kinase activity – thus PKC can mediate a negative feedback control of receptor activity.

The tyrosine kinase domain is the most highly conserved portion of all PTKs, and contains both an ATP and a substrate binding site. The kinase domain of the FGF and PDGF receptors is divided into two halves by a kinase insertion (KI) sequence of up to 100 amino acids; in the case of the PDGF receptor the KI contains an autophosphorylation site at Tyr 751, which may be crucial to the interaction between the activated receptor and other cellular substrates. The carboxy-terminal tail sequences are quite divergent between the receptor tyrosine kinases, but in the case of EGFR contains at least three tyrosine autophosphorylation sites. Phosphorylation of these sites is necessary for the activated receptors to act as docking sites for tethering downstream signalling proteins at or near the plasma membrane. Following the interaction of ligand with receptor, down-regulation occurs through internalization *via* coated pits (see Fig. 5.10), resulting in either the proteolytic destruction of both, or in some cases the recycling of the receptor following dissociation of the ligand at acid pH within the internal vesicles. This process is probably vital for normal mitogen signalling.

Activated receptors trigger multiple signalling pathways

Growth factor binding triggers an array of cellular responses including stimulation of Na^+/H^+ exchange, Ca^{2+} influx, Ras activation, and the stimulation of phospholipase C-γ1 (PLC-γ1). PLC-γ1 catalyses phosphatidyl inositol 4,5-bisphosphate (PIP_2) hydrolysis, generating both water soluble inositol 1, 4, 5-triphosphate (IP_3) which causes the release of calcium from intracellular compartments, and diacylglycerol (DAG), which remains at the plasma membrane and activates PKC. It is assumed that numerous intracellular substrates are phosphorylated by PKC, while some others may require phosphorylation of tyrosine by the action of the receptor tyrosine kinases.

As a general rule, ligand binding to receptor PTKs results in *receptor dimerization* which increases the catalytic activity of the respective tyrosine kinases. It has been suggested that not only does this provide a mechanism for regulation of the tyrosine kinase activity, but that autophosphorylation really occurs by cross-phosphorylation of these homodimers, thus perhaps making the receptors themselves the most import-

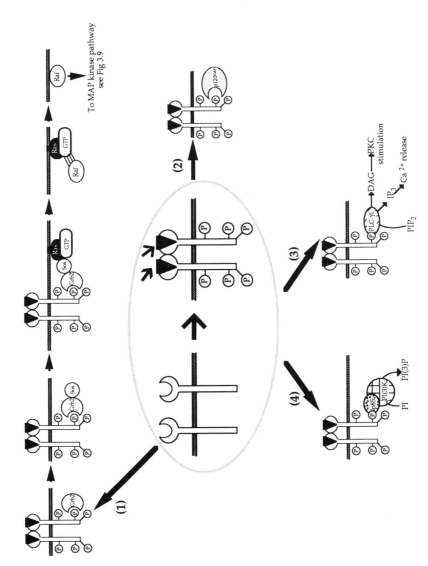

Fig. 5.15 A model of the recruitment of cytosolic enzymes with SH2 domains to ligand-activated receptor tyrosine kinases. Receptor occupancy triggers dimerization, cross-phosphorylation and recruitment of cytosolic enzymes with SH2 domains such as (1) Grb2 which leads to Ras and Raf activation, (2) p120^{GAP} which promotes Ras inactivation through GTP hydrolysis, (3) PLC-γ1 which catalyses PIP$_2$ hydrolysis, and (4) PI(3)K which phosphorylates phosphatidyl inositol. PLC-γ1 , phospholipase C-γ1; PIP$_2$, phosphatidyl inositol, 4,5-bisphosphate; PI(3)K, phosphatidyl inositol 3-kinase.

ant tyrosine kinase substrates (Fig. 5.15). Further transmission of the ligand-induced signal involves recognition of the phosphorylated tyrosines on the receptor kinase by various cytoplasmic enzymes such as PLC-γ1, GTPase-activating protein (GAP) and phosphatidyl inositol 3-kinase (PI(3)K). Thus, the tyrosine-phosphorylated receptors are acting as a 'magnet' for enzymes whose substrates are plasma membrane-associated, and the enzymes in turn are generating more 'downstream' signalling molecules. Each of these enzymatic proteins has in common a distinctive domain of approximately 100 amino acids known as a Src-homology-2 (SH2) region, and it is this region which localizes the protein to the tyrosine-phosphorylated receptors; the SH2 domain recognizes short peptide motifs bearing phosphotyrosine. The SH2 region is so-called, of course, because of its homology with a conserved domain (SH2) in the Src family of nonreceptor protein kinases. The prototype molecule for this family is pp60[c-src] a protein generally associated with the inner surface of the plasma membrane (see Fig. 3.10), while the gene responsible for the transforming activity of Rous sarcoma virus was, in fact, derived from the normal cellular gene, c-*src*.

The enzyme PI(3)K, which phosphorylates inositol lipids at the 3 position, also binds to other tyrosine-phosphorylated receptors such as the PDGF receptor. Here, the 85 kDa regulatory subunit has two SH2 domains, though only the C-terminal SH2 domain is considered crucial for binding to a phosphotyrosine in the kinase insert region. In contrast to SH2 domains, Src-homology-3 (SH3) domains bind to short stretches (~10) of amino acids which are rich in proline residues. Grb2 is composed almost entirely of SH2 and SH3 domains, and so is able to bind not only to phosphotyrosine, but also to the guanine nucleotide exchange factor Sos because this has proline-rich motifs within its C-terminal tail. Thus the receptor forms a heterotrimeric complex with Grb2 and Sos and this can lead to Ras activation (see Fig. 3.8).

Cytokines (CSFs, interleukins, EPO, interferons) interact with receptors of the cytokine receptor superfamily, however, these receptors *lack* kinase domains yet they can still trigger tyrosine phosphorylation. This is achieved by the receptors associating with cytoplasmic PTKs termed the *Janus kinases* (Jaks), and these are catalytically activated after ligand binding. The term 'Janus' refers to the ancient, two-faced, Roman god of gates and doorways, and the four family members (Jak1, Jak2, Jak3, Tyk2) all have two kinase domains. Receptor occupancy leads to receptor dimerization and Jaks are rapidly phosphorylated, possibly by each other, along with the receptors themselves (Fig. 5.16). This enables the receptors to bind SH2-containing proteins such as PLC-γ1 and PI(3)K and activate the Ras pathway, but the PTK substrates most directly involved in cytokine signalling are the transcription factors termed Stat proteins (signal transducers and activators of transcription). Much of our knowledge about Stats comes from the study of the chain of events following stimulation by interferon-α. Here we get activation of Jak1 and Tyk2, and tyrosine phosphorylation of Stat1α (p91), Stat1β (p84) and Stat2 (p113) – Stat2 forming heterodimers with either Stat1α or Stat1β through mutual interactions between phosphotyrosines and SH2 domains. In turn, these heterodimers complex with a DNA-binding protein known as the 48 kDa protein to form a factor called ISGF-3 (interferon-stimulated gene

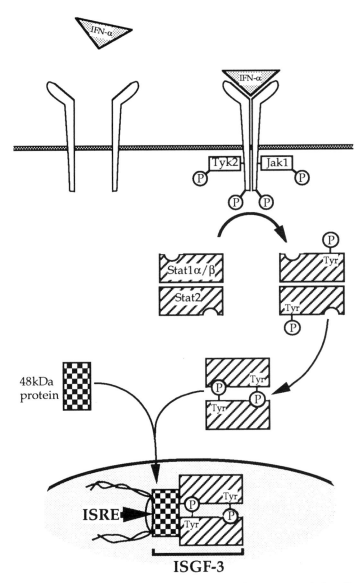

Fig. 5.16 A model for interferon (IFN)-α activation of gene transcription. Receptor occupancy leads to dimerization, the binding of Tyk2 and Jak1 and phosphorylation. The phosphorylated complex can phosphorylate Stats which form heterodimers through association of phosphotyrosines and SH2 domains. The heterodimers bind to a 48 kDa protein which allows binding to DNA and hence altered gene expression. ISRE, interferon-stimulated response element; ISGF-3, interferon-stimulated gene factor-3; Stat, signal transducers and activators of transcription.

factor-3); an association necessary to allow the binding protein to enter the nucleus and bind to DNA at the interferon-stimulated response element (ISRE). Some cytokines phosphorylate Stat proteins which form homo- or heterodimers which can bind to DNA regulatory elements without forming associations with other proteins.

The connection to cancer

We have already discussed how cells can modify their response to growth factors (Fig. 5.9), and there is good evidence that many malignant cells not only produce higher than normal levels of growth factors, but they also upregulate (over-express) the appropriate cell surface receptors. High levels of receptor expression could bestow a growth advantage upon malignant cells (Fig. 5.17), and may be achieved through gene amplification or more often, increased transcriptional activity. Over-expression of EGFR occurs commonly in squamous carcinomas; and in breast, lung and bladder tumours over-expression of EGFR may be an indicator of poor prognosis. C-erbB-2 over-expression is a prominent finding in many breast carcinomas, and this can be readily demonstrated by immunocytochemistry (Fig. 5.18), and quantitative measurements can be made by techniques such as Western blotting and radioligand binding assays. In the rat, the c-*erbB-2* gene is called *neu* because it was found that when pregnant rats were treated with ethylnitrosourea, then the offspring rapidly developed neuroblastomas. This was due to a point mutation in the c-*erbB-2* gene, resulting in the substitution of a glutamic acid residue for a valine in the transmembrane region; the mutation stabilizes the receptors in a dimeric form in which they are catalytically active. In humans, activating point mutations of c-*erbB-2* seem quite rare, and the chief mechanism for elevated protein expression appears to be through gene amplification. We have already discussed the phenomenon of autocrine stimulatory loops in cancer, and sections 3.2 and 3.3 (Chapter 3) have indicated the role of the protein

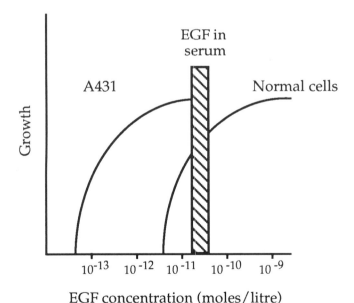

Fig. 5.17 How cancer cells (in this case A431 vulval cancer cells over-expressing epidermal growth factor receptor-EGFR) could gain a proliferative advantage over their normal counterparts in a situation where the availability of binding ligand was limited. (Based on a idea by Professor Bill Gullick.)

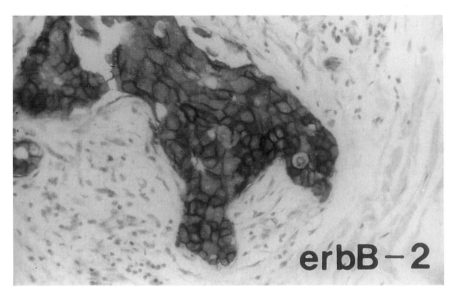

Fig. 5.18 Photomicrograph illustrating very prominent membranous expression of the c-erbB-2 protein on breast cancer cells. (Kindly supplied by Nick Lemoine, ICRF.)

products of v-*oncs* and c-*oncs* in either mimicking, perpetuating or otherwise sub-verting normal cellular processes initiated by growth factor receptor occupancy. These would include v-*erbB* production of a shortened oncogenic version of EGFR, and the oncogenic activation of *int-2* (encoding FGF-3) through insertional mutagenesis by mouse mammary tumour virus in mice.

Through recombinant DNA technology the synthesis of various growth factors in sufficient quantities to allow their introduction into clinical practice has been achieved. In particular, haematopoeitic growth factors have been used in the management of patients with myeloid and other malignancies, where many deaths have been due to infections caused by chemotherapy-induced neutropenia. Recombinant SCF, GM-CSF, G-CSF and EPO are all now used to promote the growth of myeloid and eryth-roid precursor cells.

Tumour cell receptors for growth factors and hormones act as growth regulators, thus, they are ideal targets for new forms of cancer therapy. Approaches have included using neutralizing antibodies against growth factors and antibodies against the extra-cellular domains of growth factor receptors. Such antibodies could potentially be useful *per se* to down-regulate surface receptors, to inhibit ligand binding or to act as vehicles for localizing toxic molecules to the sites of tumours. Other experimental approaches have targeted the receptor signalling pathways, including the design of inhibitors of receptor dimerization and inhibitors of tyrosine kinases. The treatment of hormone-dependent tumours (e.g. breast and prostate) often targets the cytosolic receptor-hormone interaction. Much of this treatment is palliative, simply blocking the binding of the naturally occurring active steroid using a synthetic analogue. The best known example of this is the treatment of oestrogen-dependent breast cancer by tamoxifen since the tamoxifen-oestrogen receptor complex fails to act as a transcription factor for oestrogen-dependent gene expression, and currently tamoxifen is being used prophylactically in a large clinical trial in the hope of reducing the incidence of breast cancer.

5.3 Cell death (necrosis and apoptosis)

Introduction

Cell death is a common enough occurrence in both healthy and diseased tissues. In the embryo, genetically controlled cell death occurs at precise developmental stages in the process of organogenesis, while in the adult, cell death (or loss) must keep pace with cell production in the cell renewal systems (bone marrow, gastrointestinal tract, skin) if the tissues are not to expand. It is also a prominent feature of lymph node germinal centres, and is responsible for the collapse of the endometrium at the end of the menstrual cycle. In tumours, cell death and cell loss are major determinants of the rate at which tumours grow (see Chapter 5, section 5.4). Cell death is the end-result of the unwanted toxicity of many compounds such as paracetamol in the liver and of many anti-cancer cytotoxic drugs which target proliferating cells, not only in tumours, but also in the continually renewing cell populations. If the mechanism of cell death was the same in all these cases and all dead cells underwent the process of *necrosis*, an essentially passive phenomenon, then a less than enthusiastic approach to the topic would be readily understandable. However, following the pioneering work of Andrew Wyllie and his colleagues in Edinburgh, we now recognize at least two types of cell death separable by both morphological and mechanistic criteria. This new classification of cell death separates the degenerative phenomena known as necrosis, characterized by cell and organelle oedema, from a second pattern in which the dying cell undergoes a progressive contraction of cellular volume, widespread chromatin condensation, but preservation of cytoplasmic organelles. The affected cells then fragment into a number of membrane-bound bodies which are rapidly phagocytosed by neighbouring cells. This latter type of cell death was termed *apoptosis*, since it was initially observed in a variety of normal physiological states where it appeared to complement mitosis in maintaining tissue size.

Necrosis

Necrosis is not cell death, but may be defined as the morphological changes that *follow* cell death. Inciting agents either directly damage the plasma membrane (e.g. by complement, heat, physical trauma) or interfere with mitochondrial oxidative phosphorylation (e.g. by poisons, ischaemia) causing a failure of the plasma membrane ATP-dependent ion pumps. The net result is the same – a loss of plasma membrane volume control. The earliest changes are reversible and can be summarized as mild cell and organelle oedema with dilation of the rough endoplasmic reticulum (RER), collapse of the Golgi apparatus, slight mitochondrial swelling, and the margination of

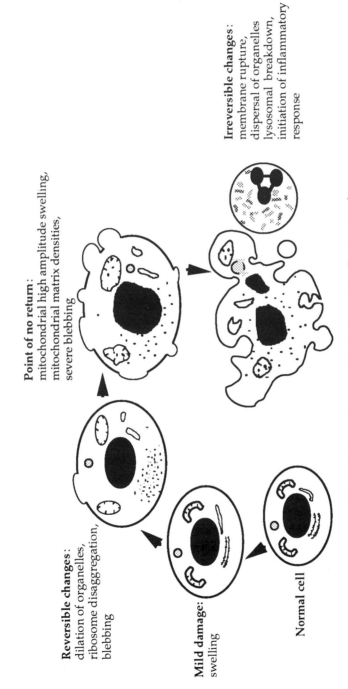

Reversible changes:
dilation of organelles,
ribosome disaggregation,
blebbing

Point of no return:
mitochondrial high amplitude swelling,
mitochondrial matrix densities,
severe blebbing

Irreversible changes:
membrane rupture,
dispersal of organelles
lysosomal breakdown,
initiation of inflammatory
response

Mild damage:
swelling

Normal cell

Fig. 5.19 The major morphological events leading to necrosis.

heterochromatin around the nuclear membrane. 'Blebs' also start to appear in the plasma membrane, probably because of excess cytosolic calcium interfering with the integrity of microtubules and microfilaments which maintain cell shape; in particular increased calcium causes a dissociation of actin microfilaments from α-actinin which serves as an intermediate in the association of microfilaments with actin-binding proteins in the plasma membrane. The cisternae of the RER become readily dilated through the action of abnormal osmotic forces, and protein synthesis suffers as ribosomes become detached and polyribosomes disaggregate into monoribosomes. Many toxic compounds (e.g. cancer chemotherapeutic agents) interfere with protein synthesis and the processing of secretions, leading to the collapse of the Golgi cisternae. Mitochondria are very sensitive indicators of sub-lethal cell damage since many injurious agents (e.g. hypoxia, chemicals, bacterial toxins) inhibit mitochondrial energy generation, leading to progressive swelling and disruption of the internal structure of cristae. The influx of sodium and water leads to swelling which gives the cell an irregular contour, and further localized blebbing occurs through cytoskeletal disruption. Surface specializations such as microvilli and cilia also become deranged or even lost; these events are summarized in Fig. 5.19.

Cell and organelle oedema have in the past been variously called 'cloudy swelling', 'vacuolar degeneration' and 'hydropic degeneration', names now obsolete, though the term 'balloon cells' used by histopathologists to describe such affected cells as viewed by light microscopy seems wholly appropriate. Initially such changes are reversible, but the cell then reaches the 'point of no return' at which there is an irreversible commitment to necrosis. Prevailing adverse conditions send the cell on a downward spiral particularly with sustained increased levels of cytosolic calcium causing disruption of the cytoskeleton and activating membrane-located degradative phospholipases and proteases. Violent dilation of mitochondria called 'high amplitude' swelling is a significant event with rupture of their internal cristae and the resultant formation of flocculent densities of denatured matrix protein. Together with a switch to anaerobic glycolysis, a decrease in intracellular pH, and a reduction of macromolecular synthesis, the affected cell dies with the accompanying rupture of organelles and the plasma membrane (Fig. 5.20A), manifest at light microscopy as coagulative necrosis (Fig. 5.20B, C, see also Fig. 4.16B). As we shall see, apoptosis in contradistinction is an energy dependent process, usually requiring macromolecular synthesis which results initially in cell shrinkage rather than cell swelling.

The major biochemical pathways (Fig. 5.21) involved in precipitating cell death are:

- Interference with endogenous substrate metabolism.
- Production of reactive intermediates.
- Protein-thiol (-SH group) modification.
- Production of reactive oxygen intermediates.

(A)

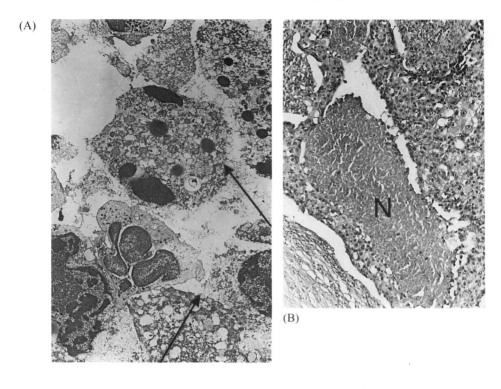

(B)

(C)

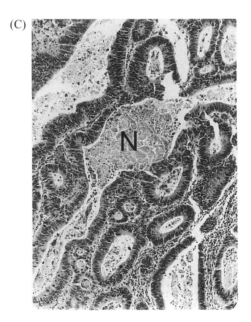

Fig. 5.20 (A) Electron micrograph of necrotic tumour cells, note the disruption of organelle membranes (arrows). Areas of coagulative necrosis (N) in a breast carcinoma (B) and (C) a colonic adenocarcinoma, note the homogeneous appearance of the necrotic tissue.

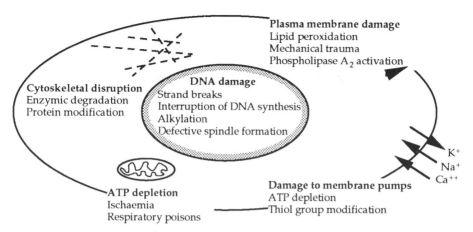

Fig. 5.21 Sites of cell injury which might cause cell death. Some cells with special attributes are prone to certain types of injury, e.g. proliferating cells are selectively killed by DNA-damaging agents.

- Lipid peroxidation.
- Protease and phospholipase activation.
- DNA damage.

Many compounds block substrate metabolism, particularly the antimetabolites (5-fluorouracil, cytosine arabinoside, methotrexate) used in cytotoxic chemotherapy (see Chapter 7, section 7.2). Methotrexate binds to the enzyme dihydrofolate reductase blocking the generation of tetrahydrofolate which is required for purine and pyrimidine biosynthesis. Many toxic compounds or their metabolites are chemically reactive, interacting with proteins and other macromolecules and binding covalently to them. A classic example is paracetamol, a widely used analgesic which is hepatotoxic at high dose. Protein-thiol modification is also important in producing cell injury; free SH-groups are critical determinants of the activity of many enzymes, and these can be readily modified. Electrophilic free radicals are produced not only from the metabolism of some compounds, but also from the radiolysis of water by ionizing radiation and by the reaction of generated free radicals with molecular oxygen. In living cells all systems concerned with oxygen transport and exchange can be sources of reactive oxygen intermediates, and include haemoglobin, cytochrome P-450 and the mitochondrial electron transport chain. However, the damage these would cause is limited by the protective mechanisms afforded by glutathione, vitamin E and enzyme systems like glutathione synthetase, glutathione peroxidase, superoxide dismutase (SOD) and catalase. Many compounds which cause cell injury are first metabolized to electrophilic free radicals which react with molecular oxygen to produce reactive oxygen intermediates, initially superoxide anion ($O_2^-\cdot$). Chemicals that can generate $O_2^-\cdot$ include alloxan, adriamycin, paraquat and quinones such as menadione. The superoxide can readily undergo dismutation to H_2O_2 by SOD, which can be further metabolized to water by glutathione peroxidase or catalase. This is normally a detoxification reaction, but at high rates of production, $O_2^-\cdot$ and H_2O_2 in the presence of transition metal ions generate hydroxyl radicals (OH·) which can cause lipid peroxidation and cell injury. Polyunsaturated fatty acids are especially susceptible to free radical attack, so possibly compromising the integrity of the plasma membrane and the membranes of organelles like lysosomes, mitochondria and endoplasmic reticulum.

Interference with calcium homeostasis can occur in a variety of ways. The functional impairment of the plasma membrane calcium transporting ATPase can occur through ATP depletion or modification of the thiol status, and will result in a rise in cytosolic calcium. Direct damage to the plasma membrane and the failure of the endoplasmic reticulum to sequester calcium (also controlled by a thiol-containing ATP-dependent enzyme) will have the same effect. The increase in cytosolic calcium has a number of consequences:

- Cytoskeletal disruption.
- Activation of proteases.
- Phospholipase activation.
- Endonuclease activation.

Disruption of the cytoskeleton readily leads to cell blebbing, and may be due to a dissociation of the actin microfilaments from α-actinin, the intermediate protein between the microfilaments and the actin-binding proteins in the plasma membrane. Alternatively, toxic reactive metabolites may cause oxidation or arylation of cytoskeletal proteins and thereby alter their integrity. Calcium activated proteases (calpains) are associated with membranes, and increased levels of calcium activate these enzymes which degrade both cytoskeletal elements and integral membrane proteins, again leading to cell blebbing. Phospholipase A_2 is also activated by elevated calcium, and its ability to degrade the plasma membrane directly by hydrolysis of membrane phospholipids suggests the enzyme has a role in cell injury. The enzyme may also be important in the detoxification of phospholipid hydroperoxides, releasing fatty acids from peroxidised membranes. A non-lysosomal endonuclease which cleaves double-stranded DNA into oligonucleosome-length fragments is also activated by increased calcium, but this seems to be a feature of some, though not all cells undergoing apoptotic cell death.

Ionizing radiation and many of the chemotherapeutic drugs used in the treatment of neoplastic disease specifically kill proliferating cells. Radiation can cause lethal double-strand breaks in DNA (see Chapter 7, section 7.3), and affected cells die at mitosis. Antimetabolites are analogues of substrates for DNA synthesis, and they rapidly cause the death of DNA-synthesizing cells. Alkylating agents such as melphalan and nitrogen mustard also target proliferating cells, causing inter- and intrastrand DNA cross-links and cross-links between DNA and other molecules. Antitumour antibiotics (e.g. actinomycin-D, adriamycin, bleomycin) kill proliferating cells by causing local DNA-unwinding and/or generating free radicals. Mitotic spindle poisons such as colchicine and vincristine cause the degeneration of cells at mitosis; these agents inhibit the polymerization of tubulin into microtubules and thereby prevent chromosome segregation after metaphase. Many of these perturbative stimuli result in necrosis of the affected cells, though equally well the affected cells can undergo apoptosis: it is often said that while mild injury provokes apoptosis, more severe injury (e.g. a higher concentration of a cytotoxic drug) results in necrosis. The evidence supporting this notion is, to say the least, flimsy, and while ischaemia seems to be a major cause of tumour cell necrosis, most anticancer drugs cause only apoptosis, irrespective of the drug dose level.

Apoptosis

Introduction

The power of cells to multiply and propel life into the world is universally appreciated, yet for over 100 years embryologists have recognized that in developmental growth cell death plays a part, for example in the sculpting of the fingers in the embryonic hand. However, until relatively recently few considered that cell death was significant later in life, regarding it more as an enemy of life and equating it with the running down of a clockwork mechanism. We know that cells can be murdered by a variety of noxious agents and undergo the series of degradative reactions known as necrosis. This accidental form of cell death supposedly results from violent injury, but many forms of injury caused by extrinsic agents may trigger a 'suicide programme' in the cells of multicellular organisms. Such cell death may be desirable for the organism as a whole since it provides a mechanism for the disposal of cells damaged by mutagenic chemicals or irradiation, and this type of cell death is called apoptosis. Thus from the outset we can be certain that apoptosis is a prominent player in the field of neoplasia. It is now clear that the seeming stability of life is only possible by grace of a fine balance between new life through cell division and cell death through apoptosis.

In contrast to necrosis, apoptosis is not a passive phenomenon but is gene-directed, usually requiring on-going protein synthesis. The dying cell is characterized by having a raised level of cytosolic Ca^{2+} and a breakdown in the organization of DNA folding which commonly, though not invariably, leads to the activation of a non-lysosomal Ca^{2+}- and Mg^{2+}-dependent endonuclease which digests the chromatin into oligonucleosome length fragments. If the DNA from these apoptotic cells is size fractionated by electrophoresis, then the so-called 'DNA laddering' pattern is seen. The dying cell may or may not fragment into a number of apoptotic bodies, but in all cases the intracellular contents are wrapped in protective protein shells preventing the leakage of potentially harmful material such as mutated DNA and pro-inflammatory molecules. Apoptotic cells are eliminated through heterophagocytosis by neighbouring cells and macrophages, and cell surface changes on apoptotic cells aid their recognition and engulfment by the phagocytosing cells. Recent work has begun to unravel the molecular mechanisms of apoptosis, and studies of the nematode *Caenorhabditis elegans* have shown that at least two cell death controlling pathways (*bcl-2/ced-9* and interleukin-1β-converting enzyme ICE/*ced-3*) are conserved through much of evolution. Members of the Bcl-2 family of proteins (Bcl-2, Bax, Bcl-x, Bak, Ced-9) interact with each other in many cell systems to control cell sensitivity to apoptotic stimuli, and the expression of a wide variety of other genes including c-*myc*, *p53*, *ced-3*, *ced-4* and *ICE*, may drive cells down the apoptotic pathway under certain circumstances. Apoptosis is widely involved in organogenesis in the embryo, and its occurrence in response to noxious stimuli such as cytotoxic drugs, irradiation and hyperthermia may be viewed as an altruistic suicide process. Apoptosis provides a safe disposal mechanism for neutrophils at inflamed sites, and within the immune system it is considered responsible for the elimination of self-reactive T-cell clones and is instrumental in the process of affinity maturation of antibody producing cells. Many normal and malignant cells will undergo apoptosis following exposure to or withdrawal of a hormone or growth factor, and a failure to undergo apoptosis through over-expression of cell survival genes may be a significant event in the development of many tumours. Apoptosis has now grabbed the scientific community by the throat, not least because it features strongly in many diseases of modern humans – i.e. in cancer where it does not occur enough and in neurodegenerative disease and AIDS where it occurs too much. Promoting apoptosis as a therapeutic strategy for cancer will be a major goal over the next few years.

Apoptosis comes of age

In 1972, John Kerr and colleagues published a paper (Kerr J.F.R, Wyllie A.H & Currie A.R., Apoptosis: a basic biological phenomenon with wide-ranging implications in tissue kinetics. *British Journal of Cancer* 1972; 68:239–57), which formally defined this mode of cell death in morphological terms. However, few scientists took an interest in the subject in the decade after its original description, but then in 1986 the laboratory of Robert Horvitz described the discovery of genes in *C. elegans* whose expression promoted cell death. This discovery of *death genes* represented a field change in apoptosis research, and now research into apoptosis is intense, even fashionable.

Morphology of apoptosis

The outstanding feature of apoptosis is its remarkably stereotyped morphology across a wide variety of tissues: an apoptotic body from the liver can be indistinguishable from an apoptotic body from a breast carcinoma. The major morphological stages of apoptosis are illustrated in Fig. 5.22

At light microscope level, where a comparatively wide field of view is available, it is easily appreciated that apoptosis is a mode of cell death in which cells may be deleted but the broad architecture of the tissue can remain undisturbed. Apoptotic cells are easily recognizable, whether in normal adult tissues, where they occur with low frequency, or normal developing tissues where their levels might be higher or in abnormal tissues such as tumours. Large apoptotic cells break up and resultant fragments, apoptotic bodies, may or may not have nuclear components; smaller cells, such as apoptotic thymocytes, do not usually fragment. With haematoxylin and eosin staining, their cytoplasm is highly eosinophilic and they have condensed (pyknotic) nuclear chromatin. Apoptotic bodies are readily identifiable with low power observation because each is situated within an unstained 'halo' of tissue (Fig. 5.23). Apoptotic

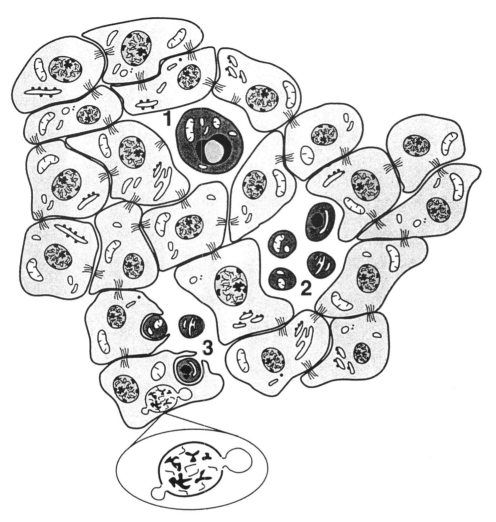

Fig. 5.22 Schematic diagram of the major stages in the apoptotic process beginning with cyto-plasmic condensation, chromatin margination under the nuclear membrane, and loss of contact from surrounding viable cells (1); fragmentation into a number of apoptotic bodies (2) and finally phagocytosis by neighbouring cells and dissolution within heterophagosomes after fusion with lysosomes (3).

bodies are rapidly phagocytosed by macrophages or neighbouring cells (neutrophils play no part in the scavenging of apoptotic debris) and it seems that the vast majority of apoptoses seen in tissue sections are already within heterophagic vacuoles.

At electron microscope level the morphological characteristics of apoptosis are clear, beginning with condensation of chromatin into typical dense crescents at the periphery of the nucleus adjacent to the nuclear membrane (Fig. 5.24). Loss of cell surface features such as cell–cell junctions, microvilli and other surface specializations are early events, and the cell progressively presents a smoother outline with the plasma membrane intact. It begins to shrink, condensation of the cytoplasm being the result

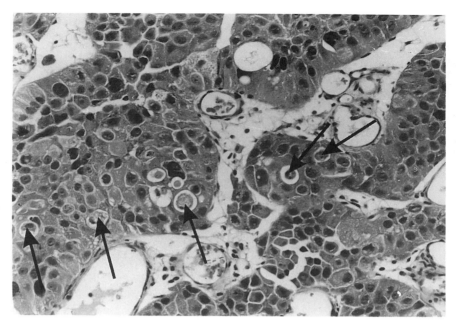

Fig. 5.23 Light micrograph of apoptotic cells in a tumour. Notice the contiguity of viable tumour cells, while the apoptotic cells (arrows) are shrunken and out of contact with their neighbours.

of reduction in the water content of the apoptotic cell. Cytoplasmic organelles are, thus, crammed closer and closer together (Fig. 5.25), although initially they remain functional and morphologically intact. In transmission electron micrographs of apoptotic cells from this stage on, the cytosol becomes progressively more electron dense as ribosomes and cytoplasmic filaments fill a higher proportion of the available volume. Mitochondria show none of the distension that is characteristic of necrotic cells, and thus remain functional late into the apoptotic process. Much of the water loss is initially into the endoplasmic reticulum (ER) of the apoptotic cell, so although overall the cell is shrinking, the cisternae of the endoplasmic reticulum dilate. The ER develops many outlets to the surface of the plasma membrane, serving to channel water away, and giving the cell a typical vacuolated, pitted surface (Fig. 5.26). Apoptotic fragments are readily engulfed by macrophages and/or neighbouring cells, and fragments are degraded enzymatically within the engulfing cells' heterophagic vacuoles. Final intracytoplasmic stages of disintegration (secondary necrosis) are similar to degradation of any cellular material within secondary lysosomes; the only unequivocal way that apoptotic debris can be identified from structures autophagocytosed in organelle turnover is by the presence of chromatin-bearing fragments. In normal organelle turnover no nuclear components appear in autophagic vacuoles.

Biochemistry and genetics of apoptosis

Irrespective of how apoptosis is caused, the DNA is always degraded to a greater or lesser extent which appears responsible for the characteristic nuclear morphological

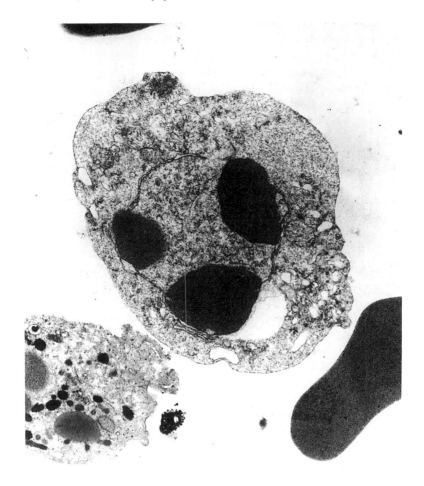

Fig. 5.24 Electron micrograph of an apoptotic lymphocyte from the peripheral blood of an AIDS patient. Prominent caps of chromatin can be seen immediately beneath the nuclear membrane, presumably due to the action of 'domain' nucleases (see Fig. 5.29).

changes. Using thymocytes or cell lines it has become very clear that one of the commonest events in apoptotic cells is the cleavage of double-stranded DNA, so resulting in the production of oligonucleosome-length fragments of DNA.

In eukaryotic cells the DNA double helix in each chromosome is folded in a highly ordered fashion; the fundamental packing unit being the nucleosome, a histone octamer consisting of two copies of each of four histones – small proteins with a high proportion of positively charged amino acids. The nucleosome forms a protein core around which the double stranded DNA helix is wrapped twice, and in apoptotic cells, a non-lysosomal endonuclease (DNase I) and possibly a lysosomal endonuclease (DNase II) become activated which digest the DNA (linker DNA) between the nucleosome beads; the rest of the DNA being protected from digestion and remaining as double stranded DNA fragments associated with one or more nucleosomes. This quite

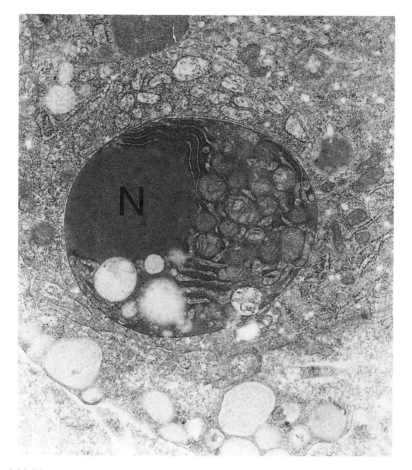

Fig. 5.25 Electron micrograph of a shrunken phagocytosed early apoptotic body. N is chromatin, flanked by rough endoplasmic reticulum, mitochondria crammed together, and smooth endoplasmic reticulum.

common pattern of DNA cleavage in apoptotic cells has been elucidated by chromatography of the partially degraded chromatin. Chromatin from apoptotic cells can be deproteinized and subjected to agarose gel electrophoresis which separates double stranded DNA molecules of different sizes. The negatively charged molecules migrate towards the positive electrode with the smallest molecules migrating furthest; DNA from apoptotic cells often separates with stepwise increments in DNA conforming to integer multiples of a subunit which corresponds to the number of base pairs associated with each nucleosome – hence the so-called *ladder-pattern* of DNA cleavage products (Fig. 5.27). DNA 'laddering', reflecting oligonucleosomal fragmentation is not a cardinal feature of apoptosis, and other studies have found that relatively large DNA fragments are transiently present in apoptotic cells *before* DNA is fragmented to 180–200 bp integers, and in some cases no internucleosomal cleavage is seen. These large fragments can be resolved by field inversion gel electrophoresis (FIGE),

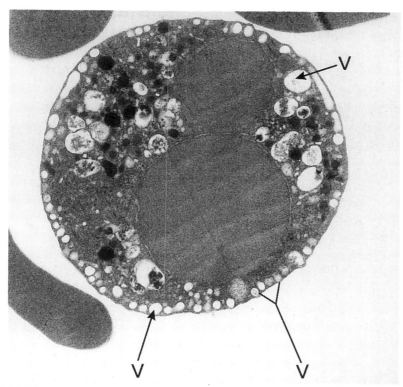

Fig. 5.26 Electron micrograph of an apoptotic lymphocyte from the peripheral blood of an AIDS patient. Two portions of dense chromatin cap are visible, the endoplasmic reticulum is dilated and the cell surface appears to be vacuolated (V). Viewed three dimensionally, in all probability these features are fully linked channels of endoplasmic reticulum, opening on to the surface of the cell.

whereas conventional gel electrophoresis used to establish DNA laddering, can only separate DNA fragments of ~20 kbp and below. These large DNA fragments correspond to ~300 and/or ~50 kbp, and it seems likely that they arise from the release of loops (50 kbp) or rosettes (300 kbp) of chromatin detached from the nuclear scaffold. The proteinases which carry out this function are referred to as the 'domain nucleases' and their activation correlates with the collapse of the chromatin outwards against the nuclear membrane ('capping' see Fig. 5.24). Therefore the release of chromatin loop domains may be a more crucial event in apoptosis, and internucleosomal DNA cleavage is a late event, commonly seen, but not essential for apoptosis.

Other common features of the apoptotic process are that *de novo* protein synthesis is usually required along with a sustained increase in cytosolic Ca^{2+} concentration. Certainly Ca^{2+} and Mg^{2+} are involved in activation of one of the endonucleases, and also calpains which degrade both cytoskeletal elements and integral membrane proteins. Calpains are expressed very early in apoptotic cells, before morphological changes are seen, and since calpains are Ca^{2+}-binding, thiol (-SH) containing proteins,

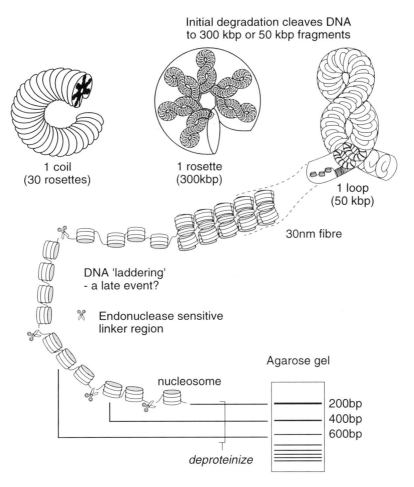

Fig. 5.27 DNA has many orders of packing, and in some apoptotic cells chromatin degradation only appears to proceed as far as the release of rosettes (~300 kbp) and loops (~50 kbp) from the nuclear protein matrix. The loop is made up of a coiled 30 nm fibre which is itself a contracted solenoid comprising six nucleosomes per turn. Further degradation involves cleavage at linker regions between nucleosomes, yielding fragments of integer multiples of the number of base pairs associated with one nucleosome, hence the 'ladder' pattern of DNA degradation products after agarose gel electrophoresis.

they may represent a step in evolution since in *C. elegans* the products of the cell death genes *ced-3* and *ced-4* are a sulphydryl-containing protease and a Ca^{2+}-binding protein respectively. Transglutaminases are another group of Ca^{2+}-dependent enzymes which appear to be activated during cell death, and it is likely that the enzyme functions to provide a highly cross-linked protein shell in apoptotic cells and bodies, so rendering the apoptotic process 'silent' in that there is no leakage of intracellular components which might provoke an inflammatory response.

bcl-2 is the acronym for the B-cell lymphoma/leukaemia-2 gene, and it is the prototype of a family of genes that regulate apoptosis. As implied by its name, this gene was first discovered because of its involvement in B-cell neoplasms, where the t(14;18) translocation activates the gene in the majority of follicular non-Hodgkin's B-cell lymphomas. In such cases, the *bcl-2* gene is translocated from its normal position on the long arm of chromosome 18 to a region adjacent to powerful enhancer elements in the immunoglobulin heavy-chain (IgH) locus on the long arm of chromosome 14. This results in deregulated *bcl-2* expression and over-production of the encoded proteins. The Bcl-2 protein is a true 'survival factor' since it rescues lymphoid and myeloid cells from an inevitable death caused by the withdrawal of the growth factor IL-3, but does so without causing them to proliferate. Expression of *bcl-2* is a key component of the affinity maturation process in lymphoid germinal centres, specifying the survival of a small minority destined to become memory cells following antigen challenge. As expected, gene transfer mediated elevations in Bcl-2 protein levels in a variety of normal and malignant cells are correlated with increased resistance to apoptotic stimuli, e.g. growth factor withdrawal or cytotoxic anti-cancer drugs. Since the Bcl-2 protein can rescue cells normally destined to die by widely dissimilar stimuli, it must mean that it acts close to the final irreversible step where the various afferent pathways converge and at which the effector processes are activated.

The Bcl-2 protein is a 25–26 kDa molecule associated with a variety of membranes, notably the nuclear membrane, parts of the endoplasmic reticulum and the mitochondrial membranes. These are intracellular sites of oxygen free radical generation, and reactive oxygen species are clearly implicated in many examples of apoptotic death, where they are involved in lipid peroxidation, oxidative damage to DNA and thiol modification of proteins. The Bcl-2 protein is probably part of an antioxidant pathway, acting as a free radical scavenger, and Bcl-2-deficient mice suffer from a range of tissue pathologies consistent with this notion. Another member of the Bcl-2 family, Bax, is a 21 kDa protein with considerable amino acid homology to Bcl-2. Bax forms homodimers, but it also forms heterodimers with Bcl-2, and when Bax predominates it accelerates apoptosis in the familiar model of apoptosis in IL-3-dependent B-cells induced by cytokine deprivation. Thus the ratio of Bax to Bcl-2 determines survival or death following an apoptotic stimulus; when Bax is over-expressed, the death repressor activity of Bcl-2 is countered and the cell is driven towards apoptosis.

The Bcl-2 family of proteins is expanding rapidly; *bcl-x* is a *bcl-2*-related gene from which two distinct *bcl-x* mRNAs result from alternative splicing. The larger mRNA, *bcl-x$_L$*, when stably transfected into an IL-3-dependent cell line, is as effective as Bcl-2 at preventing apoptosis upon growth factor withdrawal; *bcl-x$_L$* mRNA is expressed at high levels in long-lived postmitotic cells such as adult neural tissue. Bcl-x$_L$ is perfectly able to prevent apoptosis on its own, though some of its death repressor activity may be due to its heterodimerization with Bax or Bak. However, the smaller mRNA species, *bcl-x$_S$*, encodes a protein which inhibits the ability of Bcl-2 to enhance the survival of IL-3-deprived cells. Presumably these proteins dimerize with each other or another partner since they share highly conserved dimerization motifs with Bcl-2. The family members of Bcl-2 proteins share two highly conserved regions, referred to as the Bcl-2 homology 1 and 2 (BHI and BH2) domains; site-directed mutagenesis in either domain of Bcl-2 prevents the heterodimerization of Bcl-2 with Bax and abolishes its death-repressor activity in IL-3-dependent cells after IL-3 deprivation. This indicates that Bcl-2 function critically depends upon hetero-dimerization with Bax, perhaps because Bcl-2 protects cells from apoptosis by mop-ping up Bax. Bak (Bcl-2 homologous antagonist/killer) is a recently described protein which promotes cell death, perhaps also by direct interaction with survival proteins such as Bcl-2 and Bcl-x_L; Fig. 5.28 summarizes these interactions.

More evidence that specific gene expression is required for apoptosis comes from studying *C. elegans*. This microscopic worm has only 1090 cells, and 131 of the embryonic cells die at specific stages of development. By painstakingly searching for mutations in which this precisely programmed pattern of cell death was perturbed, either too few or too many deaths, it has been possible to identify the genes respon-sible. These are known as the *ced* (cell death abnormal) genes, and mutations in one of them, *ced-9*, can cause embryonic lethality, indicating that Ced-9 function is essen-

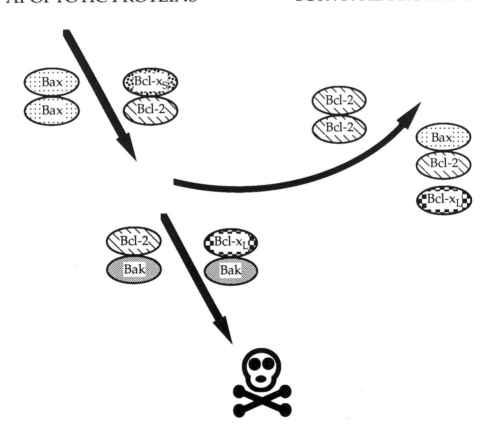

Fig. 5.28 Interactions of members of the Bcl-2 family of proteins which help determine either survival or apoptosis.

tial for development, i.e. it is a gene for life. The *ced-9* gene belongs to the *bcl-2* gene family, and shares with *bcl-2* the highly conserved BH1 and BH2 domains which are so crucial for function. A mutation (glycine-to-glutamate) at amino acid position 169 in the BH1 domain of the *ced-9* gene is a gain-of-function mutation, which causes the survival of cells which normally die during *C. elegans* development.

Studies of *C. elegans* have also found mutations in two genes called *ced-3* and *ced-4*. These two genes are essential for cell death during the development of *C. elegans*, and mutations that inactivate either *ced-3* or *ced-4* result in the survival of almost all cells that normally die during development. By the study of double mutants it appears that *ced-3* and *ced-4* act downstream of *ced-9*, since mutations in *ced-3* and *ced-4* block the lethality of recessive loss-of-function mutations in *ced-9*, which normally acts as a cell death repressor gene. It is most likely that *ced-3* encodes a cysteine protease, and this is related to mammalian interleukin-1β-converting enzyme (ICE), the first member of a new family of cysteine proteases (the Ced-3/ICE/Nedd2 family). ICE is a cysteine protease, a protein-splitting enzyme, whose known function is to cleave the 33 kDa pro-IL-1β into the 17.5 kDa biologically active IL-1β. The function of the Ced-3/ICE family of proteases is becoming clearer and one of their targets is the nuclear DNA repair enzyme poly (ADP-ribose) polymerase (PARP). PARP is massively up-regulated by chromatin fragmentation and binds to DNA breaks; cleavage by the proteinases separates the DNA binding domain (contains two zinc-finger DNA-binding motifs) of PARP from its catalytic domain, so rendering the latter insensitive to DNA damage and unable to carry out its functions of genome maintenance. The 32 kDa cysteine protease known as CPP-32, originally called prICE (protein resembling ICE), has closer homology to Ced-3 than ICE, and this is a proenzyme which requires proteolytic activation, presumably by an aspartate-specific protease, to form subunits of 17 and 12 kDa. This enzyme, named apopain, is responsible for the cleavage of PARP and probably other proteins. Cytotoxic T lymphocyte (CTL)-mediated cell killing also involves activation of CPP-32; during killing, granules containing serine proteases (the granzymes) are exocytosed, and granzyme B cleaves and activates CPP-32 in the target cell. Of course ICE itself is implicated in many instances of apoptosis, it may even activate CPP-32, and ICE-induced cell death can be blocked by Bcl-2 and by CrmA, the protein product of the cowpox virus cytokine response modifier gene. CrmA is able to prevent neuronal cell death in culture which normally occurs upon nerve growth factor withdrawal, and this is due to the ability of the *crmA* gene product to inhibit ICE's protease activity. The virus presumably uses this protein for the twin purposes of inhibiting host cell apoptosis and suppressing inflammation. Other targets for the ICE family of cysteine proteases include proteins associated with the actin cytoskeleton. Proteolytic cleavage of Gas2 (a member of the growth arrest-specific gene family) in its C-terminal region is associated with the typical cell shape changes observed in apoptotic cells. Likewise, α-fodrin, a membrane-associated cytoskeletal protein is cleaved in apoptotic cells, an event which can be blocked by Bcl-2 or an ICE inhibitor. *Nedd2* (NPC [neuronal precursor cells] – expressed, developmentally down-regulated genes) is a member of the *ICE/ced-3* gene family which appears to be involved in the high rates of apoptosis found in the developing CNS.

Another protease activated in apoptotic cells is a lamin protease (LamP) responsible for degrading the nuclear lamins, proteins which normally make up the intermediate filament network lining the inner surface of the inner nuclear membrane. This seemingly bewildering profusion of biochemical events associated with apoptosis is depicted in Fig. 5.29.

The expression of the proto-oncogene c-*myc* also appears to be intimately linked to apoptosis. Many cells in a state of high turnover, e.g. germinal centre cells and

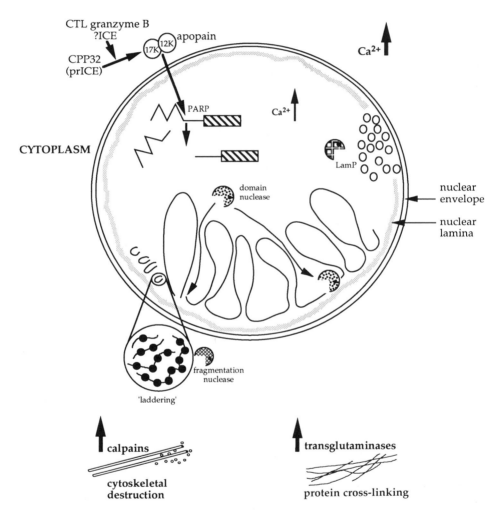

Fig. 5.29 Biochemical events which occur in apoptotic process. The activation of the Ced-3/ICE family proenzyme CPP-32 to apopain results in it being able to cleave poly(ADP-ribose) polymerase (PARP); PARP is thus unable to bind to DNA and carry out its repair function. The activation of endonucleases results in the breakdown of DNA into large ~300 and ~50 kbp fragments and then sometimes into smaller oligonucleosome fragments. Other enzymes are also activated; lamin protease degrades the nuclear lamina, calpains cause cytoskeletal destruction and transglutaminases cross-link proteins which might help in the formation of the apoptotic bodies.

intestinal crypt cells, have high c-*myc* expression. In fact, there is a series of *myc* genes, including N-*myc* and L-*myc,* first detected in neuroblastomas and small cell lung carcinomas respectively, both of which were discovered through gene amplification. The *myc* genes all encode proteins of approximately 62 kDa which are more abundant in proliferating cells. When a cell picks up the machinery to proliferate it also picks up an abort pathway, and c-*myc* expression determines either continuous proliferation or apoptosis depending upon the availability of critical growth factors. When cultured immortalized fibroblasts are induced to proliferate by the addition of growth factors, this is preceded by increased c-*myc* transcription, and when growth factors are withdrawn, c-*myc* is down-regulated as cells revert to growth arrest. If, however, cells are modified to express the c-Myc protein constitutively, then growth factor deprivation does not cause growth arrest, but instead cells remain in cycle and many die by apoptosis. Thus Myc abundance and growth factor availability determine three extreme states:

- growth arrest: c-*myc* off, growth factors absent;
- population expansion: c-*myc* on, growth factors present;
- apoptosis: c-*myc* on, growth factors absent.

It follows that cells that are in a high turnover state may be primed for apoptosis, and indeed cells in small intestinal crypts are highly susceptible to die by this means in response to a wide variety of highly toxic stimuli. The Myc protein is a transcription factor which binds to DNA, but it is inactive alone and only binds to DNA as a dimer with its partner protein, Max. It is not yet clear if the Myc-Max dimers have a common or distinct target genes for the apparently opposing pathways of cell cycle progression and apoptosis.

We have already described the functions of the p53 protein in Chapter 3, section 3.3. The function of p53 has been likened to that of a 'molecular policeman' or 'guardian of the genome'; when DNA is damaged, p53 accumulates and switches off replication to allow time for DNA repair (see Figs. 3.16 and 3.19). If repair fails, p53 may trigger apoptosis. Cells in which p53 is mutated or bound to viral proteins (see Fig. 3.18), cannot carry out this protective arrest, are more likely to accumulate genetic mutations and are, thus, more prone to malignant transformation. Indeed, the *p53* gene can be engineered out of cells, and while such 'p53 null mice' grow normally, they are highly prone to tumour development and often are quite resistant to cell-damaging agents like irradiation. If normal mice are irradiated, the p53 protein is strongly expressed in the small intestinal crypts but not in the large bowel crypts. This may explain why tumours are much more common in the human large bowel than in the small bowel; in the small bowel the damaged DNA is in some way 'sensed' resulting in increased p53, which temporarily inhibits cell cycle progression allowing time for DNA repair. In the large bowel, perhaps such minor damage is less effectively repaired so resulting in a higher incidence of mutations and malignancy. Exactly how a cell 'decides' between cell cycle arrest and apoptosis in response to p53 is not clear. A clash between growth activation (an increase in c-Myc) and growth suppression (elevation in p53) could precipitate apoptosis, or alternatively persistent damage may induce apoptosis through p53 activating *bax* gene expression, thus nullifying the protective effect of Bcl-2. In solid tumours, cells with mutated p53 appear to be best equipped to resist hypoxic death, thus bestowing mutant cells with a survival advantage over cells with intact p53.

One cell surface receptor whose activation mediates apoptosis is called Fas (CD95). Fas mediated apoptosis is one of the examples of this mode of cell death which may not depend on specific protein synthesis, and receptor occupancy can activate the Ced-3/ICE proteases. Fas belongs to a very large family of similar proteins including the TNF receptors and the nerve growth factor (NGF) receptor, all of which characteristically contain 3–6 extracellular cysteine-rich subdomains.

The Fas receptor is activated by a Fas ligand. Historically, however, the first molecules to be independently described were the anti-Fas and anti-APO-1 mouse monoclonal antibodies which induced apoptosis in cultured human lymphoid cells and were able to destroy human B cell lymphoid tumour xenografts in nude mice. Subsequently it was found that these antibodies recognized the same antigen, Fas; finally its ligand was sequenced, cloned and found (not surprisingly) to be related to TNF and NGF. Thus, the receptor Fas is related to the TNF type I receptor, and Fas ligand is related to TNF.

Not all cell types express the Fas receptor on their surfaces, but some, such as activated T and B lymphocytes, express it abundantly; in addition some specific cytotoxic T cell lines, which induce apoptosis in a Ca^{2+} independent manner, express the Fas ligand. So it seems that the normal roles of Fas receptor and ligand in the thymus, at least, are in T cell development, where apoptosis is a key regulatory mechanism. In HIV-1-infected humans, the expression of the envelope protein (env) on the surface of infected macrophages or CD4$^+$ T cells, can cause apoptosis in neighbouring uninfected T cells. This may occur because env cross-links CD4 on uninfected T cells causing them to express Fas and the Fas ligand, resulting in a form of fratricidal T-cell killing by apoptosis. Further transmission of the message upon occupancy of the Fas receptor may involve hydrolysis of sphingomyelin to ceramide, triggering a downstream ceramide-activated kinase.

Incidence of apoptosis

Substantial cell death is part and parcel of normal embryonic development, from the sculpting of tissues to the induction of immunological self-tolerance. Careful examination of any histological section of normal tissue will probably identify the occasional apoptotic cell, and one would guess that the elimination of isolated cells in normal adult tissues is a means of ridding the body of potentially harmful cells, e.g. those harbouring DNA damage. Apoptosis is vital in the resolution of inflammation since neutrophils undergo apoptosis and associated cell surface changes aid their phagocytosis by macrophages. Viral infection can trigger host cell apoptosis, which can then limit virus production. However, the inhibition of apoptosis by viral proteins will provide a selective advantage to the virus. A growing number of apoptosis-suppressing genes has now been identified which act through a variety of mechanisms to prolong the life-span of infected cells (see Fig. 3.18), and thus apoptosis may be a primary antiviral defence mechanism for cells. Epstein-Barr virus, a herpes virus responsible for infectious mononucleosis as well as being involved in Burkitt's lymphoma, prolongs the survival of infected B cells, possibly through the production of the early lytic cycle protein, BHRF 1, a viral homologue of Bcl-2. The cowpox virus gene *crmA* encodes a protein which inhibits ICE activity, at least in neuronal cells, while the expression of the *p35* gene from the baculovirus *Autographa californica* nuclear polyhedrosis virus is required to prevent mammalian neural cell death *in vitro* induced by nutrient or growth factor deprivation. The regulation of apoptosis may be of general importance in transformation; the transforming genes of adenovirus cooperate for this purpose, the E1A protein induces cell proliferation while the E1B proteins disable the p53-driven apoptotic pathway in the infected cells.

It is widely appreciated that in most experimental and human tumours there is a gross disparity between the *observed* rate of growth of the tumour population and the rate of growth we would expect from a consideration of the rate of cell production in that population. The difference is due to cell loss from the tumour, most of which is accounted for by the familiar 'lakes' of necrosis in areas most disadvantaged with respect to the afferent blood supply (see Figs. 4.16B and 5.20B) and in most, if not all solid tumours, an increasing rate of cell loss rather than a diminished rate of cell production is largely responsible for the curtailment of growth manifest by the typical sigmoid growth curve (see Fig. 5.32). However, apoptosis also occurs widely in tumours, the frequency of which is not related to the proximity of the vasculature, and it is not uncommon to find apoptotic tumour cells next to dividing cells (Fig. 5.30).

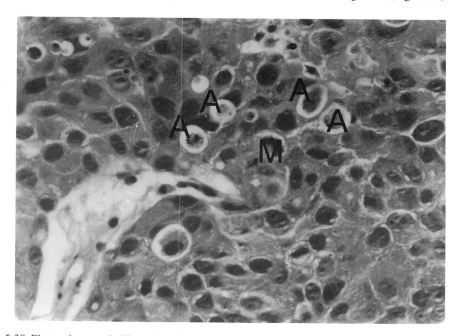

Fig. 5.30 Photomicrograph illustrating the presence of apoptotic tumour cells (A) next to a mitotic tumour cell (M), a proximity indicating that death is not due to lack of oxygen.

Why tumour cells undergo apoptosis is not clear, but there are several possibilities. A chromosomal imbalance, a lack of local growth factors or the activities of cytotoxic T lymphocytes (CTLs), natural killer- (NK-) or killer- (K-) cells could be responsible. TNF secreted by macrophages can also stimulate apoptosis, and there is also the intriguing possibility that apoptosis represents a residual attempt at autoregulation which ultimately fails, since in some tumours apoptosis is more common when they are small. In certain experimental tumours, low apoptotic rates are associated with extensive necrosis and an overall fast growth rate, while high apoptotic indices correlate with a slower net growth and little necrosis.

5.4   Tumour growth

Introduction

As tumour cells proliferate the tumour grows. However, when tumour growth rate is monitored by daily measurements, and the potential doubling time (t_{PD}) is calculated from the labelling index (see equation 2) or from a metaphase arrest technique (see equation 4), the actual growth rate and the t_{PD} are found to be very different. Tumour mass does not increase as fast as one would predict from the t_{PD} calculation, and the explanation for this is that over a given time almost as many cells can be lost as are produced. The rate of cell production in tumours can be much slower than in normal tissues, but the population of tumour cells will expand in size as long as the rate of cell production *exceeds* the rate of cell loss; in normal tissues these rates are equal to ensure no increase in size.

Cells may be lost from tumours in several ways – principally by exfoliation from exposed surfaces or through embolization into the vascular or lymphatic systems. There is a distinction between cells lost in this way, and cell death in tumours which does not immediately result in the cells' removal. In histological sections both areas of necrosis and individual dead cells can be found. There is a variety of likely causes of cell death in tumours, including non-viable chromosomal abnormalities, immune attack, and inadequate oxygenation and nutrition. Tumour cells die individually by apoptosis in areas of tissue that have a sufficient oxygen and nutrient supply, and as will be apparent from the preceding discussion (Chapter 5, section 5.3), the current fascination with apoptosis comes from its potential for manipulation as a form of cancer therapy.

Necrosis, however, maybe less controllable; as tumours grow, their cell mass outstrips tumour angiogenesis. Tumour cells produce angiogenic growth factors, stimulating vessels of surrounding normal tissues to form new blood vessels that are able to infiltrate the tumour mass. In contrast to situations in normal tissues that require angiogenesis (wound healing, for example), tumour angiogenesis is not perfectly regulated and ultimately poor neovascularization results in insufficient oxygenation and nutrient supply for all the tumour cells. Cells closest to functional blood vessels are able to proliferate, but as oxygen tension decreases downstream, hypoxic areas develop, and though these cells are alive they are unable to divide

(Fig 4.16B). In regions more distant still from a blood supply viability is lost and characteristic areas of necrosis develop; human tumours often have substantial volumes of necrotic tissue. The presence of non-proliferative hypoxic cells is also important as these cells can re-enter the proliferative pool if conditions become more favourable to them.

Measurements of tumour size

The study of human tumour growth rates has been strictly limited since therapy has to be initiated immediately after clinical detection; dispassionate measurement of a relentless increase in human tumour size is clearly unethical. Furthermore, human tumours are often deep within the body, so their initial phases go undetected, and final stages of relatively very large tumours whose cell loss rates might begin to approach proliferation rates are not representative of the whole tumour life history. Some measurements have been made by serial chest X-rays and other imaging techniques, usually applied to primary and metastatic tumours of the lung, though these are quite difficult to interpret accurately, particularly when the tumours are small. An alternative approach has been to measure the level of a tumour marker in the blood in the hope that it might reflect the tumour cell burden, and for example, the levels of circulating immunoglobulin appear to correlate with myeloma cell number.

Whatever the limitation to the method of analysis, a major feature is that most human tumours have gone through the greater part of their growth before they are detected clinically. If tumours arise from a single cell, then they will have undergone at least 30 doublings, attaining a weight of about 1 g (Fig. 5.31) before any real chance of clinical detection. Only a further 10 doublings is needed to reach a weight of 1 kg, a size likely to be lethal to the host. Therefore, the range of size that a tumour can be studied in humans only encompasses about one-quarter of its total growth history, so we are obliged to study the growth of animal tumours.

It is difficult to say how much the growth of experimental animal tumours mimics the situation in human tumours for a number of reasons. Nevertheless, general parallels can be drawn between the experimental and clinical situations, particularly in the realm of assessing the effectiveness of new drugs/therapies. Both native animal tumours and human tumours grown in animals are used. In the first case tumours that have either arisen naturally or as a result of chemical induction are passaged from one animal to another, expanding the tumour to many animals and/or keeping samples frozen for transplantation on future occasions. Tumours are excised from the original host and either transplanted as small tissue blocks or are split up into cell suspensions and cells are injected into the new hosts. Host animals are progressively brother/sister mated to ensure that the genetic constitution of the generations remains as close as possible to the original animal in which the tumour arose, to prevent tissue rejection. Transplantable animal tumours are often totally anaplastic because repeated passage means that the fastest proliferating cells (correlating with the least differentiated phenotype) soon predominate in each implanted specimen.

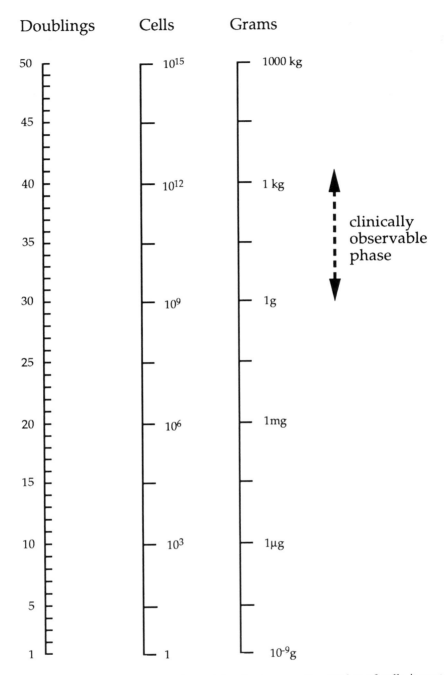

Fig. 5.31 The relationship between the weight of a tumour, the number of cells it contains (based on 10^9 cells/g), and the number of doublings achieved from a single cell.

Fig. 5.32 illustrates the *growth curve* of one such animal tumour, with the tumour weight plotted against time after subcutaneous implantation of 10^6 cells, on a logarithmic scale. Tumour growth starts slowly, sometimes with an initial lag period, before a period of rapid exponential growth followed by a plateau, where the tumour cell loss rate approaches equality with tumour cell production rate. At any point in time the growth rate (K_G) of the tumour equals the slope of a tangent drawn to the curve, at that point. From this we can calculate the doubling time (t_D) of the population from the equation:

$$t_D = \log_e 2/K_G \qquad\qquad (5)$$

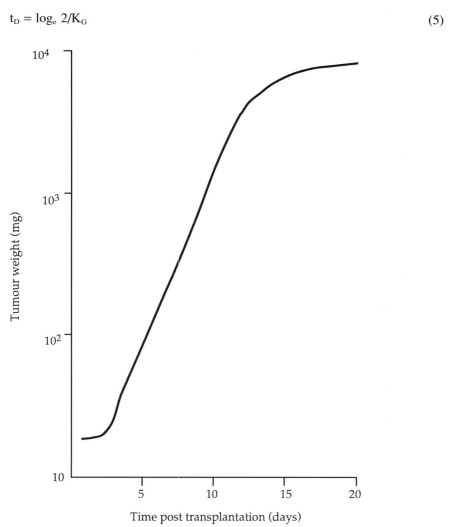

Fig. 5.32 A growth curve for a transplantable mouse sarcoma plotted on a semi-logarithmic scale. In the initial period the data show a straight line indicating growth is exponential, but after ~12 days growth rate slows and the curve begins to plateau. This retardation in growth rate is solely due to an increase in cell loss, and at 21 days ϕ (cell loss factor) is almost 1, i.e. for every 100 cells born per unit time almost 100 are lost in the same time. (Data kindly supplied by Professor Nick Wright.)

Table 5.3. *Changes in the growth characteristics of a transplantable mouse sarcoma with time after transplantation*

Time after transplantation (days)	t_D (hours)	t_{PD} (Hours)	ϕ
7	31.2	27	0.1
14	166	28	0.83
21	2376	38	0.98

Data kindly supplied by Professor Nick Wright. *Abbreviations*: t_D, tumour doubling time; t_{PD}, potential doubling time; ϕ, the cell loss factor.

Exponential growth implies that t_D is constant, and will occur when the rates of cell production and cell loss are proportional to the number of cells in the population. This type of sigmoid growth curve is typical of many experimental tumours, and it is likely that most human solid tumours have a similar life history. The Gompertz growth equation can be used to fit the data points, hence this type of growth is often referred to as Gompertzian growth. Since experimental tumours are often implanted at sites that are accessible to measurement, commonly subcutaneously, then another way of monitoring tumour size is to measure, using callipers, three diameters of the tumour at right angles to each other, and then the volume of the tumour can be calculated from the formula:

$$\text{Volume} = \pi/6 \times (\text{mean diameter})^3 \tag{6}$$

In theory, using calliper measurements, a growth curve for a tumour could be constructed from a single tumour-bearing animal, but allowances have to be made for the inclusion of skin thickness as well as having to make assumptions about the geometric form of the tumour.

From a knowledge of the LI and the duration of DNA synthesis, or by calculating the cell birth rate from a metaphase arrest experiment (see Chapter 5, section 5.1) it is possible to estimate the potential doubling time (t_{PD}) from equations (2) and (4) respectively, at any chosen point in the tumour's life history. Table 5.3 illustrates measurements made at three separate occasions on the tumour depicted in Fig. 5.32

When t_{PD} is estimated for the tumour illustrated in Fig. 5.32 at various points during its growth, it is apparent that the calculated value at day 21 is little different from that at day 7. Thus, measurements based on proliferation are *not* reliable indicators of the actual tumour growth rate. Hence the term *potential* doubling time is used with considerable justification, and simply predicts how fast the tumour will double its cell number from consideration of cell production alone. Of course in real life, cell loss occurs continually from tumours, counteracting cell production, and an increased rate of cell loss rather than diminished cell production would seem to be largely responsible for the slowing in growth rate in the expanding tumour.

It follows that the difference between the cell birth rate (K_B) and the tumour growth rate (K_G) is the cell loss rate (K_L), thus:

$$K_L = K_B - K_G \qquad (7)$$

It is customary to express the cell loss rate as a fraction of the cell birth rate, using the term the cell loss factor (ϕ), thus, $\phi = K_L/K_B$. The cell loss factor is related to the actual (t_D) and potential doubling times by the equation:

$$\phi = 1 - t_{PD}/t_D \qquad (8)$$

If $t_{PD} = t_D$ there is no cell loss, whereas a ϕ of 1.0 indicates a situation where cell production and cell loss just balance (e.g. in continually renewing systems). Like the experimental tumour at 21 days after transplantation where $\phi = 1-38/2376 = 0.98$, most human solid tumours have high cell loss factors suggesting most are almost at the plateau phase of growth when they become symptomatic.

Despite the shortcomings of growth measurements in human tumours, some general conclusions can be made:

- Carcinomas have high cell loss factors in the clinically detectable phase.
- Sarcomas have generally much lower cell loss factors than carcinomas.
- Within any histological type of tumour, there is an enormous range of tumour growth rates.
- Metastases generally grow 1.5 to 2 times faster than their primary tumours.
- Doubling times for pulmonary metastases are often between 1–3 months.
- Well differentiated tumours commonly have slower growth rates than their poorly differentiated counterparts.

The study of human tumours in an experimental situation requires the approach of *xenografting*, where human tumour tissue is grown in experimental animals. Xenografts can be used to assess treatment regimes for patients and anti-tumour activity in the xenograft correlates well with patient response; fine adjustments with drug combinations can be performed in the animal to achieve the best results in the patient. Host animals need to be immune suppressed before they will accept the transplant of human tissues. Rodents (most often mice), can have their ability to mount an immune response abolished by thymectomy followed by whole body irradiation. The former procedure removes their T cell component, and the latter kills the B cells of their bone marrow. Such animals, clearly, could not survive in normal infection laden conditions, and so are kept under sterile conditions.

Alternatively, a strain of mouse exists that is innately immune suppressed because it congenitally lacks a thymus. In addition to this genetic peculiarity these mice also have no fur and so, not unreasonably, are known as *nude* mice (Fig. 5.33). Nude mice are reared in clinically clean conditions separate from general animal house stock, with air filters over their cages. They are, however, somewhat more robust than thymectomized irradiated mice and are generally handled in the open air although handlers are required to wear gloves, be masked and gowned. As with animal tumours, human tumour xenografts can be passaged to many generations of mice, expanding the tumour stock and/or samples kept frozen and implanted at a future date.

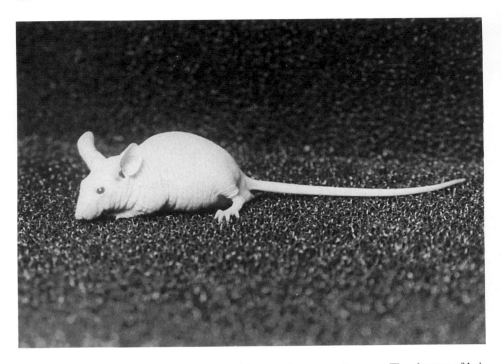

Fig. 5.33 A congenitally athymic mouse used for growing human tumours. The absence of hair has resulted in these mice being known as 'nude' mice. (Kindly supplied by Harlan-Olac Ltd, Bicester, Oxon.)

5.5   Further reading

Cell proliferation

Alison, M. R. (1995). Assessing cellular proliferation: what's worth measuring? *Human and Experimental Toxicology*, 14, 935–44.

Begg, A. C. (1993). Cell proliferation in tumours. In *Basic Clinical Radiobiology*, ed. G. G. Steel, pp. 14–22. London: Edward Arnold.

Fantes, P. & Brooks, R. (1993). *The Cell Cycle. A Practical Approach*. Oxford: IRL Press.

Hall, P. A., Levison, D. A. & Wright, N. A. (1992). *Assessment of Cell Proliferation in Clinical Practice*. London: Springer-Verlag.

Steel, G. G. (1977). *Growth Kinetics of Tumours*. Oxford: Clarendon Press.

Steel, G. G. (1993). The growth rate of tumours. In *Basic Clinical Radiobiology*, ed. G. G. Steel, pp. 8–13. London: Edward Arnold.

Wright, N. A. & Alison, M. R. (1984). *The Biology of Epithelial Cell Populations*, vols. 1 and 2. Oxford: Clarendon Press.

Growth factors and their receptors

Aaronson, S. (1991). Growth factors and cancer. *Science*, 254, 1146–53.

Alison, M. R. & Wright, N. A. (1993). Growth factors and growth factor receptors. *British Journal of Hospital Medicine*, 49, 774–90.

Gullick, W. J. (1991). Prevalence of aberrant expression of the epidermal growth factor receptor in human cancers. *British Medical Bulletin*, 47, 87–98.

Ihle, J. N. & Kerr, I. M. (1995). Jaks and stats in signalling by the cytokine receptor superfamily. *Trends in Genetics*, 11, 69–74.

Pawson, T. (1995). Protein modules and signalling networks. *Nature*, 373, 573–80.

Cell death

Alison, M. R. & Sarraf, C. E. (1995). Apoptosis: regulation and relevance to toxicology. *Human and Experimental Toxicology*, **14**, 234–47.

Bortner, C. D., Oldenburg, N. B. E. & Cidlowski, J. A. (1995). The role of DNA fragmentation in apoptosis. *Trends in Cell Biology*, **5**, 21–6.

Bowen, I. D. & Lockshin, R. A. (1981). *Cell Death in Biology and Pathology*. London: Chapman and Hall.

Earnshaw, W. C. (1995). Nuclear changes in apoptosis. *Current Opinion in Cell Biology*, **7**, 337–43.

Nicholson, D. W. *et al.* (1995). Identification and inhibition of the ICE/CED-3 protease necessary for mammalian apoptosis. *Nature*, **376**, 37–43.

Potten, C. S. (1987). *Perspectives on Mammalian Cell Death*. Oxford: Oxford University Press.

6

Tumour assessment

6.1 Introduction

When a histopathologist examines a slide of tumour tissue, he or she will be expected to provide a certain amount of information which will determine how the clinician treats the patient. This information can be summarized as follows:

- Histogenesis – what type of tumour it is (tissue of origin).
- Benign or malignant.
- Grade – how differentiated it is.
- Stage – extent of local invasion.
- Metastatic disease; yes/no; likely/unlikely.

Tumours that are benign closely resemble their parent tissue, are found in the locations where they arose, and the histopathologist is usually able to determine the histogenesis from morphological criteria. This information alone is normally sufficient for the clinician to determine the most appropriate treatment, usually curative resection without any additional treatment modalities such as irradiation or chemotherapy.

6.2 Grading

In contrast to benign tumours, malignant tumours generally merit a much more comprehensive description. One of the major exercises is to *grade* the tumour; this is a microscopic assessment of the degree of tumour differentiation. For example, gland formation by tumour cells derived from a secretory epithelium (e.g. colonic epithelium) would be considered a differentiating feature, while in a squamous carcinoma such a feature would be cells whose nuclei degenerate and whose cytoplasm fills up with keratin (anuclear squames being the terminally differentiated cells of the epidermis, see Fig. 4.17). Malignant tumours are usually graded as either 'well', 'moderately' or 'poorly' differentiated, but if there are no signs of differentiation the tumour is said to be *anaplastic*. As a general rule, well differentiated tumours are less aggressive than their poorly differentiated counterparts, so sometimes the well differentiated tumours are referred to as 'low grade' and the poorly differentiated as 'high grade'. In a well differentiated adenocarcinoma of the stomach almost all the tumour cells are organised into glandular structures (Fig. 6.1A), whereas in a poorly differentiated adenocarcinoma very few cells would be organized into glands and most of the cells would be in sheets or occurring singularly (Fig. 6.1B). Moderately differentiated tumours would be intermediate between these two extremes, but since this is a subjective assessment, what is poorly differentiated to one pathologist can easily be described as moderately differentiated by another. Normal prostatic cells form secretory acini, so a carcinoma of the prostate is graded from well differentiated (low grade) when the tumour cells form a uniform glandular pattern (Fig. 6.2A) to poorly differentiated (high grade) when there is no or minimal gland formation (Fig. 6.2B).

Since well differentiated tumours more closely resemble the parent tissue than do poorly differentiated ones, their classification is usually made from the routinely stained tissue section, while poorly differentiated tumours are more likely to require further diagnostic tests (special stains, electron microscopy, immunocytochemistry) for the histogenesis to be determined (see Chapter 1, section 1.3). This is particularly so for anaplastic tumours – i.e. those which have no recognizable differentiated features. For example, a well differentiated thyroid carcinoma is readily identified by the presence of colloid (Fig. 6.3A), whereas the so-called large cell anaplastic variant has

(A) (B)

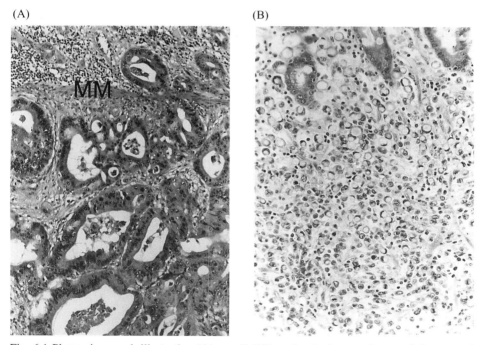

Fig. 6.1 Photomicrograph illustrating (A) a well differentiated adenocarcinoma of the stomach in which most of the tumour cells are forming glands beneath the muscularis mucosa (MM) contrasting with (B) a poorly differentiated gastric tumour in which the tumour cells form a sheet with no gland formation; note the individual cells are distended with mucin giving the cells a signet ring shape, hence signet cell carcinoma.

(A)

(B)

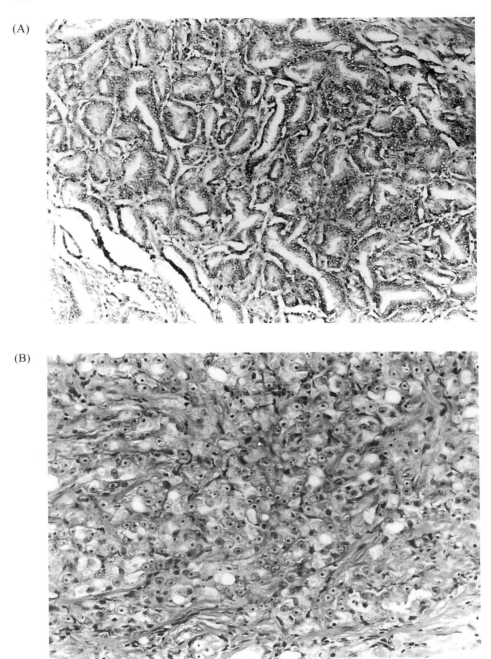

Fig. 6.2 Photomicrograph illustrating (A) a well differentiated adenocarcinoma of the prostate in which most of the tumour cells are forming glands lined by a single layer of epithelial cells, contrasting with (B) a poorly differentiated tumour from the same tissue in which there is minimal gland formation.

(A)

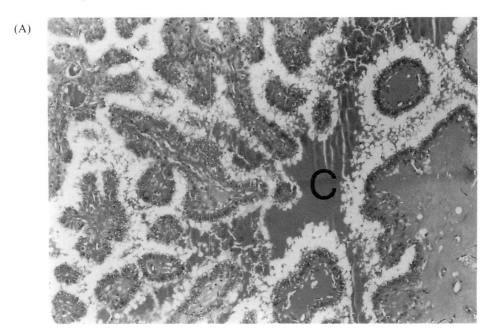

(B)

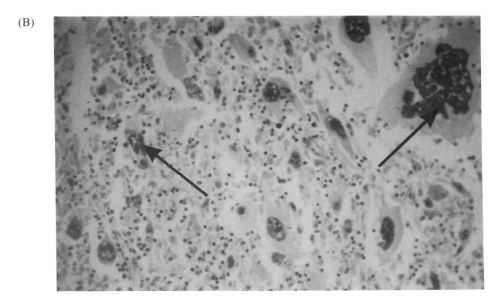

Fig. 6.3 Photomicrograph illustrating (A) a well differentiated papillary adenocarcinoma of the thyroid in which colloid (C) can be clearly seen between the cell fronds whereas in (B) an anaplastic thyroid tumour there are no recognizable thyroid features and there are many multinucleated tumour giant cells (arrows).

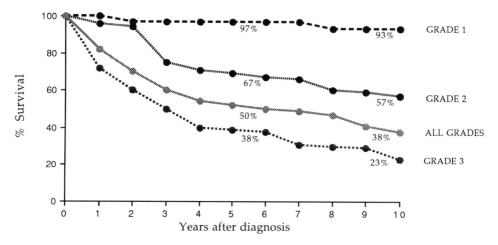

Fig. 6.4 Survival curves for patients with various grades of soft tissue sarcoma. (Data from Myhre-Jensen, O. *et al.*, 1983. Histopathological grading in soft tissue tumours. Relation to survival in 261 surgically treated patients. *Acta Pathologica Microbiologica Immunologica Scandanavia A*, **91**, 145–50.)

no recognizable thyroid features (Fig. 6.3B). The vast array of antibodies reactive with formalin-fixed tissues has resulted in few tumours remaining unclassifiable, and terms such as 'spindle cell' or 'round cell' tumour are now rare on histopathology report forms.

The grading of malignant connective tissue tumours (sarcomas) is somewhat different to that of carcinomas. Normal epithelial cells often form well defined glandular structures such as crypts (see Fig. 5.3) or have a clearly demarcated cell hierarchy as in squamous epithelia (see Fig. 5.2B) – easily recognisable differentiated features. In contrast, normal connective tissue cells can be widely separated from one another (fibroblasts) or just form bland sheets of cells (adipocytes). Therefore the grade of

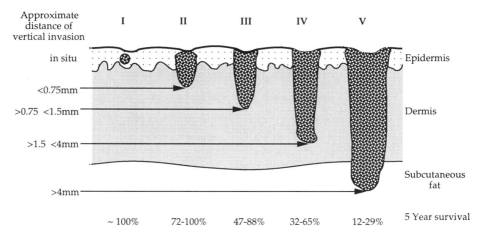

Fig. 6.5 Clark's levels in malignant melanoma are indicators of five-year survival.

(A) **(92-99%)**

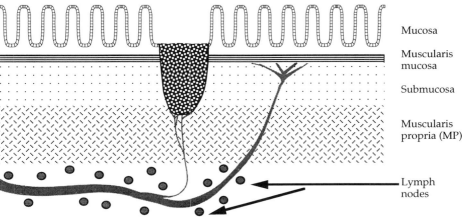

Mucosa

Muscularis mucosa

Submucosa

Muscularis propria (MP)

Lymph nodes

(B) **(72-78%)**

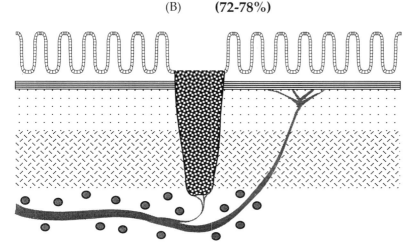

Fig. 6.6 Dukes' classification of large bowel carcinoma with five-year survival rates. In (A) the tumour is confined to the bowel wall, in (B) the tumour extends through the muscularis propria but no lymph nodes are involved. In (C1) proximal nodes are involved, but in (C2) more distal nodes are affected.

malignancy of sarcomas is generally determined by a combined assessment of several histological features, namely:

- Cellular pleomorphism and anaplasia.
- Mitotic activity (frequency and abnormality).
- Occurrence of cell death.
- Degree of cellularity.
- Expansive or infiltrative growth.

(C1)   **(45%)**

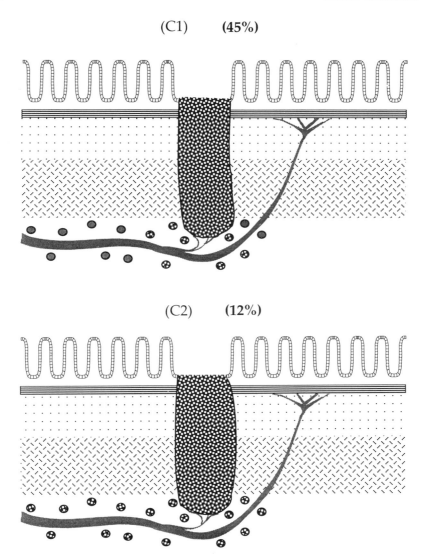

(C2)   **(12%)**

More aggressive growth would be expected to be associated with increased cellular pleomorphism, a lack of differentiated characteristics in the cells, greater mitotic activity, the occurrence of bizarre mitotic figures, more cell death, more cellular lesions and an infiltrative growth pattern. There are various grading systems in use, most have three or four grades, and Fig. 6.4 shows how grading has a profound discriminating power on predicting survival, with 10-year survival rates of 93%, 57% and 23% for grades 1–3 respectively.

6.3   Staging

Tumour *staging* is a semi-quantitative assessment of the clinical gravity of the disease. In some tumours a complete profile can be given which describes the mass of

Table 6.1. *The Jass classification of rectal carcinoma*

Feature	Numerical value
Tumour limited to bowel wall	
Yes	0
No	1
Invasive margin	
Expanding	0
Infiltrating	1
Number of lymph nodes containing metastases	
0	0
1–4	1
>4	2
Conspicuous peritumoral lymphocytic infiltrate	
Yes	0
No	1

Stage	Total numerical value (5-year survival as %)
I	0–1 (94%)
II	2 (83%)
III	3 (56%)
IV	4–5 (27%)

From Jass, J. R., Love, S. B. & Northover, J. M. A. (1987). A new prognostic classification of rectal cancer. *Lancet,* **1**, 1303–6.

the primary tumour, the extent of local lymph node involvement and the presence or absence of distant metastases. This TNM staging usually has the following scales:

    T: 1–4 = size of local tumour.

    N: 0–3 = number of involved local nodes.

    M: 0–1 = presence or absence of distant metastasis.

There are numerous pathological staging systems that are useful in predicting prognosis. In malignant melanoma, a tumour derived from melanocytes, which is certainly the most aggressive of all skin tumours, 'Clark's levels' of vertical invasion are strong prognostic indicators; the five-year survival rate decreases dramatically with increasing level of invasion (Fig. 6.5). This is obviously because the more invasive tumours have had a greater opportunity to metastasize through encountering dermal lymphatic vessels. Likewise the 'Dukes' classification' of large bowel cancer is a good indicator of prognosis (Fig. 6.6). Of course, almost all major organ systems have more than one staging classification, and the large bowel is no exception. Table 6.1 summarizes the Jass classification of rectal carcinoma, which, as might be expected puts emphasis on the extent of local invasion, the nature of the tumour margin, the number of lymph nodes with tumour and the presence of a lymphocytic infiltrate. Each stage has a statistically significant difference in prognosis, and as is usual, claims and counter-

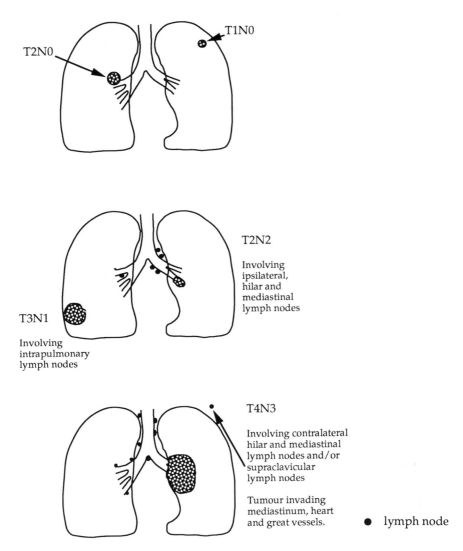

Fig. 6.7 Examples of the TNM (tumour, node, metastasis) classification in the lung.

claims have been made concerning the superiority of one classification system over another. Whatever the respective merits of each system they broadly look for the same features, and the survival data clearly indicate that these are important to the clinical outcome.

In the lung, the TNM classification has been adopted as the basis for staging lung cancer patients, and once again these stages have a prognostic significance. Broadly speaking the size of the primary tumour (T) is graded on a scale of 1–4, the degree of nodal (N) involvement is graded on a scale of 1–3 and the presence (M1) or absence (M0) of distant metastases is recorded. Examples of these tumours are schematically illustrated in Fig. 6.7, and when they are classified into stages (Table 6.2) then the

Table 6.2. *Stage grouping of lung tumours excluding small cell lung carcinoma*

Stage	Stage grouping		
I	T1	N0	M0
	T2	N0	M0
II	T1	N1	M0
	T2	N1	M0
IIIA	T1	N2	M0
	T2	N2	M0
	T3	N0-2	M0
IIIB	Any T	N3	M0
	T4	Any N	M0
IV	Any T	Any N	M1

From Hansen, H. H., Goldstraw, P., Gregor, A. & Vindelov, L. (1995). Tumours of the trachea and the lung. In *Oxford Textbook of Oncology*, vol. 2, ed. M. Peckham, H. M. Pinedo & U. Veronesi, pp. 1533–57. Oxford: Oxford University Press.
Abbreviations: T 1–4, size of primary tumour; N 0–3, degree of nodal involvement; M 0–1, absence or presence of distant metastases.

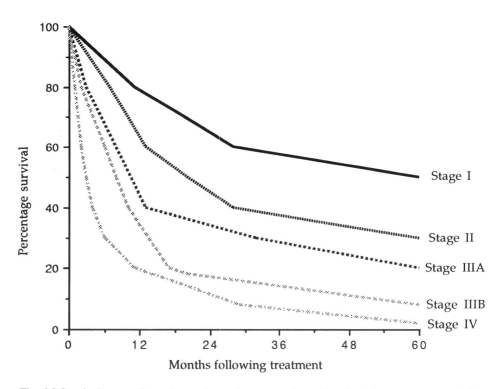

Fig. 6.8 Survival curves for patients with various stages (see Table 6.2) of lung cancer excluding small cell lung carcinoma. (Data from Hansen, H. H., Goldstraw, P., Gregor, A. & Vindelov, L., 1995. Tumours of the trachea and the lung. In *Oxford Textbook of Oncology*, vol. 2, ed. M. Peckham, H. M. Pinedo & U. Veronesi, pp. 1533–57. Oxford: Oxford University Press.)

correlation between survival and stage is quite clear (Fig. 6.8). Thus in summary, information regarding the appearances of a tumour, its local spread, local nodal involvement and the presence or absence of metastases all contribute to assessing the likelihood of recurrence of disease after surgery (if this is possible), and high-risk groups can be identified and treated appropriately.

6.4   Further reading

Enzinger, F. M. & Weiss, S. W. (1995). *Soft Tissue Tumors*, 3rd edn. St. Louis: Mosby.
Fletcher, C. D. M. (1995). *Diagnostic Histopathology of Tumours*, vols. 1 and 2. Edinburgh: Churchill Livingstone.
Sternberg, S. S. (1992). *Histology for Pathologists*. New York: Raven Press.
Sternberg, S. S. (1994). *Diagnostic Surgical Pathology*, vols. 1 and 2, 2nd edn. New York: Raven Press.
Underwood, J. C. E. (1981). *Introduction to Biopsy Interpretation and Surgical Pathology*. Berlin: Springer-Verlag.
Wheater, P. R., Burkitt, H. G., Stevens, A. & Lowe, J. S. (1991). *Basic Histopathology*, 2nd edn. Edinburgh: Churchill Livingstone.

7

Cancer treatment

7.1 Available strategies

Successful treatment of neoplastic disease largely depends on inflicting the *maximum* damage on the tumour stem cells and the *minimum* damage on normal tissue stem cells (Fig. 7.1). A single dose of a cytotoxic drug or combination of drugs may inflict comparable stem cell damage on a tumour cell population and normal renewing tissues, but if the rate of regeneration of stem cell numbers is much more rapid in the normal tissues then this is exploitable therapeutically. If drugs are administered continuously, there is no opportunity for stem cell recovery and hence differences between normal and tumour tissue will not be apparent. However, if a series of treatments is given, with appropriate intervals for recovery of normal tissue between treatments, then in theory it should be possible to eradicate the tumour stem cells while at the same time sparing the normal stem cells (Fig. 7.1A). By contrast, too short an interval will progressively deplete normal stem cells (Fig. 7.1B), and too long an interval between treatments will allow the tumour stem cells to recover in number and even increase (Fig. 7.1C). The mainstay of treatment is usually surgical resection combined with systemic chemotherapy or localized irradiation. The use of multiple treatment modalities, e.g. surgery + chemotherapy is known as *adjuvant* therapy, and the simultaneous use of a number of anticancer drugs is referred to as *combination* therapy. The all too familiar unwanted side-effects of chemotherapy (myelosuppression, hair loss, gastrointestinal toxicity) occur because most of the conventional drugs are effective at killing all proliferative cells, not just proliferative tumour cells. The age of molecular biology promises a revolution in the oncology clinic as ways of specifically targeting tumour cells come into use; the presently available drugs are perfectly good at killing cells, but their use is limited by the toxic side-effects.

Of course, we cannot witness the sterilization of tumour stem cells *in situ* with a particular treatment, but we can perform a clonogenic assay. We have already discussed *in vitro* colony assays (see Fig. 4.22), and the fact that the plating efficiency of a transplantable experimental tumour can be reduced by a cytotoxic drug, to a degree which is consistent with the effect that drug has on the tumour *in situ* (e.g. growth retardation, cure), then it seems that the cells which are clonogenic under test

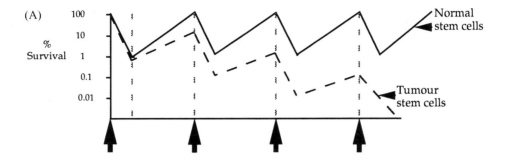

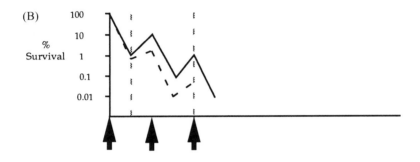

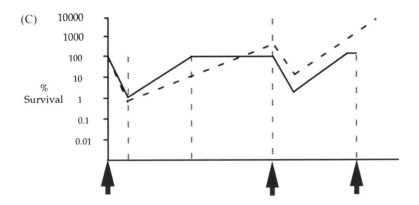

Fig. 7.1 The rationale of cancer chemotherapy. (A) If regeneration of tumour stem cells is slower than normal (haematopoietic) stem cells then appropriately timed chemotherapy could lead to a 'cure'. (B) Too short an interval between treatments can lead to a potentially lethal decimation of normal stem cell numbers. (C) Too long an interval between treatments can result in an expansion of tumour stem cell numbers. (↑ Indicate treatment times.)

conditions are the same cells which are stem cells *in situ*. This sort of approach can be carried out on experimental tumours that are growing subcutaneously, where size can be serially monitored by calliper measurements. A group of animals with similarly sized tumours are divided into two groups, one group left untreated and the other treated. Tumour volume is then measured at regular intervals thereafter as shown in Fig. 7.2, and typically treatment results in regression followed by regrowth. In order to measure the *growth delay*, an end-point such as the time to reach a fixed multiple (usually 2–4 ×) of the size at the time of treatment is selected. The extra time the treated tumour takes to reach this size is the 'growth delay'. Results with increasing drug doses can then be plotted as a dose-response curve; increasing dose causing more clonogenic cell kill and hence more growth delay.

Much of the regrowth after treatment is due to repopulation by surviving clonogenic cells, and Fig. 7.3 illustrates how in malignant melanoma cells growth delay (which was dependent on drug dose) is correlated with clonogenic cell survival in these same populations when they are plated in a soft agar assay (see Fig. 4.23). However, for a given level of clonogenic cell survival, e.g. 1%, the growth delay was ~5 days after the nitrosourea (CCNU), but ~13 days after cyclophosphamide. Therefore growth delay after treatment is probably a function of not only the level of clonogenic cell survival, but also the rate of regrowth.

A number of *in vivo* clonogenic assays exist for testing the effects of novel anti-cancer compounds or new treatment regimes, the best known being the *spleen colony*

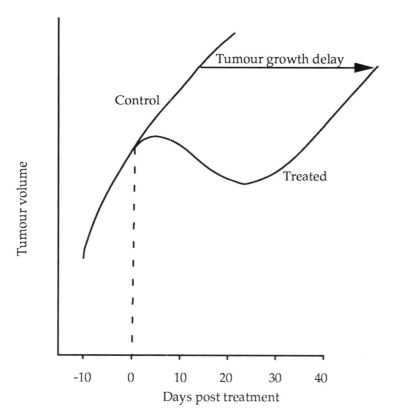

Fig. 7.2 Tumour growth delay is the extra time required for the treated tumours to reach a multiple of the tumour size at the time of treatment compared to untreated tumours.

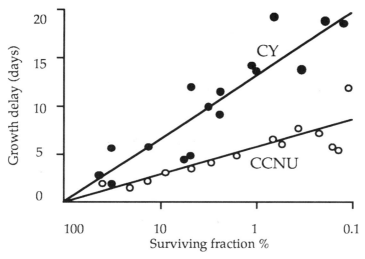

Fig. 7.3 In B16 mouse melanoma cells there is a linear relationship between tumour growth delay and clonogenic cell survival after either cyclophosphamide (CY) or the nitrosourea (CCNU). However, for a particular level of stem cell killing, growth delay is much greater after CY. (Data from Steel, G. G. 1993. *Basic Clinical Radiobiology*. London: Edward Arnold.)

assay, which can investigate bone marrow stem cells and the survival of stem cells in experimental leukaemias and lymphomas. A cell suspension is prepared and injected intravenously into mice that have received a dose of irradiation sufficient to destroy all endogenous bone marrow stem cells. The injected cells grow in various sites but principally in the spleen where they form macroscopic colonies; an estimate of the stem cell fraction can be made from simply counting the number of colonies visible on the spleen surface at about 10 days after injection – the CFU-S (colony forming units in the spleen). Analogous to the spleen colony assay is the *lung colony assay* which is applicable to any transplantable mouse tumour that readily forms colonies in the lung after intravenous injection of a single cell suspension: in practice the colonies are only scored on the surface of the lung.

There are many ways of treating cancer and Table 7.1 lists some of the common and some of the more novel (and largely still experimental) approaches to cancer treatment. Surgery was the first treatment for cancer, and remains the predominant method of removing primary tumours and the locally involved lymph nodes. Surgery is often accompanied by a course of systemic chemotherapy, to mop-up any of the primary tumour cells accidentally dislodged during resection and/or to treat known or suspected metastatic disease.

7.2   Chemotherapy

Introduction

Conventional chemotherapeutic drugs can be broadly divided into those which are cell cycle phase-specific and those which can kill all proliferative cells. Cell cycle

Table 7.1 *Possible ways of treating neoplastic disease*

Surgery
Systemic chemotherapy
Local chemotherapy
Irradiation
Antibody-guided chemotherapy and radiotherapy
Antibody-directed enzyme prodrug therapy (ADEPT)
Antibodies to growth factors and their receptors
Antibody-dependent cellular cytotoxicity
Genetic prodrug activation therapy (GPAT)
Hormonal therapy
Differentiation therapy
Stabilization of the extracellular matrix
Cytokine therapy
Apoptosis induction
Antisense oligodeoxynucleotides

---

phase-specific drugs are widely used and include the antimetabolites and antimitotic drugs, while most of the rest, including the anti-tumour antibiotics, alkylating agents and platinum-related compounds are simply cell cycle-specific. At the outset it is important to emphasize that most anti-cancer agents induce apoptosis (see Chapter 5, section 5.3) rather than necrosis, illustrating the fundamental importance of this mode of cell death to the whole topic of neoplasia. Other compounds are palliative rather than potentially curative, notably the antiandrogens and antioestrogens which do not actually kill cells, but rather they occupy the respective cytosolic receptors and so block the action of the normal trophic hormones. Though chemotherapeutic drugs are often given systemically, more localized treatment is possible, e.g. intraperitoneal chemotherapy for ovarian cancer. Table 7.2 lists the major categories of compounds used to treat neoplastic disease.

The antimetabolites

Before a cell can divide it must duplicate its DNA and build up protein. These synthetic processes require smaller molecules to be assembled and incorporated into the macromolecules. The antimetabolites can be analogues of nucleic acid precursors and thus incorporated in their place, or alternatively they can bind tightly to vital enzymes and inhibit their biological function.

Methotrexate exerts its cytotoxicity through binding tightly to the enzyme dihydrofolate reductase (DHFR), the enzyme responsible for the conversion of dihydrofolate to tetrahydrofolate (Fig. 7.4). The reduced folate is required for one-carbon transfers in purine ring biosynthesis and for thymidylate (dUMP) synthesis; the methylation of dUMP to dTMP being solely responsible for oxidation of the reduced folate. Cytosine arabinoside (Ara-C) is an analogue of the naturally occurring nucleoside deoxycytidine (Fig. 7.5), it is actively taken up and converted by a succession of phosphorylation

Table 7.2 *The major categories of anti-cancer drugs*

Class	Examples
Antimetabolites	Methotrexate, cytosine arabinoside 5-fluorouracil, purine analogues, hydroxyurea
Anti-tumour antibiotics	Bleomycin, daunomycin doxorubicin, mitomycin C actinomycin D
Alkylating agents	Nitrogen mustard, cyclophosphamide melphalan, chlorambucil nitrosoureas
Platinum compounds	Cisplatin, carboplatin
Plant derivatives	Vinca alkaloids, epipodophyllotoxins, taxol
Hormonal therapy	Tamoxifen, cyproterone acetate goserelin acetate, octreotide

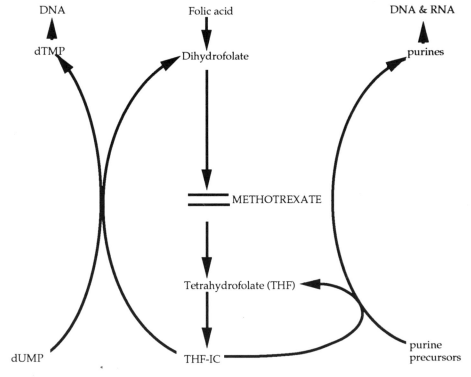

Fig. 7.4 The folic acid pathway, methotrexate binds to the enzyme dihydrofolate reductase.

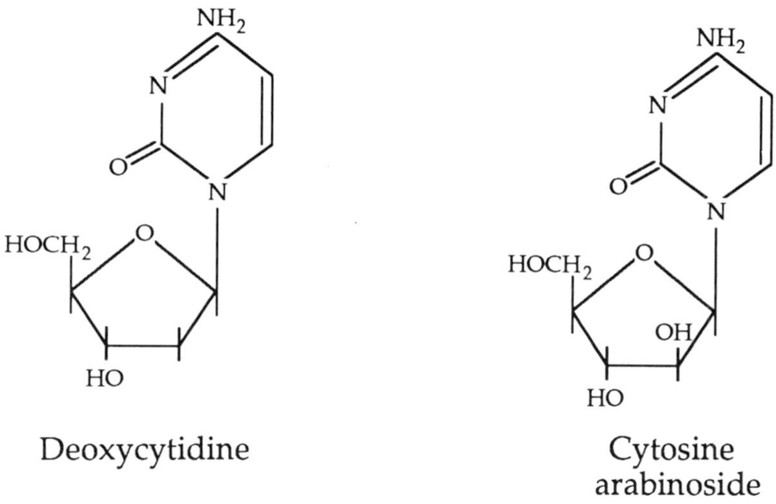

NH$_2$

Deoxycytidine

NH$_2$

Cytosine
arabinoside

Fig. 7.5 The structure of the nucleoside deoxycytidine and its analogue cytosine arabinoside.

steps to the triphosphate whose incorporation into DNA produces termination of the nascent DNA strand. An important point about antimetabolites like Ara-C is that they are self-limiting in that cells in the S phase at the time of administration are killed, but other cells are prevented from entering the sensitive S phase, being blocked at the G$_1$-S boundary. Increases in tumour cell kill are possible if the tumour cells can be synchronized (perhaps by the use of a recombinant growth factor) in S phase, *but out of synchrony* with normal S phase cells in the renewing tissues. This may be particularly appropriate for certain leukaemias using colony stimulating factors. 5-Fluorouracil (5-FU) is a monosubstituted analogue of the pyrimidine, uracil. The phosphorylated derivative binds tightly to thymidylate synthetase and inhibits its activity, competing successfully for the catalytic site of the enzyme concerned with the production of thymidine nucleotides from dUMP; this leads to a depletion of deoxythymidine triphosphates (dTTPs) which are crucial for DNA synthesis (Fig. 7.6).

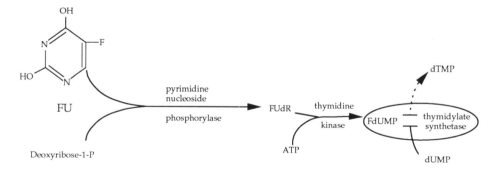

Fig. 7.6 Part of the metabolism of 5-FU. The deoxyribonucleoside derivative 5-fluoro-2′-deoxyuridine (FUdR), is further metabolized to the nucleotide form by thymidine kinase. FdUMP forms a stable complex with thymidylate synthetase.

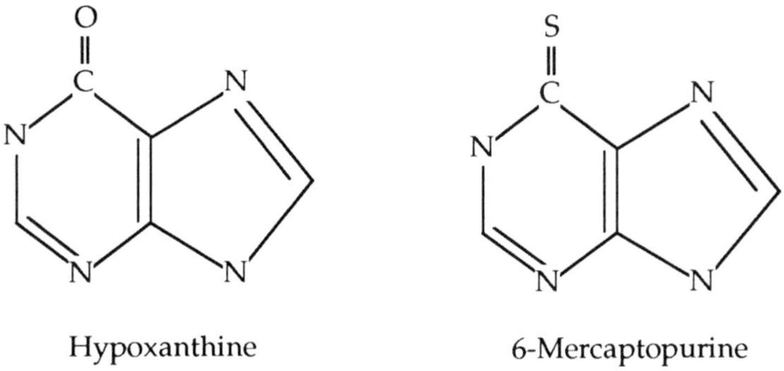

Hypoxanthine   6-Mercaptopurine

Fig. 7.7 The purine hypoxanthine and its analogue 6-mercaptopurine.

6-Mercaptopurine (6-MP) is an analogue of the purine hypoxanthine (Fig. 7.7) whose activity is related to its metabolism *via* hypoxanthine-guanine phosphoribosyl transferase (HGPRT) to 6-thioinosine monophosphate (6-thio-IMP). This monophosphate blocks the essential first step in the construction of the purine skeleton, the condensation of phosphoribosylpyrophosphate (PRPP) with glutamate, as well as inhibiting the conversion of inosinic acid (IMP) to the adenine and guanine nucleotides AMP and GMP. The build-up of PRPP promotes the activation of 6-MP to its active nucleotide form through the action of HGPRT, and this is further aided by other inhibitors of purine biosynthesis, e.g. methotrexate, which expand the PRPP pool thereby also activating 6-MP. The triphosphate of 6-MP (6-thio-GTP) gets into DNA, resulting in DNA strand breaks and hence cytotoxicity. Hydroxyurea (HU) is a relatively simple molecule which inhibits ribonucleotide reductase, leading to a depletion of deoxyribonucleotide triphosphates. Like Ara-C, hydroxyurea causes the death of cells in the S phase and blocks cells at the G_1-S boundary. Fig. 7.8 summarizes the loci of action of these antimetabolites during the formation of the nucleotide triphosphate precursors of DNA.

Anti-tumour antibiotics

Most of the anti-tumour antibiotics are derived from *Streptomyces* species, and can cause local DNA unwinding through intercalation, and by forming tight adducts with DNA can also block transcription. Bleomycin is a 1.5 kDa peptide isolated from the fungus *Streptomyces verticillus*. By virtue of having an iron-binding fragment at one end of the molecule and a DNA-binding fragment at the other, bleomycin exposes DNA to the action of radicals by binding an oxidizable substrate close to DNA. Bleomycin binds to divalent cations, in particular Fe^{2+}, and then binds to DNA. Ferrous iron undergoes spontaneous oxidation to the Fe^{3+} state and the released electron is accepted by molecular oxygen and highly toxic oxygen intermediates are formed. These can attack the 4'-H of deoxyribose leading to cleavage of the sugar resulting in release of free bases, particularly thymine and cytosine, hence leading to DNA strand breaks (summarized in Fig. 7.9). As expected, the action of bleomycin is

PURINE SYNTHESIS

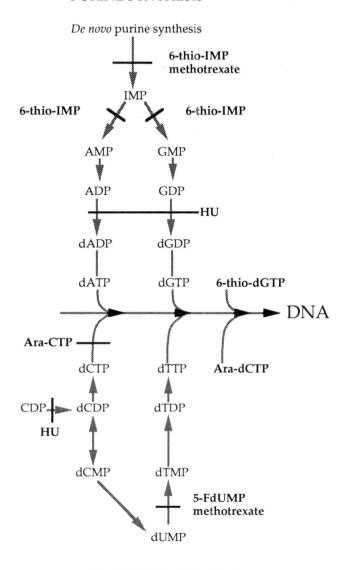

PYRIMIDINE SYNTHESIS

Fig. 7.8 The pathways leading to the formation of the nucleotide triphosphates of DNA and the sites of inhibitory action of some of the major antimetabolites.

inhibited by the removal of oxygen, or the presence of free radical scavengers or iron chelators. Cells in G_2 are particularly sensitive to bleomycin, and pulmonary fibrosis is a common side-effect due to the destruction of type I pneumocytes. The anthracyclines, daunorubicin and doxorubicin (adriamycin) are produced by a large number of *Streptomyces* species. The antibiotics belong to a group of highly coloured products

(i)   BLM + Fe^{2+}
(ii)   BLM—Fe^{2+} Iron - binding
(iii)   DNA—BLM—Fe^{2+} DNA - binding

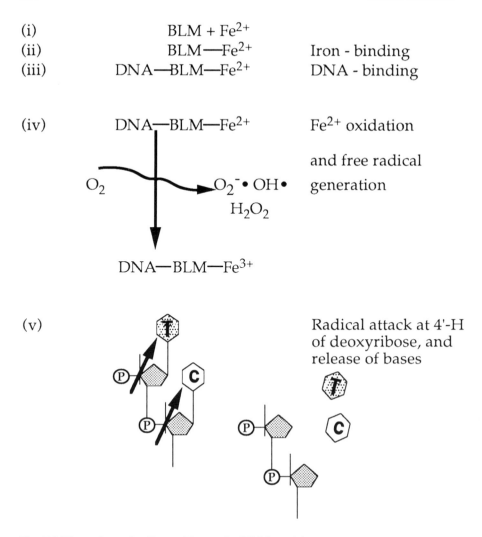

(iv)   DNA—BLM—Fe^{2+} Fe^{2+} oxidation

                                                and free radical

O$_2$ O$_2^-$• OH•   generation
                               H$_2$O$_2$

                  DNA—BLM—Fe^{3+}

(v)   Radical attack at 4'-H
                                                 of deoxyribose, and
                                                 release of bases

Fig. 7.9 The pathway leading to bleomycin (BLM) toxicity.

known as the *rhodomycins*. These compounds have a planar tetracyclic ring attached to an amino sugar and may intercalate into DNA parallel to the base pairs; this could lead to local unwinding of the sugar-phosphate backbone and trigger strand breaks. Anthracyclines may also bring about iron-mediated free radical formation, or indeed they themselves may undergo a one-electron reduction to the corresponding free radical and this extra electron is rapidly donated to molecular oxygen, resulting in the formation of superoxide. Through DNA intercalation anthracyclines may also be promoters of topoisomerase II-associated DNA fragmentation, but they prevent the enzyme from finishing its cycle by inhibiting religation of the broken strands. Cardiac toxicity is a noticeable side-effect, and is probably due to the free radical formation. Unlike most anti-tumour antibiotics, mitomycin C can not only be reduced to a radical species, but it is also activated to an alkylating agent, able to bind to DNA, causing cross-links and inhibiting DNA synthesis and function.

Alkylating agents

Alkylating agents were among the first chemicals to be identified as being useful in cancer chemotherapy and they exert their toxicity through covalent binding to intracellular molecules, principally DNA. Nitrogen mustard, first studied for its potential in chemical warfare, has two chloroethyl groups, thus it is a *bifunctional* alkylating agent like melphalan and chlorambucil (Fig. 7.10), and exerts its toxicity either through the formation of simple DNA adducts, or DNA-protein cross-links or DNA interstrand cross-links. The most lethal event is a DNA interstrand cross-link, and only bifunctional agents are able to form these.

Platinum compounds

The platinum complexes, cisplatin and carboplatin (Fig. 7.11), are extremely useful anticancer agents, usually employed in combination with other compounds. Inside the cell, positively charged platinum complexes are formed which are highly reactive with DNA, and interstrand cross-links and intrastrand guanine-guanine cross-links appear to be the most cytolethal events.

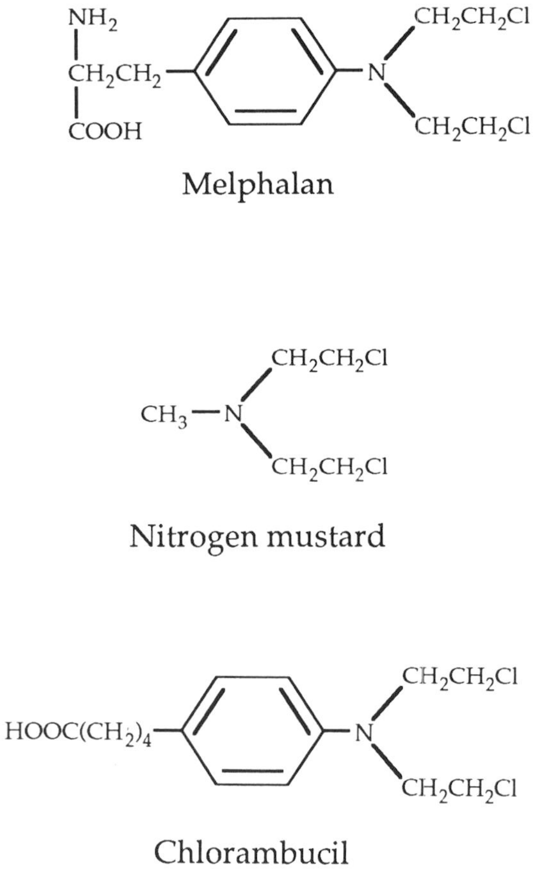

Melphalan

Nitrogen mustard

Chlorambucil

Fig. 7.10 Structure of some of the bifunctional alkylating agents.

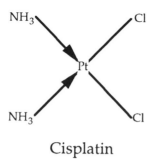

Cisplatin

Carboplatin

Fig. 7.11 The structure of cisplatin and carboplatin.

Plant derivatives

A great deal of effort has been expended on screening plant extracts for cytotoxicity against mammalian cells, though relatively few have had a clinical impact. The epipo-dophyllotoxins etoposide (VP-16) and teniposide (VM-26) are derived from extracts of the roots of the May apple (mandrake) plant, and are most effective against late S and early G_2 phase cells. They exert their cytotoxicity through interrupting the 'breakage reunion reaction' of DNA topoisomerase II. The vinca alkaloids, vincristine and vinblastine, are present in the common periwinkle plant, and are lethal to mitotic cells. These alkaloids bind tightly to tubulin so preventing the polymerization of tubu-lin subunits into microtubules, resulting in mitotic cells being arrested in metaphase from which death rapidly ensues. This metaphase-arresting property of the vinca alka-loids is exploited in the metaphase arrest technique for estimating the potential doub-ling times of tumours (see Fig. 5.5).

Hormonal therapy

Hormone-dependent tumours can be treated by surgical removal of the gonads (ovariectomy or castration), but this is a somewhat drastic step. Apart from conventional chemotherapy, another approach is to treat with a synthetic analogue of the natural stimulating hormone which successfully competes for the cytosolic receptor, but fails to elicit the normal cellular response. Tamoxifen is weakly oestrogenic and is capable of tight competitive binding to oestrogen receptors (ERs), however despite binding to DNA, the tamoxifen-ER complex is not an effective transcription factor to promote the normal cellular response to oestradiol. Tamoxifen is useful in improving the life expectancy of patients with advanced breast cancer, and its use has been advocated as a chemopreventitive agent for women at high-risk of developing breast cancer. A similar approach can be used in the palliative treatment of androgen-dependent prostate cancer. Cyproterone acetate binds to the prostatic receptor for the active metabolite of testosterone, 5α-dihydrotestosterone, so reducing the stimulatory effects of testosterone.

Another approach has been to reduce gonadotrophin secretion from the anterior pituitary, commonly adopted for the treatment of breast cancer in premenopausal women. The release of gonadotrophins (LH and FSH) is under the control of gonado-trophin releasing hormone (GnRH) which is delivered in pulses to the anterior pituitary from the hypothalamus (Fig. 7.12). GnRH reacts with receptors on pituitary gonadotrophs and is internalized, but by the time the next pulse arrives the receptors have been recycled. GnRH agonists such as goserelin acetate (Zoladex®) lead to a more permanent down-regulation of receptors, so in effect desensitizing the pituitary to further GnRH pulses. Octreotide (Sandostatin®) is an analogue of the 14 amino acid peptide known as somatostatin. It has a longer half-life than somatostatin and exerts its effect by inhibiting the release of GH from the pituitary. This analogue is useful in the management of benign and malignant neuroendocrine tumours of the gut, where it may suppress growth as well as reducing hormonal secretion which is responsible for so much of the symptomatology associated with such tumours (see Table 1.3)

Drug resistance

One of the major obstacles to the ultimate success of cancer chemotherapy is the ability of malignant cells to develop resistance to cytotoxic drugs. This may be resistance to a single agent, e.g. DHFR gene amplification confers resistance to methotrexate; but more important is the phenomenon of multi-drug resistance (MDR) which confers upon cells the ability to withstand exposure to lethal doses of many structurally unrelated agents. Figure 7.13 summarizes the main biochemical mechanisms of drug resistance.

Reduced drug uptake can be a cause of resistance to methotrexate which utilizes the reduced folate transporter system to enter cells efficiently. Many drugs exert their cytotoxic effects only after metabolic activation. As we have seen this includes anti-metabolites such as Ara-C and 5-FU, and even some alkylating agents, e.g. cyclophos-phamide. Tumour cells may acquire resistance to anti-cancer agents by alteration of the intracellular target. Quantitative and qualitative changes in DHFR, thymidylate synthetase and DNA topoisomerase II have been associated with resistance to the

Normal cell   Zoladex® treated cell

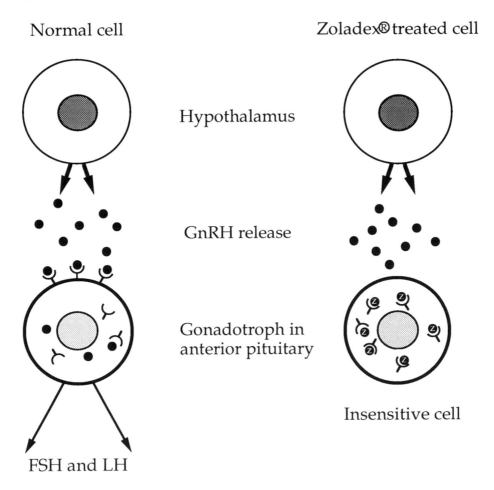

Fig. 7.12 The mode of action of goserelin acetate (Zoladex®) which down-regulates the receptors on pituitary gonadotrophs for gonadotrophin-releasing hormone (GnRH) thus desensitizing them to further stimulation by GnRH.

inhibitors of these enzymes. Point mutations in the gene encoding DHFR can reduce the enzyme's affinity for methotrexate, but more commonly methotrexate resistance is due to over-production of the enzyme caused by the presence of multiple copies of the gene – gene amplification. Gene amplification can occur through unscheduled duplication of already replicated DNA, and as these regions are somewhat unstable, double minute chromosomes can be formed.

MDR is caused by the overexpression of a membrane-associated energy-dependent drug efflux pump, the P-glycoprotein, p170, (Fig. 7.14). The P-glycoprotein is encoded by the *mdr1* gene, and cells with MDR often show amplification of this gene. Typically the affected cells show resistance to a wide range of seemingly unrelated drugs,

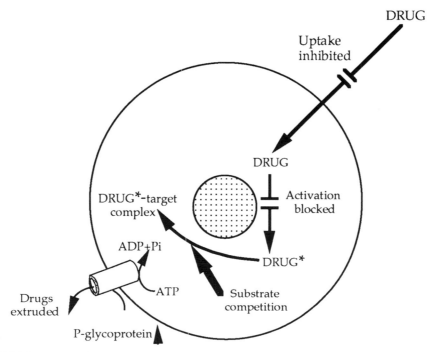

Fig. 7.13 Summary of the major mechanisms of drug resistance.

including vincristine, vinblastine, actinomycin-D and adriamycin. Possible strategies against MDR include using monoclonal antibodies against the P-glycoprotein.

Acquired drug resistance invariably results from genetic alterations in the tumour cells, thus resistant cells are mutant cells, and of course most of the anti-cancer drugs are mutagenic. It has been predicted that drug-resistant mutations occur at the rate of one every 10^6 cell divisions, so a clinically detectable tumour ($>10^9$ cells, see Fig. 5.31) will probably harbour many resistant cells. Therefore the treatment of large tumours with single agents is, not surprisingly, not very effective, and combinations of drugs with no overlapping resistances are much more useful.

7.3   Radiotherapy

Besides surgery and chemotherapy, radiotherapy is the other major treatment modality. Ionizing radiation damages DNA and thus is a method of killing proliferative cells. What is broadly covered by the term 'ionizing radiation' falls into two distinct groups – streams of subatomic particles, and the spectrum of electromagnetic radiation. Each is separately characterised by its *linear energy transfer* (LET) between the beam and the tissue under consideration, a measure of the rate at which a beam of radiation gives energy to the material through which it is traversing. The absorbed dose is measured in grays named after Hal Gray the prominent radiation therapist of

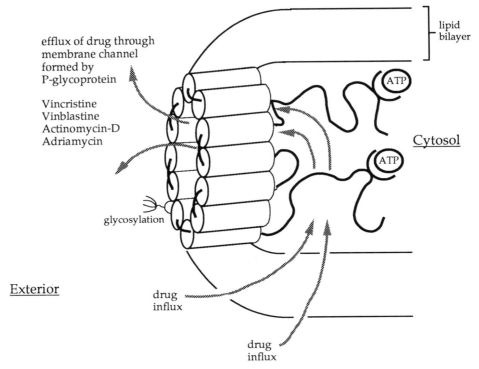

efflux of drug through
membrane channel
formed by
P-glycoprotein

Vincristine
Vinblastine
Actinomycin-D
Adriamycin

lipid
bilayer

ATP

ATP

Cytosol

glycosylation

Exterior

drug
influx

drug
influx

Fig. 7.14 Schematic diagram of the P-glycoprotein which functions as an energy-dependent drug efflux pump for a variety of anti-cancer agents.

the first half of this century; 1 gray = 1 joule of energy absorbed per kilo of tissue (1 j/kg); in earlier terminology 1 Gy is equivalent to 100 rads.

High LET radiation is associated with particulate streams such as neutrons and α-particles. Low LET radiation is mostly associated with the electromagnetic spectrum. Wavelengths from the ultraviolet and shorter have enough energy to cause ionizing events; γ rays are spontaneously emitted from sources, in the breakdown of unstable radioactive elements such as [137]caesium and [60]cobalt, whereas X-rays are produced when non-radioactive heavy elements such as tungsten are bombarded with electrons across an electrical potential difference. The energy of any radiation is inversely proportional to its wavelength, i.e. the shorter the wavelength the higher the energy of the radiation. The dose ratio of different quality LET beams to produce the same biological effect is called the *relative biological efficiency* (RBE). In general the RBE falls as the dose increases, since the probability of low LET radiation causing a lethal double strand break in DNA increases with dose (Fig. 7.15).

There are two critical cellular targets for radiation: (i) DNA, to cause a double strand break, and (ii) water, the main constituent of living tissues, causing the formation of free radicals in the cell and in the aqueous environment. Both of these events are more likely with high LET radiation. Since irradiation damages DNA, the different phases of the cell cycle have differing sensitivities to the effects of radiation; cells in mitosis die, post-synthetic cells are sensitive but S-phase cells seem to be resistant.

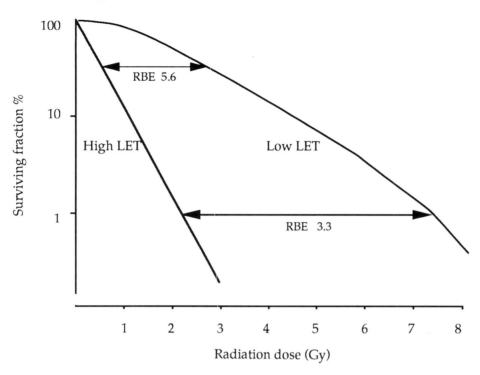

Fig. 7.15 Clonogenic cell survival curves for cultured mammalian tumour cells irradiated with increasing doses of different quality LET (linear energy transfer) beams (diagrammatic). The relative biological efficiency (RBE) decreases with dose. The surviving fraction is measured in a soft agar assay (see Fig. 4.22 and 4.23).

Many malignant cells are in G_0, sometimes as the result of hypoxic conditions in large solid tumours (see Fig. 4.16) and such hypoxic cells are radioresistant. Air, or preferably oxygen alone, 'grabs' electrons, thus making actively proliferating tumour cells more sensitive to the therapy. Oxygen mimetic drugs such as metronidazole and misonidazole are often used to increase radiosensitivity. The relative efficiency of this mode of treatment is the *oxygen enhancement ratio* (OER) which is the ratio of dose required for equivalent cell killing in the absence of O_2 compared with in its presence. Generally speaking, three times as much radiation is required under hypoxic conditions compared to under oxic conditions for the same level of kill (Fig. 7.16). Free radical scavengers can be used to protect normal tissues from radiation, thus glutathione and cysteine render tissues *radioresistant*. These molecules have reactive sulphydryl groups which can repair radicals by reduction:

$$X\cdot + RSH \rightarrow XH + RS\cdot$$
free radical   protector

After a large dose of irradiation most aerobic cells in a tumour will be killed, and the survivors will be the hypoxic fraction. These cells could well be reoxygenated after treatment because the dead cells will be resorbed, leading to tumour shrinkage

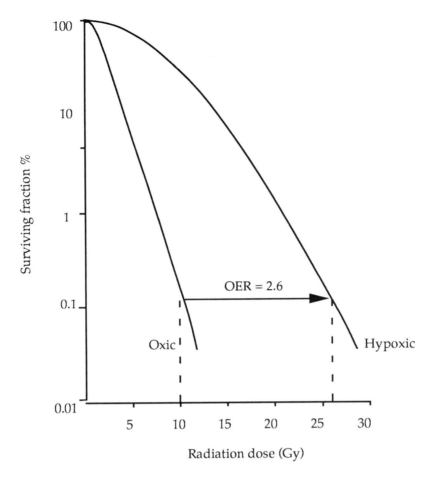

Fig. 7.16 Clonogenic cell survival curves for cultured mammalian tumour cells irradiated with X-rays under either oxic or hypoxic conditions (diagrammatic). The surviving fraction is measured in a soft agar assay (see Fig. 4.22 and 4.23).

and a reduction in intercapillary distances. Therefore effective treatment often involves multiple treatments, so-called *fractionated radiotherapy*, which allows for reoxygenation of hypoxic (radioresistant) cells after each treatment.

Treatment of body surface lesions by radiotherapy is preferentially performed with high LET modalities, α particles or low voltage X-rays which impart all their energy to the top millimetres of the tissue, thus avoiding damage to underlying organs. In contrast, the penetrative properties of low LET radiation are required to treat deep-seated organs. High doses of radiation need to arrive at the tumour site without damaging the overlying tissues and this is achieved by attacking the tumour from several different angles so that the surface dose is divided between different areas of skin and underlying organs. In the future, radiolabelled antibodies may significantly improve radiotherapy and reduce the effects on normal tissues.

The effect of radiation on normal tissues is a significant dose-limiting factor.

Exposure of the skin, whether accidental or during the course of radiotherapy is very important, as quite small doses produce a reaction which is not only uncomfortable but potentially dangerous. Initially the affected epidermis sloughs off, this might be mild as in the case of a sunburn, or a severe desquamation painfully exposing the dermis. When the affected areas are large they present significant exposure to subsequent infection; this and resultant dehydration can become potentially lethal. Cells which are irradiated harbour what is known as 'potential lethal damage'. If post-irradiation conditions suppress cell division then moderate damage only may be repaired and the cells survive. Damage to any particular tissue is dependent upon when the irradiated cells reach mitosis. If the gut is irradiated with 20 Gy, then within four to five days all the epithelial lining cells will be destroyed as all the crypt cells will have died at mitosis, thus failing to replenish the post-mitotic villous cells which have been sloughed off in the normal course of events. An individual with such a high dose of irradiation would suffer from the 'gastrointestinal radiation syndrome', and death due to infection and dehydration would inevitably result. Cell death at mitosis occurs in all heavily irradiated tissues and is therefore clearly linked to the turnover rate of the population. Tissues which have a slow turnover rate, e.g. endothelial cells lining blood vessels, typically suffer from the 'late effects' of irradiation, and it is not unusual for irradiated tissues to suffer oedema many months after irradiation because of the delayed cytotoxic effects on the vasculature.

7.4   Newer approaches to treatment

Anti-tumour antibodies

A major obstacle to the successful treatment of cancer is the inability to selectively destroy metastatic tumour cells by the use of systemic agents. The best way, in theory at least, of localizing a drug to tumour tissue is by using a tumour-specific antibody to carry the drug, this is known as *drug targeting*. A highly tumour-specific antibody linked to a tumouricidal drug would offer a perfect system for drug delivery. The term *magic bullet* was coined to describe the hopeful combination of a successful chemotherapeutic agent with a highly specific antibody to a tumour antigen, and these antigens would be either:

* Histocompatibility antigens.
* Tumour-specific transplantation antigens.
* Viral antigens.
* Tumour-specific differentiation antigens.

These immunotoxins are cell-binding monoclonal antibodies (or their fragments) conjugated to drugs, radionuclides or toxins (e.g. diphtheria toxin, ricin). Unfortunately this type of therapy has encountered many problems, not least the fact that there are very few truly tumour-specific antigens, therefore even using specific antibodies just to image tumours has not met with much success. The heteroconjugates are also somewhat unstable, and loss of antibody specificity can occur through coupling of the antibody to the toxin. In addition most monoclonal antibodies are raised in the mouse and are recognized as 'foreign' by the human patients; this immunogenicity though, can be reduced by constructing 'humanized' monoclonals where the antibody variable domains of the appropriate specificity are ligated to human antibody constant domains. Enzymes which convert drugs to their active metabolites can also be targeted to tumour cells by monoclonal antibodies, an approach known as antibody-directed enzyme prodrug therapy (ADEPT). Once targeting is complete, a prodrug is administered which is metabolized by the targeted enzyme releasing a toxic metabolite in the tumour environment – alkylating agents can be delivered by this means. Anti-tumour antibodies may also be used to recruit complement, which apart from its cell lytic and opsonic effects, also generates anaphylatoxins (C3a and C5a) which increase vascular permeability – this could facilitate the entry of new immunoconjugates to the tumour. The binding of anti-tumour antibodies will also lead to antibody-dependent cell-mediated cytotoxicity (ADCC) with the recruitment of killer, natural killer and cyto-toxic T lymphocytes, and this is likely to be a significant natural event. The therapeutic possibilities of monoclonal antibodies are summarized in Fig. 7.17.

Other possibilities

An alternative to ADEPT is genetic prodrug activation therapy (GPAT). For example, some tumours, notably breast and pancreatic cancers, over-express c-erbB-2, thus a gene construct of the c-*erbB-2* promoter and a gene encoding an enzyme which converts a prodrug into its activated form will be over-expressed in these cells with abundant transcription factors for the c-*erbB-2* promoter region. This approach is being evaluated in pancreatic cell lines using the c-*erbB-2* promoter and the gene

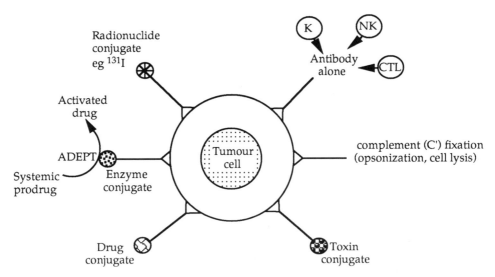

Fig. 7.17 Schematic diagram of the therapeutic potential of monoclonal anti-tumour antibodies. K, killer cell; NK, natural killer cell; CTL, cytotoxic T lymphocyte; ADEPT, antibody-directed enzyme prodrug therapy.

encoding *Herpes simplex* virus- thymidine kinase (HSV-TK), the enzyme which selectively phosphorylates the antiviral agent ganciclovir to a highly cytotoxic form (Fig. 7.18). Gene therapy is a rapidly advancing field and cancer being a 'genetic disease' would seem an obvious candidate. However, there are significant problems unique to cancer besides the general ones of choosing a suitable vectoring system and achieving stable integration for long-term expression. These include the necessity for 'hitting' all the malignant stem cells, and the fact that established cancers have multiple gene defects makes for more complication. However, there may be scope for genetic intervention in cases where a single gene defect exists in the early stages, for example in patients with familial adenomatous polyposis.

Retinoic acid is a vitamin A (retinol) metabolite that can induce differentiation and/ or suppress cell proliferation in malignant cells. As such, retinoids may have a role in the management of malignant disease, and so might inhibitors of enzymes which destabilize the extracellular matrix. Inhibitors of matrix metalloproteinases (e.g. Marimastat) and urokinase plasminogen activator might well impair tumour invasion and metastasis, either directly or indirectly by impeding the process of neovascularization.

The growth factor binding and signalling pathways are obvious candidates for therapeutic manipulation, though perhaps more as palliative measures rather than being curative. Antibodies to growth factors and their receptors are being developed, along with inhibitors to receptor dimerization and tyrosine kinases. Small cell lung cancer

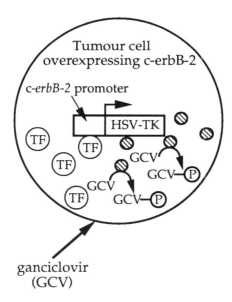

Fig. 7.18 Schematic diagram of genetic prodrug activation therapy (GPAT). A construct of the *c-erbB-2* promoter and the gene encoding Herpes simplex virus thymidine kinase (HSV-TK) introduced into a tumour which over-expresses c-erbB-2 will lead to overexpression of HSV-TK because of the abundance of transcription factors (TFs) for the *c-erbB-2* promoter region. Systemically administered ganciclovir will be preferentially phosphorylated to its cytotoxic derivative in these cells.

is driven by neuropeptides through autocrine loops, notably bombesin, and a variety of bombesin antagonists have been developed which bind the receptor and inhibit growth.

Cytokines produced by recombinant DNA technology have possible benefits. Cells of the immune system undoubtedly play an important role in tumour cell recognition and destruction, so the use of cytokines to stimulate and enhance the natural anti-tumour response is an attractive proposition. So far interleukins IL-2 and IL-4 have been used extensively to stimulate the proliferation and activation of lymphokine activated killer cells (LAKs) and cytotoxic T lymphocytes, whereas interferon-γ may be of use in causing the upregulation of MHC Class I antigens in weakly immunogenic tumours. The direct induction of tumour cell apoptosis is clearly an attractive proposition, and monoclonal antibodies to the Fas antigen will kill cells which express this plasma membrane-located receptor, notably found on many lymphoid malignancies.

Another novel strategy is the use of antisense oligodeoxynucleotides (ODNs), which rely on the ability of an ODN to bind a complementary messenger RNA sequence (the sense molecule) and prevent translation of the mRNA. Antisense therapy is still in its infancy, but obviously the technique is very appealing for the treatment of a number of human diseases, and an obvious target for researchers has been the *bcr/abl* mRNA of chronic myeloid leukaemia (see Fig. 3.3) since the base sequences which code for the mutant protein are not in normal haemopoietic cells. Similar strategies could be employed against any mutant mRNA, including mutated *ras* and *p53*.

Besides all these seemingly sophisticated approaches to improving life expectancy after surgical removal of the primary tumour, in breast cancer patients, survival has been shown to be at least partly dependent upon the time at which surgery was performed. Women operated upon during the first half of the menstrual cycle fare much worse than women operated upon during the second half of their cycle. In the first half of the menstrual cycle oestrogen is being produced unopposed by progesterone, and it is believed that this unopposed oestrogen at the time of tumour handling may promote the establishment and growth of micrometastases.

Often a further complication of chemotherapy is that the profound suppression of bone marrow function often renders the patient highly susceptible to infection because of drug-induced neutropenia. Fortunately this is less of a problem these days with the widespread use of recombinant growth factors (e.g. G-CSF and GM-CSF) to promote neutrophil production. Anaemia is also common in cancer patients and this can be further exacerbated by cytotoxic chemotherapy, so here too a recombinant growth factor, erythropoietin, can be of benefit and can promote erythropoiesis to correct the anaemia.

In conclusion, the coming of age of molecular biology in the last 15 years has provided a quantum leap in our understanding of the natural history of cancer, and mankind will soon fully understand the genetic mechanisms underlying this complex disease of multifactorial origin. The new knowledge will certainly aid in the development of agents which impede growth factor-mediated signalling pathways, increase the selectivity of cytolethal compounds, and significantly lessen the toxic effects on normal renewal tissues which are often such a constraining influence on treatment regimes. All these developments will improve the quality of life and life expectancy of patients with cancer, but it is still undeniable that the most dramatic improvements in the foreseeable future will come from the abstinence of habits known to cause irreversible changes in the cell genome – mutations in critical growth regulatory genes – combined with improvements in the early detection of cancer to reduce the likelihood of metastatic disease.

7.5   Further reading

Deonarain, M. P. & Epenetos, A. A. (1994). Targeting enzymes for cancer therapy: old enzymes in new roles. *British Journal of Cancer*, **70**, 786–94.

Dorr, R. T. & Von Hoff, D. D. (1994). *Cancer Chemotherapy Handbook*, 2nd edn. East Norwalk, Conn: Appleton & Lange.

Fisher, D. E. (1994). Apoptosis in cancer therapy: crossing the threshold. *Cell*, **78**, 539–42.

Harrisson, D. J. (1995). Molecular mechanisms of drug resistance in tumours. *Journal of Pathology*, **175**, 7–12.

Haskell, C. M. (1995). *Cancer Treatment*, 4th edn. Philadelphia: W. B. Saunders.

Pinedo, H. M., Longo, D. L. & Chabner, B. A. (1991). *Cancer Chemotherapy and Biological Response Modifiers Annual 12*. Amsterdam: Elsevier.

Priestman, T. J. (1993). *Cancer Chemotherapy: An Introduction*, 3rd edn. London: Springer-Verlag.

Steel, G. G. (1993). *Basic Clinical Radiobiology*. London: Edward Arnold.

Wagner, W, (1994). Gene inhibition using antisense oligodeoxynucleotides. *Nature*, **372**, 333–5.

Warr, J. R. & Atkinson, G. F. (1986). Genetic aspects of resistance to anticancer drugs. *Physiological Reviews*, 68, 1–26.

Whartenby, K. A., Abboud, C. N., Marrogi, A. J., Ramesh, R. & Freeman, S. M. (1995). The biology of cancer gene therapy. *Laboratory Investigation*, 72, 131–45.

Glossary

α-actinin   linking protein between cytoplasmic microfilaments and actin-binding proteins of the plasma membrane.

actin   cytoskeletal protein, member of a family represented in all cell types. In cells of grossly non-contractile tissues it is a microfilament ~ 5 nm in diameter particularly associated with the sub-plasma membrane and perinuclear web; in muscle it is localized in the I band of myofibrils and when acting with myosin is responsible for the contraction and relaxation of muscle.

actinomycin-D   (dactinomycin), antibiotic; member of a family of antibiotics from various species of *Streptomyces* used as anti-cancer drugs, can cause local DNA unwinding through intercalation, and also form tight adducts with DNA and thus block transcription; also generates free radicals.

ADCC   *see* antibody-dependent cellular cytotoxicity.

adduct   product of a reaction of association between molecules, e.g. carcinogenic agent and DNA base.

adeno   *prefix* (Gr.) gland.

adenocarcinoma   malignant tumour of glandular epithelium: when well differentiated, tumour cells form recognizable glandular structures.

adenoma   benign tumour of glandular epithelium.

adenoma-carcinoma sequence   disease continuum starting with (sometimes multiple) adenomas; a stepwise accumulation of genetic errors occurs. One mutation in one cell of the adenoma confers a proliferative advantage on this cell and its progeny; a further mutation in one of these cells once more confers a further advantage and so on, until the frankly malignant phenotype emerges.

ADEPT   *see* antibody-directed enzyme prodrug therapy.

adipose   of fat.

adjuvant therapy   cancer therapy regime in which there is a combination of modalities; e.g. surgery supplemented with chemotherapy.

adriamycin®   anti-tumour antibiotic based on doxorubicin hydrochloride, can cause local DNA unwinding through intercalation, and by forming tight adducts with DNA can block transcription; also generates free radicals.

aetiology   assignment of a cause, science of the causes of disease.

aflatoxin   toxin $C_{17}H_{12}O_6$, produced by the fungus *Aspergillus flavus*, commonly a contaminant of stored ground nut seeds in producing countries, implicated in the initiation of hepatocellular carcinoma.

AFP   *see* alphafoetoprotein.

AIDS   acquired immunodeficiency syndrome that emerged in the 1980s as a novel and epidemic form of immunodeficiency disease resultant from defective cell-mediated defence. It was initially associated with young, previously fit homosexual men, then more fully acknowledged in the wider heterosexual population, particularly in parts of Africa.

albumin any protein of the class that dissolves in water without the addition of salt and, unlike a globulin, stays in solution on half saturation with ammonium sulphate. Protein of egg whites.

alkylating agent cancer chemotherapeutic agent that causes the substitution of an alkyl (usually ethyl or methyl) group for an active hydrogen atom in an organic compound such as a DNA base, causing inter- and intrastrand DNA cross-links and cross-links with other macromolecules, e.g. nitrogen mustards, melphalan, chlorambucil.

allele one of two or more alternative forms of a gene at corresponding sites (loci) on homologous chromosomes, which determine the inheritance of alternative characteristics.

alphafoetoprotein (AFP), protein produced by foetal liver, yolk sac and gastrointestinal tract. Also associated with hepatocellular carcinoma and germ cell neoplasms in adults; expressed by regenerating hepatocytes.

alpha particle (α^{2+}), positively charged particle with atomic mass of 4 and charge of 2^+; composed of 2 protons + 2 neutrons.

alpha radiation stream of alpha particles, comparatively low energy and high energy transfer.

Ames test bacterial mutagenicity test; a strain of *Salmonella typhimurium* that lacks the enzyme necessary for histidine synthesis is cultured in the absence of histidine and in the presence of the suspected mutagen. If the substance causes DNA damage resulting in appropriate mutations (i.e. is mutagenic) some of the bacteria will regain the ability to synthesize histidine and will proliferate to form colonies.

amine organic compound containing nitrogen – aromatic compound with a resonance-stabilized ring or aliphatic straight chain compound.

amplification compartment compartment of continuously renewing epithelial tissues, between stem cell compartment and maturation compartment, where a limited number of cell divisions occurs increasing the overall number of cells.

anaphase third phase of mitosis in which one set of the newly synthesized chromosomes separates from the other on the metaphase plate and each set begins to draw away from the other; preceded by metaphase and followed by telophase.

anaphylatoxin substance produced in blood serum during complement fixation, which serves as a mediator of inflammation by inducing mast cell degranulation and histamine release; when injected causes anaphylactic shock.

anaplastic tumours those which have no recognizable differentiated features; disrupted orientation of cells towards each other and also in their normal polarity with respect to blood supply.

aneuploid a cell whose DNA content is an inexact multiple of the normal (diploid) content, common in malignant tumours.

angiogenesis new development of blood vessels, seen in the embryo, wound healing and tumour expansion.

angiography X-ray examination of blood vessels after introduction of a contrast medium.

angiosarcoma malignant tumour of vascular endothelial cells.

aniline dyes bladder carcinogens. Colorants from coal tar and indigo or alternatively prepared by reducing nitrobenzene; also cause bone marrow cell depression and haemoglobinaemia.

anoxia absence of oxygen supply to tissues, despite adequate overall blood perfusion.

anthracyclins anti-cancer antibiotics (rhodomycins), cause local DNA unwinding through intercalation and promote DNA fragmentation by inhibiting topoisomerase II activation; also generate free radicals, e.g. daunorubicin and doxorubicin (adriamycin).

antibiotics *see* anti-tumour antibiotics.

antibody immunoglobulin molecule that recognizes a specific antigen. *In vivo* produced by plasma cells (activated B lymphocytes) in immune system defensive strategy. Laboratory or industrially produced from appropriate hybridomas; used extensively as tools to demonstrate localization of antigens. *See* immunocytochemistry, monoclonal antibody, polyclonal antibody.

antibody-dependent cell-mediated cytotoxicity   (ADCC), a natural event leading to recruitment of T lymphocytes.

antibody-directed enzyme prodrug therapy   (ADEPT), anti-cancer therapy in which an enzyme is delivered to a tumour by being linked to a tumour-specific antibody. The patient is then treated with an inactive prodrug. Only the prodrug in the vicinity of the tumour/enzyme can be metabolized into the active agent.

antibody-guided chemotherapy   anti-cancer therapy in which a chemotherapeutic agent is directed specifically at a tumour with the aid of antibody recognizing specific tumour antigen.

antibody variable domain   variable portion of immunoglobulin molecule, gene-directed variation, enabling vast numbers of antibodies to be produced each recognizing a specific antigen.

antigen   a substance capable of inducing a specific immune response and of reacting with the products of the response, such as specific antibody, specifically sensitized T cells or both. In immunocytochemistry, the target of the exploratory antibody.

antimetabolite   cancer chemotherapeutic agent; can be analogues of DNA precursors which exert their effects by replacing the normal substrate and thus blocking nucleic acid synthesis, e.g. Ara-C. Alternatively, antimetabolites may bind to vital enzymes thus inhibiting their functions, e.g. methotrexate, 5-fluorouracil.

anti-oncogene   alternative name for a tumour suppressor gene, the loss or mutation of which is involved in neoplastic development.

anti-PCNA   antibody to proliferating cell nuclear antigen, used as a proliferation marker of the late G_1 to M fraction of cycling cells.

antisense oligodeoxynucleotides   (ODN), short synthetic nucleotide sequences made to be complementary to specific RNA sequences. Therapeutic strategy to prevent translation of mRNA into proteins that promote tumour growth.

anti-tumour antibiotics   cancer chemotherapeutic agents, frequently rhodomycins derived from *Streptomyces* species; cause local DNA unwinding through intercalation and by forming tight adducts with DNA; can also block transcription, e.g. bleomycin, anthracyclins such as daunorubicin and doxorubicin (adriamycin).

AP-1   (activator protein-1), transcription factor commonly a heterodimer of protein products of c-*fos* and c-*jun*. Confers tetradecanoylphorbol acetate (TPA) inducibility: heterodimers join by leucine zipper domain.

APC   (adenomatous polyposis coli), tumour suppressor gene, often mutated or lost in familial and sporadic colorectal cancer; protein product forms cytoplasmic complex with α- and β-catenins.

APO-1/Fas antigen   (CD95), cell surface antigen which when stimulated mediates apoptosis in some tissues, particularly lymphoid tissues although mRNA is also found in heart, lung, liver and ovary.

apopain   cleavage product of CPP32, itself cleaving poly(ADP-ribose) polymerase (PARP) which is active in apoptosis.

apoptosis   gene-directed mechanism of active cell death particularly associated with tissue sculpting in the embryo and tissue cell population size control in the adult. Important mechanism both in tumour behaviour and tumour therapy.

Ara-C   *see* cytosine arabinoside.

aromatic hydrocarbon   organic compound with a resonance-stabilized ring structure, e.g. benzene, naphthalene.

asbestos   fibrous incombustible magnesium and calcium silicate widely used for its insulating properties but implicated in industrially associated lung diseases.

Aspergillus flavus species of fungus (mould) that can be an opportunistic endoparasite of humans. Common contaminant of stored ground nuts.

astrocytoma tumour of astrocytes, neuroglial cells of ectodermal origin.

ataxia telangiectasia severe hereditary progressive failure of muscle co-ordination, transmitted as an autosomal recessive trait possibly leading to malignancy through defective DNA repair.

bak member of the large *bcl-2* family of related genes that regulate apoptosis, including *bax*, *bcl-x* and *ced-9*.

basal cell carcinoma (rodent ulcer), epithelial cell-derived malignant neoplasm of the skin, usually locally invasive but rarely metastasizing.

basement membrane extracellular matrix upon which all epithelial cells reside, and to which they have specific orientation and polarity, synthesized jointly by epithelial cells and underlying connective tissue cells. Typically composed principally of type IV collagen, laminin, fibronectin and heparan sulphate proteoglycans.

bax member of the large *bcl-2* family of related genes that regulate apoptosis, including *bcl-x*, *bak* and *ced-9*.

B-cell clone B lymphocyte expansion after antigen stimulation of the single B cell that fortuitously produces the most avid binding antibody to the antigen under consideration.

bcl-2 oncogene originally described from B cell lymphoma, prevents cell death by apoptosis. Chromosomal translocation t(14;18) translocates the gene from chromosome 18, and juxtaposes it to the actively transcribed immunoglobulin heavy chain junctional locus on chromosome 14, resulting in increased *bcl-2* expression. Member of a large family of related regulators of apoptosis including *bax*, *bcl-x*, *bak* and *ced-9*.

bcl-x member of the large *bcl-2* family of related genes that regulate apoptosis, including *bax*, *bak* and *ced-9*.

bcr (breakpoint cluster region), associated with chronic myeloid leukaemia. In this condition breaks on chromosome 22 are restricted to a relatively small region of DNA of 5–6 kilo base pairs giving rise to the region's specific nomenclature. *See c-abl.*

benign tumour non-malignant neoplasm; non-invasive, non-metastasizing, increasing in size locally. New growth is confined within normal tissue boundaries; not generally life-threatening unless arising within a confined space, e.g. skull.

benzo(*a*)pyrene active carcinogenic constituent of coal tar; polycyclic hydrocarbon which covalently binds to cellular macromolecules including DNA, the extent of binding correlates with carcinogenic potential.

beta particle (β^-), subatomic particle, electron, of negligible atomic weight but negative charge equal but opposite in sign to that of a proton.

betel evergreen plant of which nut and/or leaf might be chewed, retaining the pellet in the mouth for extended periods of time; associated with carcinogenesis in buccal epithelia.

BHRF 1 Epstein-Barr virus-encoded protein, homologue of Bcl-2; both proteins abrogate apoptosis.

biopsy removal of tissue, from the living body, for examination and disease status determination.

bleomycin polypeptide anti-tumour antibiotic, can cause local DNA unwinding through intercalation; forms tight adducts with DNA which block transcription and also generates free radicals. Action inhibited by the removal of oxygen.

Bloom's syndrome a rare hereditary disorder characterized by stunted growth and facial erythema. Cancer-prone condition thought to involve defects in the BLM protein – a helicase responsible for the separation of the two DNA strands during replication. There is a strong tendency to develop leukaemia in the second and third decades of life.

bombesin neuropeptide growth factor, produced by the cells of small cell lung carcinoma, which augments tumour growth in an autocrine manner.

Bowen's disease   skin condition which can develop full thickness epidermal dysplasia (carcinoma *in situ*).

BRCA1   tumour suppressor gene which, when mutated, is implicated in the development of cancers of the breast and of the ovary, located on chromosome 17q. The protein product has a zinc finger, which may indicate a function in transcription.

BRCA2   tumour suppressor gene which, when mutated, is implicated in the development of cancers of the breast (particularly in the male) and of the ovary, located on chromosome 13q.

bromodeoxyuridine   methylated synthetic analogue of the DNA nucleoside thymidine. In cell proliferation studies, if bromodeoxyuridine is supplied in place of thymidine in the nucleoside pool, DNA synthesizing cells will incorporate it into DNA. It can then be localized as the antigen by immunocytochemistry with an anti-bromodeoxyuridine antibody.

Burkitt's lymphoma   malignancy of lymphatic tissue with usually insignificant lymph node involvement, e.g. jaws, orbit, abdominal viscera and ovaries; the cells have basophilic cytoplasm and contain lipid filled vacuoles. The tumour is endemic to Africa and further warm-to-temperate climates, and is closely associated with the Epstein Barr virus and stability of falciparum malaria.

c-*abl*   proto-oncogene translocated from chromosome 9, in chronic myeloid leukaemia, to the breakpoint cluster region (*bcr*) of chromosome 22; gene product has constitutive tyrosine kinase activity.

cachexia   catabolic clinical state caused by a combination of endocrine, metabolic and immunological disturbances resulting from tumour-host interactions.

cadherin   calcium-dependent family of transmembrane cell–cell adhesion molecules.

calcitonin   polypeptide hormone secreted by C cells of thyroid gland (and also thymus and parathyroids to some extent); lowers calcium and phosphate concentration in plasma and inhibits bone resorption.

calpain   calcium activated protease.

cancer   day-to-day term for disease caused by presence of a malignant tumour.

capsule   (as in tumour capsule) fibrous/membranous/cellular structure covering the tumour, which presents a well-defined boundary between normal tissue and tumour tissue; characteristic of benign tumours.

carcinoembryonic antigen   (CEA), oncofoetal glycoprotein; antigen associated with colonic adenocarcinoma and other carcinomas of endodermal origin, although also expressed at other (and normal) sites. Member of the IgG superfamily of cell adhesion molecules.

carcinogen   a substance which causes cancer.

carcinogenesis   process of cancer development.

carcinoid tumour   tumours with a 'carcinoma-like' (i.e. sheets of cells) structure, arising from cells of the diffuse neuroendocrine system which may produce and release serotonin (5-hydroxytryptamine), kallikrein, somatostatin, glucagon, gastrin or other hormones of this nature.

carcinoma   malignant tumour of epithelial tissue, characterized by nests or cords of cells in close proximity to blood vessels, separated from each other by stromal elements.

catalase   enzyme present in all aerobic tissues in which there is catalysis of hydrogen peroxide into water and molecular oxygen. Its activity does not depend on an oxygen acceptor, and thus is a protective mechanism acting as a free radical scavenging system.

Cdk   *see* cyclin-dependent kinase.

CEA   *see* carcinoembryonic antigen.

ced-3   cell death modulator related to genes coding for mammalian CPP32 and ICE. The protein product is a member of the family of cysteine proteases that instigate apoptosis. Described in the nematode *Caenorhabditis elegans*.

ced-4 cell death modulator that instigates apoptosis. First described in the nematode *Caenorhabditis elegans*.

ced-9 cell survival modulator, member of the large *bcl-2* family of related genes that regulate apoptosis, including *bax*, *bak* and *bcl-x*. First described in the nematode *Caenorhabditis elegans*.

cell adhesion molecules (CAMs), e.g. selectins, integrins, immunoglobulin-related adhesion molecules and cadherins that specifically mediate cell–cell and cell–matrix adhesions.

cell birth rate (K_B), rate at which new cells are born, usually expressed as cells born/100 cells/hr.

cell loss factor (ϕ), cell loss expressed as a fraction of the cell birth rate: $\phi = K_L/K_B$; also $\phi = 1 - t_{PD}/t_D$ (t_{PD}, potential doubling time; t_D, actual doubling time).

cell loss rate (K_L), difference between the cell birth rate and the tumour growth rate.

cell progeny cells deriving from a common ancestor.

cellular atypia morphological abnormalities at a cellular level; considered relevant to neoplastic development.

c-erbA proto-oncogene encoding the thyroid hormone receptor. Name from chicken erythroblastosis – erythroid leukaemia.

c-erbB-1 proto-oncogene coding for the normal epidermal growth factor receptor (EGFR): amplified in squamous carcinomas, breast, lung and bladder cancers. Name derived from chicken erythroblastosis – erythroid leukaemia.

c-erbB-2 proto-oncogene related to c-*erbB-1*; particularly over-expressed in aggressive breast cancer; corresponds to the rat gene *neu*.

cervical intra-epithelial neoplasia (CIN), grading system used for dysplastic changes in the uterine cervix.

c-fms proto-oncogene and cellular homologue of the transforming gene v-*fms* of feline sarcoma virus; it encodes the receptor for macrophage-colony stimulating factor (M-CSF).

c-fos proto-oncogene and cellular homologue of transforming gene v-*fos*, present in the genome of the FBT (mouse osteosarcoma), FBJ or FBR murine sarcoma viruses. Product is a 55 kDa protein which with the product of the c-*jun* gene forms a DNA binding complex.

CFU-S *see* colony forming units in the spleen.

chalone hypothesis largely outmoded theory which stated that through a negative feedback mechanism, differentiated cells produced an inhibitory humoral molecule (chalone) which would prevent cell proliferation. Chalone concentration would be reduced after damage and reduction in number of differentiated cells, releasing proliferation control until the full complement of mature cells was re-instated, thus full concentration of chalone once more.

chemotherapy treatment of disease by chemical agents, particularly cancer chemotherapy – i.e. treatment of tumours by specific drugs, often those that prevent generalized cell proliferation.

chicken erythroblastosis form of chicken red cell precursor leukaemia, caused by virus carrying the v-*erb* gene (erythroblastosis).

chlorambucil nitrogen mustard derivative, causes substitution of an alkyl group for an active hydrogen atom in an organic compound such as a DNA base, resulting in inter- and intrastrand DNA cross-links and cross-links with other macromolecules.

cholangiocarcinoma malignant tumour of bile duct cells.

chondroma benign tumour of cartilage.

chondrosarcoma malignant tumour of cartilage.

chromogranin non-hormonal acidic glycoprotein associated with hormone storage in secretory granules, and calcium homeostasis in endocrine cells and endocrine neoplasms.

chromosomal translocation change of location of a gene either on the same chromosome or to a different chromosome; when aberrant can cause proximity of genes that influence each other with overall deleterious effect.

chronic atrophic gastritis   chronic stomach damage involving the loss of specialized glands in the deeper zone of the body mucosa; followed by regenerative hyperplasia and possibly intestinal metaplasia.

chronic myeloid leukaemia   (CML), malignant disease of granular leukocytes

cirrhosis   (Gr. tawny), end-stage liver disease characterized by permanent fibrosis and regenerative nodules.

c-*jun*   proto-oncogene whose product complexes with that of c-*fos* to form transcription activator protein (AP-1) and confers tetradecanoylphorbol acetate (TPA) inducibility. The protein product forms a heterodimer with Fos *via* a leucine zipper domain.

CKI genes   genes encoding proteins, e.g. p21^{Cip1}, p15^{Ink4B}, p16^{Ink4A}, p27^{Kip1} (named according to their molecular weights), which are inhibitors of cyclin-Cdk complexes.

c-*kit* ligand   *see* stem cell factor (SCF).

Clark's levels   assessment of depth of invasion of a malignant melanoma of the skin. Level 1: confined to epidermis; level 2: invasion into papillary dermis; level 3: reaching junction of papillary and reticular dermis; level 4: extension into reticular dermis; and level 5: extending subcutaneously. Useful as a prognostic indicator.

clonal derivation   arising from successive mitotic divisions of a single cell.

clonogenic assay   assay to determine the proportion of tumour cells capable of producing a macroscopically visible clone of cells either *in vitro* or *in vivo*.

Clonorchis sinensis   liver fluke; parasite of humans associated with the development of cholangiocarcinoma.

c-*mos*   proto-oncogene associated with virus induced mouse sarcomas, encoding a protein kinase which phosphorylates serine and threonine residues on substrate proteins.

c-*myb*   proto-oncogene encoding a DNA-binding protein; viral homologue v-*myb* responsible for avian myeloblastosis.

c-*myc*   proto-oncogene whose protein product, Myc, is a DNA-binding molecule, implicated in growth control; has short half life ~20 minutes. Myc normally forms heterodimers with Max to act as a transcription factor: over-expressed in breast and stomach cancers as well as Burkitt's lymphoma. Name from chicken myelocytoma.

c-N-*ras*   proto-oncogene, whose mutated form is associated with neuroblastoma. *See ras* proto-oncogene family.

colcemid   cancer chemotherapeutic agent, derivative of colchicine, blocking cells in metaphase of mitosis because it disrupts mitotic spindle formation, results in death of arrested cells.

colchicine   a naturally occurring alkaloid from the plant *Colchicum autumnale* used as a cancer chemotherapeutic agent; *see* colcemid.

colectomy   resection of part or all of the large intestine.

collagen   general term for a family of strong, fibrous proteins of connective tissue. There are different types of collagen in which the overall chemical constitution varies.

collagenase   enzyme that permits the hydrolysis of collagen.

colony forming units   (CFU-S, CFU-L), a method of assessment of survival of tumour stem cells, particularly from leukaemias and lymphomas, in the spleen and lung respectively.

colony stimulating factors   (CSFs), cytokine glycoproteins produced by several cell types including macrophages, fibroblasts and endothelial cells in response to stimulation, including by TNFα and IFNγ. Growth factors for granulocytes (G-CSF), and macrophages (M-CSF).

colorectum   colon and rectum of the gastrointestinal system.

combination therapy   cancer chemotherapy with simultaneous use of a variety ('cocktail') of anti-cancer drugs.

computer-assisted axial tomography   (CT scan), radiograph composed of information from numerous small X-ray beams digitally integrated to form the final image.

c-*onc* gene   proto-oncogene; a normal cellular gene which when mutated or over-expressed can promote neoplastic development. c-*onc* genes are the probable ancestors of viral oncogenes to which they have close DNA sequence homology; origin of the viral oncogene probably results from previous capture of the cellular gene by the virus.

conditional renewal populations   tissue in which there is a stable cell population, but where cell proliferation can occur, for example in response to injury, e.g. liver after partial resection.

conformal therapy   radiotherapy geometrically tailored to maximize dose at the deep target tissue *only*, with the aid of precise information provided by 3-dimensional tomographic data sets.

contact inhibition   in culture, normal cell proliferation proceeds when the cell density is low; when this increases to a stage where the cells touch each other (are in contact) proliferation spontaneously ceases. This is not the case for malignant or transformed cells which ignore the inhibitory effects of cell–cell contact.

continually renewing system   tissue hierarchy in which there is constant cell turnover and renewal, e.g. skin, bone marrow, gastrointestinal tract.

CPP-32   32 kDa cysteine protease which resembles ICE. Cleaved to apopain which then cleaves PARP (poly(ADP-ribose) polymerase) in the process of apoptosis.

c-*raf*   proto-oncogene whose protein product is activated by tyrosine phosphorylation under the influence of Src, the activated protein kinase (MAPKKK) phosphorylates serine and threonine residues on substrate proteins

CREB   (cAMP response element binding protein), a transcription factor.

CrmA   protein product of the cowpox virus cytokine response modifier gene. Activity prevents neuronal cell death in culture upon removal of nerve growth factor (NGF).

cross-linking fixative   fixative solutions for routine histological tissue preservation, e.g. formaldehyde, glutaraldehyde.

CSF   *see* colony stimulating factor.

c-*src*   family of proto-oncogenes (sarcoma-related) which code for related 55–60 kDa non-receptor protein tyrosine kinases, e.g. pp60$^{c\text{-}src}$.

Cushing's syndrome   hypersecretion of corticosteroid hormones associated with adrenocortical hyperfunction including that due to the development of adenoma or carcinoma. Symptoms include: truncal obesity, muscular wasting, hirsutism, hypertension, weakness and emotional disturbance.

cyclin   family of regulatory molecules which act at specific points of the cell cycle and govern the progression of cell replication.

cyclin-dependent kinase   (Cdk), catalytic subunit of the cyclin/Cdk complex, which phosphorylates molecules fundamental to a cell's transition from stage to stage of the cell cycle.

cyclophosphamide   anti-tumour chemotherapeutic alkylating agent activated by cytochrome P450 enzyme system, frequently used in the treatment of lymphomas and leukaemias, bronchial, breast and ovarian carcinomas.

cyproterone acetate   steroid synthetic analogue, progestogenic anti-androgen. Decreases testosterone synthesis by inhibiting secretion of pituitary gonadotrophins. It also displaces and competes with dihydrotestosterone for its cytoplasmic and nuclear receptors.

cysteine   sulphur-containing amino acid used in its capacity of free radical scavenger to protect normal tissue during radiotherapy.

cytochrome P450-dependent mono-oxygenase system   energy-dependent oxidative reaction important in the metabolism of carcinogens. P450 defines the absorption wavelength of the cytochrome involved, which is an iron containing, electron accepting molecule that mediates oxidation-reduction reactions.

cytogenetics   study of chromosomal abnormalities and their relationship to pathological conditions.

cytokeratins   family of proteinaceous intermediate filaments characteristic of epithelial cells. There are two major categories: Type I (acidic) and Type II (basic), all having an alpha helical backbone. The members differ from each other in variable regions located at the head and tail of each molecule.

cytokines   generally low molecular weight glycoproteins including CSFs, interleukins, EPO, TNF and interferons (produced largely by lymphocytes, monocytes and macrophages); locally acting hormones involved in the regulation of cellular responses.

cytokine therapy   cancer chemotherapy with the aid of cytokines such as interferon.

cytology   the study of isolated cells (as opposed to tissues), their origin, structure, function and pathology.

cytosine arabinoside   (Ara-C), antimetabolite, cancer chemotherapeutic agent active in the S phase of the cell cycle; analogue of deoxycytidine. It is actively taken up and converted by a succession of phosphorylation steps to the triphosphate whose incorporation into DNA produces termination of the nascent DNA strand.

cytoskeleton   structural component of cellular cytoplasm consisting of microfilaments and intermediate filaments (beneath the plasma membrane and of the cytoplasmic web), and of microtubules.

cytosol   liquid medium of the cytoplasm which surrounds organelles and non-membranous insoluble components.

cytotoxic   poisonous to cells.

DAG   *see* diacylglycerol.

DCC   tumour suppressor gene often mutated or deleted in colorectal carcinoma and other tumours, codes for a transmembrane cell adhesion molecule (CAM) related to neural cell adhesion molecules (N-CAMs).

delayed hypersensitivity   a slowly developing increase of cell-mediated (T lymphocyte) immune response to a specific antigen, e.g. in heterologous graft rejection.

dense core granules   intracellular endocrine granules containing polypeptide hormones – electron dense thus giving rise to the name.

desmin   intermediate filament of adult smooth muscle, cardiac muscle and skeletal muscle.

desmoplasia   the promotion of connective tissue synthesis by adjacent tumour cells, probably by growth factors, prominent around basal cell carcinoma.

desmosome   cell surface adaptation to form focal site of attachment between adjacent epithelial cell membranes, analogous to 'rivets'; providing structural strength to the union of cells through the tissue. Readily identifiable as face-to-face adherent plaques, with tonofilaments and associated cell adhesion molecules inserted from the body of each contributing cell.

desquamation   shedding of epithelial cells, often applied to epidermis.

DHFR   *see* dihydrofolate reductase.

diacylglycerol   (DAG), activator of protein kinase C. When a growth factor binds at the plasma membrane it stimulates phospholipase C-γ1 (PLC-γ1), which hydrolyses phosphatidyl inositol 4,5-bisphosphate to DAG plus inositol trisphosphate.

diagnosis   determination of the nature of a disease.

diethylstilboestrol   synthetic non-steroidal oestrogenic agent, used to relieve vasomotor symptoms associated with oestrogen dependent conditions. Palliative treatment for breast carcinoma and prostatic cancer.

differentiation   progressive diversification of embryonic/stem cell progeny to post-mitotic fully mature, often terminal forms.

dihydrofolate reductase   (DHFR), enzyme through binding of which methotrexate exerts its cytotoxicity, responsible for the conversion of dihydrofolate to tetrahydrofolate.

dimethylhydrazine   nitrogenous compound (hydrazine) metabolized to the active carcinogen methyl diazonium hydroxide; known to cause tumours in rodent lung, liver, kidney and intestine.

DNase   enzyme with the ability to cleave DNA.

DP   forms a heterodimeric transcription factor composed of one E2F and one DP chain, bound to by the p105^{Rb} nucleoprotein (product of the tumour suppressor gene, *Rb*); it has an important role in control of progression from G_1 phase to S in the cell cycle.

DPC4   gene located on chromosome 18q which is commonly homozygously deleted or one allele is missing and one is mutated in pancreatic cancer. The *DPC4* gene has sequence similarity with *Drosophila mad* gene (<u>m</u>others <u>a</u>gainst <u>d</u>pp). In *Drosophila, mad* mutants have similar phenotype to *dpp* mutants. DPC4 protein may be involved in TGFβ mediated growth suppression.

dpp   decapentaplegic gene of *Drosophila*, which encodes a member of the TGFβ superfamily; *dpp* mutants have similar phenotype to *mad* mutants.

ductal carcinoma *in situ* (DCIS)   preinvasive condition of the breast in which malignant cells are still confined to ducts.

Dukes' classification   assessment of the clinico-pathological stage of colorectal carcinoma according to microscopic examination of extent of tumour invasion through the surrounding tissue, and local node involvement, useful as a prognostic indicator.

dysplasia   alterations in size, shape and organization of cells, common antecedents of neoplasia.

dysplasia-carcinoma sequence   identification of a phenotypic progression from normal cells through dysplasia to frank malignancy as seen, for example, in the development of colorectal carcinoma.

E1A   oncoprotein of adenovirus which when complexed with pRb inactivates its function.

E1B   oncoprotein of adenovirus that binds to and inactivates p53 protein.

E2F   forms a heterodimeric transcription factor composed of one E2F and one DP chain, bound to by the pRb nucleoprotein (product of the tumour suppressor gene, *Rb*); it has an important role in control of progression from G_1 phase to S in the cell cycle.

E6   oncoprotein of human papillomavirus (HPV) that binds to and inactivates p53 protein.

E7   oncoprotein of human papillomavirus which when complexed with pRb inactivates its function.

ectopic hormone production   production of hormone by tissue not normally credited with producing that hormone, e.g. ACTH produced by oat cell carcinomas of the lung.

EGFR   *see* epidermal growth factor receptor.

elastin   yellow scleroprotein, essential component of elastic connective tissue; brittle when dry but flexible and elastic *in vivo*.

electromagnetic radiation   non-particulate energy transfer, by radiation travelling in electric and magnetic fields; including the whole spectrum of X-, gamma and ultraviolet radiation, visible light and infra-red radiation.

electron   negatively charged subatomic particle – beta (β⁻) arranged in shells of specific numbers around the atomic nucleus.

electron microscope   microscope producing high energy electrons to illuminate a specimen in a specially designed vacuum chamber. Capable of high quality resolution, thus high order of magnification.

electron microscopy   high resolution observation of specimens when they are illuminated by electron bombardment in a vacuum. Images can be produced: directly by the electrons impinging on a fluorescent screen, for photography when directed on to a photographic negative and/or for TV monitor viewing.

electrophoresis   the movement of charged particles, suspended in a liquid, gel or porous medium, under the influence of an electric field.

embolism   the process in which matter, called an embolus (e.g. thrombus, clumps of tumour cells, bacteria or fat cells; or gas) gets impacted in the vascular system.

embolization   the process or condition of becoming an embolus. In metastasis tumour cell emboli may colonize distant sites.

embryology   the science of development of the body from the fertilized egg to infant.

endocrine   secreting internally; endocrine glands secrete hormones directly into the blood system or intercellular fluid. Chemical messengers of the diffuse neuroendocrine system have their target cells at (more or less) distant locations.

endocrine system   system of glands and diffuse specialized groups of cells (diffuse neuroen-docrine system – DNES), that synthesize hormones to be released directly into the blood stream and then produce their effect on distant target cells and organs.

endometrium   epithelial lining of the uterus.

endothelium   single layer of flattened specialized epithelial cells that lines the vascular and lymphatic vessels.

endotoxin   heat-stable, lipopolysaccharide toxic bacterial products; pyogenic and augment endothelial permeability.

enhancer sequences   regulatory sequences of DNA which can be located either $5'$ or $3'$ to a transcriptional start site – binding sites for transcription factors.

env   one of the three essential genes of retroviruses. *env* encodes the envelope spike glyco-protein responsible for target cell specificity. The other two genes are *gag* and *pol*.

enzymatic reaction   chemical reaction enabled by the presence and participation of a specific enzyme, which itself is unaltered by the change that it facilitates.

enzyme   polypeptide biological catalyst whose activity neither alters nor degrades itself. Potentiates and/or accelerates chemical reactions with its specific substrate.

ependymoma   usually benign tumour of differentiated ependymal (glial) cells.

epidemiology   the study of the relationships of disparate factors that determine the frequency and distribution of occurrence of disease through the general population.

epidermal growth factor   (EGF), polypeptide growth factor originally described for its mitog-enic stimulation of epidermal tissues, but now recognized to be of widespread significance in many tissues, particularly as a pan mitogen.

epidermal growth factor receptor   (EGFR), transmembrane receptor which is recognized by both epidermal growth factor and transforming growth factor alpha; the extracellular por-tion of the molecule binds the growth factor ligand while the intracellular portion initiates transduction of the growth factor's effect.

epipodophyllotoxins   family of mandrake plant root-derived cancer chemotherapeutic agents; prevent topoisomerase II breakage reunion activity in DNA, e.g. VP-16 and VM-26.

epithelium   major category of body tissues; formative tissue of some organs (e.g. glands, liver) and covering tissue of internal and external body surfaces – body's first line of defence against the outside world; as such most tumours (~90%) arise from such tissue.

epitope   antigenic determinant of a known structure – the portion that is recognized by a specific antibody.

EPO   *see* erythropoietin.

epoxide   derivative of a ring structured (i.e. aromatic) organic molecule in which an oxygen molecule forms a bridge across an opened double bond between two carbon atoms. Such a metabolite can react with DNA after polycyclic hydrocarbon metabolism.

epoxide hydrase   enzyme which acts on an epoxide substrate by breaking its oxygen bridge and then adding one molecule of water. This forms a diol derivative which then has the potential for an addition of nitrogen to become the amine final metabolite and ultimate carcinogen from a polycyclic hydrocarbon.

Epstein-Barr virus   (EBV), herpes virus associated with Burkitt's lymphoma, nasopharyngeal carcinoma and some B cell lymphomas.

erythropoietin   (EPO), 165 amino acid glycoprotein, produced in the kidney, which acts in concert with other growth factors to stimulate proliferation and maturation of bone marrow erythroid cells.

excision repair   repair of mutagen-damaged DNA strand by 'unscheduled DNA synthesis'.

exocrine   secreting externally; the products of exocrine glands are released *via* ducts, as opposed to the secretions of endocrine glands which are secreted directly into the blood system or intercellular fluids.

exophytic tumours   tumours arising from lining epithelia bulging outwards from the surface.

exponential   mathematical function describing an increase of a quantity raised to a power determined by the variable on which the function depends, e.g. logarithmic increase.

factor VIII   plasma coagulation factor whose inherited deficiency is responsible for classic haemophilia.

factor VIII-related antigen   (von Willebrand's factor), non-coagulant stabilizing portion of the factor VIII/factor VIII-related antigen complex; it is responsible for platelet adherence to subendothelial collagen.

familial adenomatous polyposis   (FAP), hereditary condition in which multiple adenomas develop in the colon or rectum; predisposes to large bowel cancer as a further mutation in a single cell of any of the adenomas might bestow a proliferative advantage to that cell over its neighbours and is thus a step nearer malignancy.

Fanconi's anaemia   hereditary, often fatal anaemia with hypocellular or aplastic bone marrow and accompanied by leukopenia, thrombocytopenia, skeletal anomalies and growth retardation; thought to involve defects in DNA repair.

Fas/APO-1 antigen   cell surface receptor which when ligated mediates apoptosis; particularly in lymphoid tissues, although mRNA also found in heart, lung, ovary and liver.

fast-transforming viruses   viruses which induce tumours in infected animals in a matter of days or weeks.

FBT   mouse osteosarcoma virus bearing the v-*fos* viral gene.

fibroblast growth factor (FGF)   a family of growth factors FGF 1-9, prototypes are acidic (aFGF, FGF-1) and basic (bFGF, FGF-2), initially described after production by fibroblasts.

fibroma   benign tumour of fibroblasts.

fibronectin   high molecular weight cell adhesion glycoprotein found in basement membranes and interstitial connective tissue.

fibrosarcoma   malignant tumour of fibroblasts; histological appearance of densely cellular interlacing fascicles of spindle-shaped cells often forming a herringbone pattern.

FIGE   field inversion gel electrophoresis.

filling defect   a region of a radiograph (X-ray) or scan with absence of medium or isotope; often due to the presence of a tumour.

FITC   fluorescein isothiocyanate; fluorescent dye with excitation wavelength of 490 nm and emission wavelength 525 nm; can be conjugated to immunoglobulin.

fixative   preservative solution that promotes formation of stable chemical complexes in tissues thus preventing decomposition and permitting examination of samples in conditions closest to life; hence 'to fix' and 'fixed tissue'.

flow cytometry   automated technique for quantitative measurement of a variety of physical and fluorescence associated parameters; e.g. (a) cell surface markers in immunology, (b) DNA content and cell proliferation, (c) cell sorting.

5-fluorouracil (5-FU)   pyrimidine antimetabolite chemotherapeutic agent, monosubstituted analogue of uracil which it replaces in nucleic acid biosynthesis and thus affects RNA processing and function; when activated inhibits DNA synthesis.

formalin   (H-CHO), highly reactive aqueous solution of formaldehyde, used as a tissue fixative cross-linking proteins and thus preventing their degradation; effects are to some extent reversible.

free radical   unstable molecular fragment, resulting from the breakage of a chemical bond in a molecule. Injurious to cells as they react with molecular oxygen to produce reactive oxygen intermediates such as the superoxide anion.

free radical scavenger   compounds that protect tissues, particularly during radiotherapy, by the reduction of oxygen radicals with the aid of reactive sulphydryl groups, e.g. glutathione, cysteine.

5-FU   *see* 5-fluorouracil.

G_0 phase of the cell cycle characterized by cells that are temporarily not cycling, but from which they can be recruited to recycle in appropriate conditions.

G6PD   *see* glucose-6-phosphate dehydrogenase isoenzymes.

Gadd45   (growth arrest and DNA damage gene), transcriptionally activated by p53, that blocks DNA replication and enhances nucleotide excision of damaged DNA.

gag   one of the three essential genes of retroviruses. *gag* (group antigen) encodes for virus core protein, which has specific antigenic determinants used to define particular groups of retroviruses.

gamma (γ) rays   short wavelength electromagnetic radiation spontaneously emitted from naturally occurring radioactive sources.

GAP   GTPase activating protein, recognizes phosphorylated tyrosines on receptor tyrosine kinases and influences Ras catalytic activity. $p120^{GAP}$ stimulates the GTPase activity of Ras several thousand-fold.

Gas2   member of the growth arrest-specific, gene family; proteolytic cleavage of the encoded protein in its C-terminal region is associated with the typical cell shape changes observed in apoptotic cells.

gastrin   gastrointestinal hormone, stimulating gastric acid secretion. Produced in G cells of gastric antrum; and less commonly in small and large intestinal endocrine cells as well as delta cells of pancreatic islets.

gastrinoma   tumour of gastrin producing neuroendocrine cells; most often in the pancreas but also in duodenum or (rarely) stomach. Morphologically resembling carcinoid tumours, with benign to malignant spectrum of occurrence.

gene   segment of DNA that precisely codes for a specific protein which is transcribed then translated *via* the appropriate mRNA and tRNA molecules.

gene amplification   increase in gene copy number.

gene transcription   synthesis of the appropriate RNA from the template DNA base sequence of the gene.

genetic disease   a disease which is heritable as a result of genetic defect/s that are passed on from generation to generation through the germ line.

genetic prodrug activation therapy   (GPAT), where a gene is over-expressed in a tumour, e.g. c-*erbB-2* in breast and pancreatic tumours, a construct of the promoter and a gene encoding an appropriate enzyme (e.g. *Herpes simplex* virus thymidine kinase which phosphorylates ganciclovir) can specifically convert a prodrug into the active form in the tumour cells only.

genome   total genetic information present in a cell; in one chromosome set of a diploid cell or in the haploid gamete.

genotoxic (mutagenic) agents   damaging agents that act on DNA (genes).

germ cell tumours   tumours supposedly derived from germ cells. Many human germ cell tumours are mixed tumours, e.g. teratomas, composed of a variety of cell types indicative of an origin from a pluripotential stem cell.

germ line mutations   mutations, which because of their presence in the germ line become hereditary, which as the first step in multi-stage carcinogenesis, predispose the individual to development of cancer.

glial fibrillary acidic protein (GFAP), intermediate filament of glial (nervous tissue) cells.

glucagonoma islet cell tumour of alpha, glucagon-secreting cells of the pancreas; can exist in a spectrum of forms from benign to malignant.

glucose-6-phosphate dehydrogenase isoenzymes (G6PD), used in tumour clonality determination in women only. The isoenzymes, A and B, are randomly expressed in the cells of a heterozygous woman: when tumour cells are examined for this enzyme type, if all the cells bear the one isoenzyme only, it indicates that they are all progeny of one sole initial cell, i.e. the tumour is monoclonal.

glutaraldehyde cross-linking fixative solution, most commonly used in electron microscopy.

glutathione free radical scavenger which can protect tissue during radiotherapy.

glutathione peroxidase enzyme that contributes to the protective mechanism afforded by glutathione.

glutathione synthase enzyme that contributes to the protective mechanism afforded by glutathione.

glycoprotein polypeptide with covalently bound oligosaccharides.

Gompertz growth equation mathematical representation of the sigmoid exponential growth curve which is typical of many experimental tumours.

gonadotrophin secretion of the anterior pituitary gland; follicle stimulating hormone (FSH) and luteinizing hormone (LH).

gonadotrophin releasing hormone (GnRH), hormone delivered from the hypothalamus in pulses, to the anterior pituitary, resulting in the release of follicle stimulating hormone (FSH) and luteinizing hormone (LH).

goserelin acetate (Zoladex®), GnRH agonist which permanently down-regulates pituitary receptors, effectively desensitizing the gland to further pulses of GnRH.

GPAT *see* genetic prodrug activation therapy.

grade/grading microscopic assessment of the degree of tumour cell differentiation.

granulocyte colony stimulating factor (G-CSF), growth factor whose activity promotes granulocyte production and differentiation.

granulocyte/macrophage colony stimulating factor (GM-CSF), growth factor whose activity promotes production and differentiation of cells which are precursors of both granulocytes and macrophages; can be used therapeutically to promote neutrophil and macrophage production after chemotherapy.

granuloma chronic inflammatory lesion characterized by an accumulation of macrophages (which may have undergone epithelioid transformation) – lymphocytes and multinucleate giant cells may or may not be present.

granzyme granules containing serine proteases, produced and exocytosed by cytotoxic T lymphocytes. Granzyme B cleaves and activates CPP32 in target cells, leading to apoptosis.

gray (Gy) measurement of absorbed dose of radiation, 1 gray = 1 joule of energy absorbed per kilo of tissue (1 j/kg); equivalent to '100 rads' of earlier terminology.

Grb2 intracellular protein which plays a part in activation of Ras proteins.

growth curve graphical representation of actual increase in tumour size (e.g. weight or volume) over a period of time.

growth factor member of a series of molecules, mostly polypeptides, which are directly and specifically involved in stimulating cell activity, e.g. division, differentiation, motility.

growth factor receptor specific for the appropriate growth factor/s; after receptor occupancy they facilitate signal transduction through downstream effector molecules which ultimately cause cell stimulation.

growth fraction (GF), proportion of cells of a tissue that are cycling. GF = number of proliferating cells, N_P/ total cell number (quiescent N_Q + N_P).

GTPase enzyme activity associated with the *ras* proto-oncogene product, hydrolyses GTP to GDP.

guanosine diphosphate and guanosine triphosphate   (GDP and GTP), purine nucleotides (nucleoside phosphates) made up of base, sugar and two or three phosphate groups respectively.

haemangioma   tumour-like lesion composed of proliferated blood vessels.

haemopoietic tumour   tumour of the blood-forming tissues.

hamartoma   a local defect in tissue histogenesis, commonly an over-production of blood vessels (haemangioma) or lymphatic vessels (lymphangioma) producing a tumour-like lesion.

Harvey sarcoma virus   (H-*ras*), oncogene originally found in two mouse (Harvey and Balb strains) sarcoma viruses, whose protein product has GTPase activity. It is a member of a multigene family, including K-*ras* and N-*ras*, whose mutated forms are commonly found in tumours. *See ras* oncogene family.

HCC   *see* hepatocellular carcinoma.

hepatic portal vein   vein that transports absorbed nutrients directly from the gut to the liver.

hepatitis B   inflammation of the liver caused by the hepatitis B (HBV) DNA hepadna virus; may be acute, chronic, symptomatic or asymptomatic. Virus persists in the blood for up to years, and may be transmitted by minute inoculations of blood, blood products or bodily secretions through the skin or mucosae.

hepatocellular carcinoma   malignant tumour of liver parenchymal cells. Tumour cells are characteristically arranged in trabeculae although acinar or scirrhous patterns do occur, frequently associated with cirrhosis in adults.

hepatoma   benign tumour of the liver.

heterogeneous cell populations   tissue or tumour consisting of cells of more than one phenotype.

heterozygote   individual in which opposing alleles in homologous chromosomal locus/loci are different from each other, one having been derived from each parent.

high-grade   poorly differentiated tumour in which the cells do not closely resemble those of the parent tissue.

histogenesis   the cellular origin of a tissue or tumour.

histology   science of the study of tissue and tissue cells, their composition, structure and function, performed with the aid of a microscope on appropriately preserved and presented tissue.

Hodgkin's disease   malignant tumour of lymphoid tissue principally affecting lymph nodes and spleen, characterized by altered architecture of tissues and infiltration by lymphocytes, monocytes, plasma cells, eosinophils, fibroblasts and Reed-Sternberg cells.

homogeneous cell populations   tissue or tumour cell populations composed of cells of the same phenotype.

homozygote   individual in which opposing alleles in homologous chromosomal locus/loci are the same as each other, one having been derived from each parent.

hormone   substance secreted by specialist cells/organs directly into the bloodstream, and acting upon specific target tissues distant from the site of origin.

human chorionic gonadotrophin   glycopeptide hormone, closely related to follicle stimulating hormone and luteinizing hormone; synthesized and secreted from the placenta – maintains the secretory integrity of the corpus luteum in pregnancy, when it is found in plasma. Antigen associated with trophoblastic tumours and tumours of germ cells.

human immunodeficiency virus   (HIV), retrovirus first described in 1984 as the probable aetiological agent of acquired immune deficiency syndrome (AIDS). Enveloped virus, 80–110 nm diameter which infects and kills T cell subsets, resulting in severe immunodeficiency. Sexually transmitted from person to person and also by blood transfusion. It is distributed in bodily fluids of infected people.

human papillomaviruses   (HPVs), small, ether-resistant icosehadral viruses with circular double stranded DNA, responsible for the development of warts in humans by causing proliferation of cells of the malpighian layer of the skin. Some papillomaviruses are associated with human neoplasia, notably in the cervix. The E6 and E7 proteins are the most important ones involved in transformation, interacting with p53 and pRb respectively.

human stomach cancer gene (*hst*), proto-oncogene commonly amplified in human tumours encodes a protein product member of the fibroblast growth factor family (FGF-4).

human T cell leukaemia virus (HTLV), retrovirus closely associated with human T cell malignancies. Enveloped virus, 80–110 nm diameter and like HIV also attacks certain T cell subsets; also can infect transformed B cells *in vitro*. Endemic in regions of Africa, Caribbean, Southern Japan and Eastern USA, causes T cell leukaemias and lymphomas often with lesions in skin and bone.

hybridoma cell artificially formed by the fusion of two cell types. Commonly used to produce specific monoclonal antibodies, in which the cell types are lymphocytes from the appropriately immunogenic spleen and a cell from a malignant B cell neoplasm.

hydroxyurea antimetabolite cancer chemotherapeutic agent, inhibitor of ribonucleotide reductase, active in the S phase of the cell cycle; commonly used to treat granulocytic leukaemia, malignant melanoma and malignancies of the ovary.

hyperbaric oxygen oxygen pressure above that of air, formally used in radiotherapy to stimulate hypoxic, quiescent tumour cells back in to the cell cycle and thus become sensitive to the damaging effects of radiation.

hyperchromatism increased or excessive staining capacity of a structure, e.g. commonly the nuclei of malignant cells are hyperdiploid thus stain darkly with routine haematoxylin because of the elevated levels of nucleic acid.

hyperdiploid a cell whose DNA content is greater than the normal (diploid) quantity.

hyperplasia stimulus-induced increase in the number of cells in a tissue or organ, resulting in an overall increase in its size, which reverts to normal when the stimulus is removed.

hypodiploid a cell whose DNA content is less than the normal (diploid) quantity.

hypoxia inadequate oxygen concentration in bodily tissues.

ICE *see* interleukin 1β converting enzyme.

IFN *see* interferon.

immunocytochemistry technique to identify the location and distribution of specific antigens in cells and tissues, with the use of specifically raised and targeted antibodies. Word used often interchangeably with 'immunohistochemistry'.

immunoglobulin (Ig), large family of related proteins: antibodies are gamma (γ) globulins that bind with high specificity to antigenic determinants of antigens. Specific activity is dependent on their tertiary form, consisting of two identical heavy chains and two identical light chains, linked together by disulphide bonds. There are five major classes of immunoglobulin, IgA, found in saliva, mucus and other external secretions; IgD, found on the surface of lymphocytes; IgE, found in low concentrations in human plasma; IgG, and the commonest form of immunoglobulin – it fixes complement: IgM, a pentamer, which can use two or three of its binding arms simultaneously, thus resulting in strong binding of repeating identical determinants of such antigenic sites that possess them. Some cell adhesion molecules are also members of the immunoglobulin superfamily.

immunohistochemistry technique to identify the location and distribution of specific antigens in tissues and cells, with the use of specifically raised and targeted antibodies. Word sometimes used interchangeably with 'immunocytochemistry'.

immunophenotype definitive specification of cell type with regard to specific antigens.

immunoreactivity degree of interaction between an antigen and its specific antibody.

immunotoxin heteroconjugated moiety which combines an antibody to a target with an agent toxic to that target, e.g. anti-tumour antibody conjugated to an anti-cancer drug. In this way drugs could be specifically aimed at tumours thus avoiding damage to non-tumour tissue (the 'magic bullet').

infiltration/infiltrative growth pattern local spread of a malignant tumour amongst and between cells of the surrounding normal tissue.

inflammatory bowel disease e.g. ulcerative colitis. There is superficial inflammation with chronic damage and regenerative hyperplasia; associated increased risk of colorectal tumour formation.

inflammatory cells the cells (granulocytes and mononuclear cells) which are involved in the response to injury of vascularized living tissue.

informative pattern difference in length of restriction fragment length polymorphism which is sufficient to be clearly separable by electrophoresis in an agarose gel, thus detectable.

inositol 1,4,5 trisphosphate (IP_3), generated, with DAG, by PLC-γ1 hydrolysis of phosphatidyl inositol 4,5-bisphosphate (PIP_2); causes the release of calcium from intracellular compartments.

insertional mutagenesis retroviral mechanism of cellular transformation, e.g. by long latency (slow transforming) leukaemia viruses and murine mammary tumour viruses. Virus RNA is the template for provirus double-stranded DNA and this, in its entirety, is inserted into the host genome, causing the mutation.

in situ (L. in place), in its normal position – when applied to carcinomas implies not yet invasive; when applied to histological techniques, indicates in the histological location.

in situ **hybridization** pairing of labelled probes with investigated RNA or DNA strands in tissue samples, so that the localization of the strand of interest can be demonstrated.

insulinoma tumour of insulin-producing beta cells of pancreatic islets; often benign and secreting large amounts of insulin.

int-1 mouse proto-oncogene encoding a putative growth factor, which has homology to *wingless* in *Drosophila*. Inappropriately activated by insertional mutagenesis following integration of mouse mammary tumour virus (MMTV).

int-2 gene encoding fibroblast growth factor 3 (FGF-3), inappropriately activated by insertional mutagenesis following integration of mouse mammary tumour virus (MMTV), commonly amplified in human tumours.

integrins large family of generally extracellular matrix receptors that mediate cell–matrix adhesion. Interact with collagens, laminin, fibronectin, vitronectin and von Willebrand's factor.

intercellular adhesion molecule (ICAM), cell adhesion molecule member of the immunoglobulin superfamily (Ig-SF).

interferon (IFN), three classes (α, β, γ) of antiviral, antibacterial and antipathogen cytokines coded by a multigene family. In addition, interferons α and β inhibit the growth of malignant cells, while all three regulate further cytokine expression and are responsive to these molecules. Major immunomodulatory functions include activation of macrophages, cytotoxicity of T cells, NK cells and granulocytes.

interferon stimulated gene factor 3 (ISGF-3), complex of Stat protein heterodimers and the 48 kDa DNA-binding protein, that allows regulatory proteins to enter the cell nucleus.

interferon-stimulated response element (ISRE), region of DNA where regulatory proteins may bind.

interleukin (IL-), a large family of cytokines, often acting as 'short range hormones' influencing the activity of other specific cell types such as lymphocytes, macrophages, fibroblasts, endothelium and malignant cells. For example, IL-1 is produced by monocytes and in the immune response modulates antigen presentation by antigen-presenting cells to T lymphocytes; IL-2 stimulates the proliferation of thymus-derived cells, activates lymphokine activated killer cells (LAKs) and cytotoxic T lymphocytes; IL-3 is a factor which stimulates growth of early multilineage haemopoietic cells.

interleukin 1β converting enzyme (ICE), mammalian member of a family of cysteine proteases involved in the progression of events in apoptosis. Related to CPP32, which is more closely related to the protein product of the *ced-3* gene of the nematode *Caenorhabditis elegans.*

intermediate filaments subcellular cytoskeletal elements, around 10 nm diameter; intermediate in size between actin filaments (5 nm) and microtubules (20–25 nm).

interphase the phase of the cell cycle between cell divisions, during which synthesis of cell constituents occurs. Taken from immediately following mitosis the stages are: G_1, in which there is no DNA synthesis; S, the synthetic phase for DNA; G_2, the phase following DNA synthesis and preceding mitosis.

interstitial collagenase enzyme with specific ability to degrade collagen, in an extracellular location.

in vitro (L. in glass), i.e. in culture.

in vivo (L. in life), in animal or human tissues.

ionizing radiation particulate or electromagnetic radiation with sufficient energy to institute ionization by displacing orbital electrons, in atoms or molecules upon which it impinges or passes through.

IP$_3$ *see* inositol 1,4,5 trisphosphate.

ischaemia reduction of blood supply to a tissue, organ or tumour leading to impairment of cellular function and possibly cell death.

ISGF-3 *see* interferon stimulated gene factor.

ISRE *see* interferon-stimulated response element.

Jaks Janus kinase family; cytoplasmic protein tyrosine kinases (PTKs) which associate with cytokine receptors lacking kinase domains. Jaks are catalytically activated after ligand binding and ultimately trigger tyrosine phosphorylation.

Jass classification semi-quantitative assessment of the extent of invasion of rectal carcinomas.

Kaposi's sarcoma sarcoma (possibly related to angiosarcoma) composed of spindle-shaped cells with irregular vascular channels; there are usually multiple lesions of the skin (often on lower legs and feet) and viscera: may be associated with additional lymphoma. Formally an uncommon condition but associated with some racial groups and geographical locations, but now more widespread amongst sufferers of AIDS.

kappa (κ) immunoglobulin light chain gene gene coding for one of the two varieties of Ig light chain (the other is the lambda (λ) chain).

karyotypic abnormality abnormality in chromosome structure, e.g. due to translocation.

keratinocyte keratin-producing epidermal cell.

Ki-67 proliferation associated protein active throughout the cell cycle; antibody to this is a proliferation marker originally raised in Kiel University, Germany (hence Ki), labelling thus facilitates the assessment of the growth fraction of a tissue composed of mixture of proliferative and non-proliferative cells.

Kirsten sarcoma virus (K-*ras*), member of the *ras* oncogene family (H-*ras*, N-*ras*) originally identified in a mouse sarcoma virus and which is commonly found in mutated form in tumours. Its protein product has GTPase activity. *See ras* proto-oncogene family.

labelling index (LI), percentage of cells expressing a given label, frequently used in cell proliferation studies.

lambda (λ) immunoglobulin light chain gene gene coding for one of the two varieties of Ig light chain (the other is the kappa (κ) chain).

laminin one of the largest known proteins (~1,000 kDa) found exclusively in basement membranes. Constituent of all recognized basal laminae, e.g. of epithelia, endothelia, striated muscle and smooth muscle cells. Binds to further laminin, cell surfaces, type IV collagen and heparan sulphate.

lamin protease (LamP) enzyme activated in apoptosis, responsible for the degradation of nuclear lamins which are the cytoskeletal elements of the nucleus

LamP *see* lamin protease.

latent period period of time in which there is no apparent activity, e.g. the time between exposure to a carcinogen and the actual development of the tumour.

leiomyoma benign tumour of smooth muscle, whose cells show little variation in their form. There is extensive collagen formation which may obscure the muscle cell histogenesis of the neoplasm.

leiomyosarcoma malignant tumour of smooth muscle; when well differentiated resembles a leiomyoma; higher relative mitotic index indicates malignancy.

lesion pathological alteration in the structure or function of a tissue or organ.

LET *see* linear energy transfer.

leukaemia malignant tumour of bone marrow haemopoietic cells characterized by the presence of malignant cells in the blood. A variety of types is recognized, including: acute lymphocytic, acute myelogenous, acute monocytic, acute myelomonocytic, acute promyelocytic, erythroleukaemia, chronic myelogenous, and chronic lymphocytic, depending on the predominant cell type involved.

leukocyte white blood cell; there are various types including lymphocyte, monocyte, neutrophil, basophil and eosinophil. All are nucleate, but while lymphocytes and monocytes have large rounded nuclei ('mononuclear') and are agranular, neutrophils, basophils and eosinophils have lobed nuclei and specific, distinctive granules.

leukocyte common antigen (CD45), common to all white blood cells and their malignancies; widely employed as an immunocytochemical marker of lymphomas.

Li-Fraumeni syndrome hereditary genetic error (*p53* mutation) that leads to the disposition to develop tumours in a variety of organ systems including striated muscle, brain and breast.

ligand a molecule that binds to a specific entity; e.g. a growth factor is the ligand for its specific receptor, and through this it initiates its signal transduction.

linear energy transfer (LET), rate of transfer of energy between a beam (either particulate or electromagnetic) and the medium through which it travels; measured in kiloelectron volts/micron.

lipoma benign tumour of mature adipose tissue, showing no evidence of cellular atypia.

lipopolysaccharide (LPS), molecule consisting of lipid and polysaccharide moieties, which is a main constituent of the cell wall of Gram-negative bacteria.

liposarcoma malignant tumour of adipose tissue with atypical lipoblasts in varying stages of differentiation. Frequently found in soft tissue and particularly in the retroperitoneum.

L-*myc* member of the *myc* multi-gene family, active in some small cell lung carcinomas and identified with gene amplification techniques.

LOD logarithm of odds. Ratio describing the odds for or against linkage between genes on a chromosome. LOD score >3 equivalent to 1000:1 in favour of positive linkage.

long latency viruses viruses which lack v-*onc* sequences, e.g. the mouse mammary tumour virus (MMTV).

long terminal repeat (LTR), region of provirus DNA in which the U5 region is duplicated at the 3' end and U3 at the 5' end.

loss of heterozygosity (LOH), normal cells may be heterozygous at a particular gene locus due to a restriction fragment length polymorphism. LOH occurs when one of the two chromosome segments is lost; used to detect consistent chromosomal losses in tumours, thus implicating the region as a site of a tumour suppressor gene.

low grade well differentiated tumour in which the cells resemble the tissue of origin.

LPS *see* lipopolysaccharide.

lymphoma malignant tumour of lymphoid tissue including lymphocytic lymphoma, histiocytic lymphoma and Hodgkin's disease.

Lyonization embryonal random inactivation of one X-chromosome in every somatic cell in females, resulting in equal X-linked gene activation across the sexes (males having one X- and one Y-chromosome); thus all females are genetic mosaics, with some cells retaining activity in the paternally derived X-chromosome, while others retain activity in the maternally derived X-chromosome.

macrophage phagocytic cell of bone marrow origin (monoblast), ubiquitously found in organs and tissues although it might have different names, e.g. Kupffer cell – liver sinusoid macrophage; microglial cell – CNS macrophage; histiocyte – connective tissue macrophage. Macrophages not only phagocytose bacteria and cellular debris, but also produce cytokines and have crucial roles in immune responses.

macroscopic of, or relating to, studies that are of sufficient size as to be visible without the aid of a microscope.

magnetic resonance imaging diagnostic procedure which utilizes the magnetic dipole properties of protons, nuclear magnetic resonance (NMR).

malignant tending to destroy, harm or kill, e.g. malignant hypertension. In the case of tumours, malignancy has a specific meaning, distinguishing 'benign' tumours from the vastly more damaging malignant ones – the latter often being characterized by high cell proliferation rates, anaplasia, local invasion and metastatic spread.

malignant fibrous histiocytoma malignant tumour of fibroblasts in which some of the cells resemble histiocytes.

malignant melanoma highly malignant tumour of melanocytes of the skin (or rarely, eye), which metastasizes widely; appears most frequently in light skinned people exposed to excessive amounts of sunshine.

malignant phenotype phenotype of tumour cells – usually with the ability to invade and metastasize.

malignant schwannoma malignant peripheral nerve sheath cell (Schwann cell) tumour. Densely packed oval or spindle-shaped cells, arranged in groups or nests, with little tendency to pleomorphism.

matrix metalloproteinases e.g. Interstitial collagenase, stromelysin, and gelatinase. Enzymes which degrade extracellular matrix components including the interstitial collagens, proteoglycans and fibronectin; all require Zn^{2+} for catalytic activity. Inhibitors of these enzymes might impair tumour invasion and metastasis by stabilizing the extracellular matrix.

Mdm2 gene with p53 responsive elements, amplified in many tumours. Mdm2 is a 'zinc finger' protein that binds to p53 and abolishes its transcriptional control activity. It also binds to pRb and thus modulates the checks that both these proteins have on cell cycle progression.

MDR multi-drug resistance; ability conferred on cells to withstand exposure to lethal doses of structurally unrelated agents.

mdr-1 gene encoding P-glycoprotein, a membrane-associated glycoprotein of molecular weight 170 kDa closely associated with multi-drug resistance in chemotherapy.

medullary carcinoma of thyroid carcinoma of parafollicular (calcitonin-producing) C cells of the thyroid, may include amyloid fibrils in the stroma.

megakaryocyte progenitor cell of blood platelets, normally resident in the bone marrow. Multiple-lobed nucleus and cytoplasm divided into distinct granular entities which ultimately become detached and released as platelets.

melphalan alkylating phenylalanine analogue of the nitrogen mustards, used as a cancer chemotherapeutic agent; causes the substitution of an alkyl group for an active hydrogen atom in an organic compound such as a DNA base, causing inter- and intrastrand DNA cross-links and cross-links with other macromolecules.

6-mercaptopurine (6MP), antimetabolite cancer chemotherapeutic agent analogue of the natural purine base hypoxanthine; active in the S phase of the cell cycle exerting its cytotoxic activity principally as an inhibitor of purine nucleotide synthesis; frequently used in treatment of leukaemias.

MEN type 2   heritable tendency to develop hyperplasia(s) in C cells of the thyroid, adrenal medulla, and parathyroid; precedes multiple endocrine neoplasia.

mesothelioma   benign or malignant tumour arising from the cells of the mesothelial lining of the coelomic body cavities. Development of malignant mesothelioma of the pleura is particularly associated with exposure to asbestos fibre.

met   proto-oncogene coding for the tyrosine kinase growth factor receptor known as Met which binds hepatocyte growth factor; first identified by transfection of DNA from a human osteosarcoma cell line treated with a methylating carcinogen.

metalloproteinase   *see* matrix metalloproteinases.

metaphase   second phase of the process of mitosis, preceded by prophase and followed by anaphase and telophase. In metaphase, chromosomes arrange themselves on the mitotic spindle of microtubules, across the equator of the dividing cell.

metaphase arrest   prevention of a cell proceeding from metaphase to anaphase, brought about by treatment with specific agents that inhibit formation of the mitotic spindle so that newly divided chromosomes are unable to move apart into anaphase. This is a commonly used method of killing cells in cancer chemotherapy as well as being used experimentally to determine the birth rate, K_B, of tumour cells (measured in cells/100 cells/hour) as arrested cells are easily recognizable and quantifiable.

metaplasia   a major switch in tissue differentiation leading to an inappropriate phenotype, e.g. intestinal crypts and villi appearing in the stomach (intestinal metaplasia).

metastasis   transfer of disease from one body site to another, particularly cancers. The metastasis or secondary tumour is discontinuous with the primary tumour.

methacarn   precipitative fixative solution composed of methanol, chloroform and acetic acid; often used to protect antigens prior to immunocytochemical procedures.

methotrexate   antimetabolite cancer chemotherapeutic agent active in the S phase of the cell cycle; potent folic acid antagonist, binds to the enzyme dihydrofolate reductase (DHFR) blocking the generation of tetrahydrofolate, which is essential for both purine and pyrimidine synthesis.

metronidazole   oxygen mimetic drug used to increase radiosensitivity in radiotherapy. Also widely used in the treatment of various intestinal and liver disorders, although has been reported to be a carcinogen in rodents.

MIB   (Molecular Immunology Borstel), series of antibodies recognizing the Ki-67 antigen, that are immunoreactive in routinely processed, paraffin wax-embedded tissue. Developed at the Institute of Molecular Immunology, Borstel, Germany.

microtubule   tubular cytoskeletal structure with outer diameter of 25 nm under conditions of routine fixation; the tubule wall polymer is composed of equal numbers of α-tubulin and β-tubulin subunits. Microtubules function as rigid subcellular framework and also have specific structural roles in flagella, cilia and the mitotic spindle.

misonidazole   oxygen mimetic drug used to increase radiosensitivity in radiotherapy.

mitogenesis   activity of initiating cell division.

mitomycin C   anti-tumour antibiotic, causes local DNA unwinding through intercalation, and by forming tight adducts with DNA can also block transcription. Also can be reduced to a radical species and/or be activated to an alkylating agent.

mitotic index   (MI), proportion of recognizable cells in mitosis, expressed as a percentage of the total cell number.

monoclonal antibody   antibody generated initially by a single B cell or single hybridoma, raised against, and specifically recognizing, a single antigenic epitope. Achieved *in vitro* by cell fusion, selection and cloning.

mouse mammary tumour virus   (MMTV), tumour virus whose provirus DNA causes insertional mutagenesis.

mucosa   epithelial cells and their underlying connective tissue/basement membrane.

multi-stage carcinogenesis   development of malignancy in stages by successive single genetic mutations each time endowing one cell with a proliferative advantage over those of the previously dominant phenotype, e.g. adenoma – carcinoma progression.

mutagen   any physical or chemical agent that acts upon a cell's genes to change their composition, and thus the genetic information that they hold.

mutagenic   the activity of a mutagen.

mutation   a change in the genotype of a cell.

myb   proto-oncogene originally discovered as the transforming gene (v-*myb*) of avian myeloblastosis virus, encodes a nuclear protein involved in cell proliferation.

myc   proto-oncogene originally discovered as the transforming gene (v-*myc*) of the myelocytomatosis viruses. The gene encodes a transcription factor which is more abundant in proliferating cells – involved in the translocation found in Burkitt's lymphoma.

mycotoxin   toxin produced by a mould or fungus under specific conditions.

myelodysplasia   abnormal formation of blood cell precursors in the bone marrow.

myeloid leukaemia   malignant tumour of myeloid stem cells and their precursors. Granulocytes of all stages of maturation may be present in the blood.

myeloma   malignant tumour of plasma cells with diffuse infiltration in bone marrow and viscera; commonly multiple myeloma.

myelosuppression   suppression of formation of granulocyte white blood cells.

myoglobin   respiratory pigment found in muscle cells which binds reversibly with oxygen and acts as an oxygen transport protein.

myosin   'thick' filament component of muscle. Myosin molecules have two components, head and tail. The head protrudes from the fibril, has ATPase activity and is responsible for interaction with the 'thin' actin filament. Tails associate together and are responsible for filament formation.

naevus   localized congenital malformation of the skin, e.g. strawberry naevi. *See* haemangioma.

2-naphthylamine   aromatic amine which after metabolic activation reacts with DNA to form adducts; it is a potent human bladder carcinogen.

necrosis   passive morphological changes that occur to cells of a tissue following their death. Necrosis results from the cessation of energy-dependent processes that maintain the vital *status quo*. Typical nuclear changes include nuclear disruption (karyorrhexis), and cytoplasmic changes including organelle vacuolation and cellular swelling, protein degradation is made evident by generalized increase in eosinophilia.

Nedd   (NPC, neuronal precursor cells – expressed, developmentally down-regulated genes), a member of the *ICE/ced-3* gene family. Expression is involved in apoptosis in the developing CNS.

neoplasia   the process of tumour formation.

neoplasm   literally, benign or malignant tumour consisting of newly proliferated cells.

neovascularization   the formation of new blood vessels, e.g. to supply expanding tumour mass.

nephroblastoma   malignant tumour of the kidney (typically occurring in childhood) forming structures that resemble embryonic kidney.

neu   rat gene related to proto-oncogene c-*erbB-2* and coding for a protein of the EGF receptor family; originally identified by transfection of DNA from a rodent neuroblastoma. Single amino acid mutation results in the active c-*neu* oncogene.

neural cell adhesion molecule   (N-CAM), calcium independent cell adhesion molecule involved in cell-cell and cell-extracellular matrix interactions; particularly important in embryological development of the central nervous system.

neural crest   embryological cells of the neurosomatic junction that develop into much of the peripheral nervous system and some other tissues, including dorsal root ganglia, sympathetic ganglia, C cells of the thyroid and adrenal medullary cells.

neuroblastoma   highly malignant tumour of undifferentiated neuroblasts (often associated with the sympathetic chain). Small cells with dark-staining nuclei are arranged in groups, characteristically around tangles of fibrillary material.

neuroendocrine system   – diffuse neuroendocrine system (DNES); hormone synthesizing system of glands and/or specialized cells widespread throughout the mammalian body, particularly in the gastrointestinal tract (including islets of Langerhans), thyroid, adrenal medulla, pituitary and prostate. Cells characteristically store the polypeptide hormones and amines in distinctive granules and these substances may also act as chemical messengers in the nervous system. *See* endocrine system.

neurofibroma   benign localized or diffuse tumour, consisting of a mixture of Schwann cells and fibroblasts accompanied by loosely arranged collagen fibres and mucinous material.

neurofibromin   (p280^{NF1}), a GAP-related protein encoded by the *NF1* gene, the loss of which is responsible for disorders such as type 1 neurofibromatosis (or Von Rechlinghausen neurofibromatosis) and malignant schwannoma.

neurofilament   intermediate filament of nervous tissue cells, 10–15 nm in diameter, found in neuronal cell bodies, axons and dendrites.

neurone-specific enolase Mg^{2+}- or Mn^{2+}-dependent family of isoenzymes that catalyses the elimination of water from 2-phosphoglycerate; found in various cells including endocrine cells and endocrine neoplasms.

neutron   uncharged atomic nuclear particle, with atomic mass of 1.

NF1   gene whose protein product stimulates GTPase activity of Ras; lost or mutated in malignant schwannoma and type 1 neurofibromatosis (or Von Rechlinghausen neurofibromatosis).

NIH/3T3   mouse fibroblast line originating from the National Institute of Health in Washington DC, USA.

nitrate   anion, or salts formed with the anion NO_3^-, derived from nitric acid and forming one of the main sources of nitrogen to plants, which is ultimately essential for the synthesis of amino acids and thus proteins.

nitrite   anion, or salt with NO_2^-, derived from nitrous acid. Frequently added to foods as a preservative, particularly cooked meats. Nitrites can react with secondary amines and produce nitrosamines, which have been implicated in carcinogenesis in some circumstances.

nitrogen mustard   bifunctional alkylating agent derived from mustard gas, parent product of several anti-cancer drugs, e.g. melphalan, mechlorethamine, phenylalanine, chlorambucil. Causes the substitution of an alkyl group for an active hydrogen atom in an organic compound such as a DNA base, resulting in inter- and intrastrand DNA cross-links and cross-links with other macromolecules.

nitrosamine   nitrosylated secondary amine converted from nitrates and nitrites; an established carcinogen/mutagen in rodents.

nitrosourea   group of chemotherapeutic drugs converted into alkylating agents by a spontaneous chemical process in aqueous solution. Activity is in cross-links of two carbon atoms between two nucleophilic centres, and both inter- and intra-strand cross-links are possible.

nm23   (not in metastasis), tumour suppressor gene whose protein product may have metastasis-suppressing activity; found in rodents and man, and is probably a nucleoside diphosphate (NDP) kinase. Levels of *nm23* RNA expression are strongly inversely correlated with metastatic potential in ductal carcinoma of the breast.

N-*myc*   member of the *myc* multi-gene family, active in neuroblastomas and identified by gene amplification techniques.

Northern blotting   by analogy with Southern blotting for DNA analysis, a method of transferring denatured RNA onto a nitrocellulose or nylon filter. RNA is electrophoresed in a denaturing agarose gel, before being transferred to a membrane either by capillary action or under the action of an electrical field. A radiolabelled DNA or RNA probe is hybridized to the filter-bound RNA to detect specific sequences (tissue equivalent = *in situ* hybridization).

N-*ras*   an oncogene originally identified as a gene amplified in a human neuroblastoma and subsequently in other tumour types. It is a member of the *ras* multi-gene family which also includes H-*ras* and K-*ras* and like them is commonly found mutated in tumours.

nuclear magnetic resonance   (NMR), imaging system method which utilizes the magnetic dipole properties of protons.

nucleoside   molecule composed of purine or pyrimidine base plus ribose or deoxyribose sugar.

nucleosome   fundamental packing unit around which double stranded DNA is wound; consists of an eight-part protein core made up of two copies of each of four histones.

nucleotide   nucleoside linked to phosphoric acid which when polymerized forms a nucleic acid.

nude mouse   a strain of mouse that is innately immune suppressed because it congenitally lacks a thymus; in addition to this genetic peculiarity these mice also have sparse, or no, fur.

oat cell carcinoma   small cell anaplastic variety of lung carcinoma that can secrete hormones, e.g. ACTH, antidiuretic hormone, bombesin.

octreotide   Sandostatin®, analogue of somatostatin, inhibits release of growth hormone from the pituitary.

ODN   *see* antisense oligodeoxynucleotide.

OER   *see* oxygen enhancement ratio.

oesophagitis   inflammation of the oesophagus; when chronic there is damage to the epithelium, regenerative hyperplasia and/or metaplasia (Barrett's oesophagus).

oestradiol   steroid hormone synthesized and secreted mainly by thecal cells surrounding the developing Graffian follicle in the ovary.

oligonucleotide   a short length compound made up of nucleoside-phosphate residues joined together, obtained by partial hydrolysis of nucleic acids. Labelled oligonucleotides are used in procedures to identify DNA and RNA sequences.

oncogene   any gene involved in the initiation or progression of malignant cellular transformation; arises by mutation of proto-oncogenes (which are present in normal cells), and may have viral counterparts (viral oncogenes) that are capable of transforming eukaryotic cells.

oncogene transduction   retroviral mechanism of cellular transformation. Fast-transforming viruses have acquired new genes, often at the expense of their own replicative mechanisms; the new genes are responsible for cellular transformation in the host and are known as viral oncogenes, v-*oncs*.

oncogenic virus   virus which contains viral oncogenes; when an oncogenic virus infects normal cells it causes them to transform.

oophorectomy   surgical removal of the ovaries.

organelle   discrete subcellular structure, e.g. mitochondrion, endoplasmic reticulum, Golgi apparatus, which performs a specific function.

organochlorine pesticides   non-genotoxic carcinogens that produce their effects by means other than mutagenicity.

osteoma   benign tumour of bone, consisting of well-differentiated bone tissue, dense and ivory-like, with a predominantly lamellar structure; characterized by slow growth.

osteosarcoma   malignant tumour of bone cells whose cells produce bone or osteoid tissue to a greater or lesser extent. Age of onset is commonly 10–20 years, with males more frequently affected than females.

ovariectomy   surgical removal of the ovaries, also called oophorectomy.

oxygen enhancement ratio   (OER), the ratio of dose of ionizing radiation required for equivalent cell killing in the absence of O_2 compared with in its presence.

p15^{Ink4B}   inhibitor of cyclin-Cdk complexes

p16^{Ink4A}   protein product of tumour suppressor gene; inhibitor of cyclin-Cdk complexes, implicated in development of gliomas and cancer of the pancreas.

p21^{Cip1}   protein product of *Cip1/WAF-1* gene – universal inhibitor of cyclin-dependent kinases (Cdks).

p21^{ras}   21 kDa protein product of the *ras* proto-oncogene family.

p27^{Kip1}   27 kDa protein, inhibitor of cyclin-Cdk complexes.

p28^{sis}   protein product closely related to the B chain of platelet derived growth factor (PDGF) coded by v-*sis* gene of simian sarcoma virus.

p38   *see* synatophysin.

p53   tumour suppressor gene ('guardian of the genome'); negative regulator of cell growth coding for the transcription factor for *WAF1/Cip1*, mutated in about 70% of human cancers. One allele mutated in the Li-Fraumeni syndrome leads to predisposition to tumour formation.

p53   nuclear-acting growth suppressing protein product (53 kDa) of the *p53* gene; transcription factor for *Cip1* gene encoding p21 that causes interruption of the cell cycle to facilitate the repair of damaged DNA. Under certain circumstances, p53 induces apoptosis.

p105^{Rb} or pRb   105 kDa protein product of *Rb1*, the retinoblastoma susceptibility gene.

p120^{GAP}   ubiquitous protein which increases GTP hydrolysis by Ras by up to 20,000-fold.

p170   *see* P-glycoprotein.

P450   class of enzymes involved in oxygenating various compounds, the mono-oxygenases or mixed function oxidases. Derives its name from the characteristic wavelength of absorbed light. *See* cytochrome P450-dependent mono-oxygenase system.

palliative treatment   treatment which, while admittedly cannot cure the disease, serves to relieve the severity of its symptoms, e.g. pain.

papilloma   benign exophytic tumour of surface epithelium (skin, mucous membranes, ducts), composed of epithelial cells.

paracrine   secretion by cells with activity on their close neighbouring cells.

paraffin wax   high melting point hydrophobic alkane used to infiltrate fixed tissue to maintain it and act as a support for tissue section cutting. Tissue is infused with hot wax, which then solidifies into specifically moulded blocks as it cools; sections are then cut for light microscopy.

paraformaldehyde   polymeric fixative solution reversibly formed from formaldehyde, favoured fixative for antigen protection prior to immunolabelling at electron microscope level.

parenchyma   characteristic and functional cells and tissues of an organ.

PARP   *see* poly (ADP-ribose) polymerase.

particulate radiation   stream of charged ionizing particles commonly α^{2+} particles (2 protons + 2 neutrons), β^- particles (electrons) or β^+ particles (positrons).

passage   implantation of tumour tissue from one animal host to another in experimental situations; tumours are excised from the original host and either transplanted as small tissue blocks or split up into cell suspensions, cells then being injected into the new hosts. This can be done to many generations of mouse, expanding the tumour stock and/or samples kept frozen and implanted at a future date.

pathognomonic   characteristics of a disease that are specific and recognizable.

PC10   prototype antibody which recognizes proliferating cell nuclear antigen (PCNA); used in a method of assessing cell proliferation index.

PDGF   *see* platelet derived growth factor.

PET   *see* positron emission tomography.

P-glycoprotein (p170), membrane-associated energy-dependent drug efflux pump. When over-expressed associated with multi-drug resistance; coded for by *mdr1* gene.

phaeochromocytoma tumour (usually benign) of the adrenal medulla often with secretion of adrenalin and/or noradrenalin. The tumour cells show a strong chromaffin reaction.

phagocyte specialized cell (particularly macrophages and neutrophils) that ingests particles such as cellular debris, foreign microorganisms, etc., into the cytoplasm by engulfment. The phagocytic vacuole generates free radicals and fuses with primary lysosomes enabling further degradation of the ingestate.

phagocytosis process of engulfment, uptake and digestion of matter by specialized and non-specialized phagocytic cells.

phenotype an identifiable structure or functional characteristic of a cell or organism, that results from the combined influence of genetic activity and the environment.

Philadelphia chromosome (Ph'), shortened form of chromosome 22; karyotypic abnormality with translocation of the c-*abl* proto-oncogene from chromosome 9 to the breakpoint cluster region of chromosome 22. The hybrid transcript encodes a novel protein with enhanced tyrosine kinase activity. Associated with leukaemias, particularly chronic myeloid leukaemia.

phorbol ester variety of compounds, originally derived from plants, that can act as tumour promoters particularly in multi-stage carcinogenesis. For example, 12-o-tetradecanoyl phorbol-13-acetate (TPA) promotes skin papilloma growth, but is not DNA-damaging.

phosphatidyl inositol 3 kinase (PI(3)K), cytoplasmic enzyme which phosphorylates phosphatidyl inositol at the 3 position.

phosphatidyl inositol 4,5 bisphosphate (PIP$_2$), after growth factor binding, hydrolysis of (PIP$_2$) is catalyzed by phospholipase C-γ1 (PLC-γ1), generating both water soluble inositol 1, 4, 5-trisphosphate (IP$_3$) which causes the release of calcium from intracellular compartments, and diacylglycerol (DAG), which remains at the plasma membrane to activate PKC.

phosphoglycerate kinase gene gene with utility in tumour clonality investigations.

phospholipase C-γ1 (PLC), enzyme which hydrolyses phosphatidyl inositol bisphosphate to inositol trisphosphate and diacylglycerol.

PI(3)K *see* phosphatidyl inositol 3 kinase.

(PIP$_2$) *see* phosphatidyl inositol 4,5 bisphosphate.

pituitary gland (hypophysis), small gland at the base of the brain; cells of the anterior lobe produce hormones that control secretions of adrenals, ovary, testis, and thyroid; posterior lobe secretes hormones that are synthesized in nerve cells of the hypothalamus controlling blood pressure and water balance.

pituitary hormones hormones produced/secreted by the pituitary gland. The anterior pituitary produces adrenocorticotrophic hormone (ACTH), follicle stimulating hormone (FSH), luteinizing hormone (LH), growth hormone (GH), prolactin (PRL) and thyroid stimulating hormone (TSH), while the posterior pituitary conducts antidiuretic hormone and oxytocin from nerve cell bodies of the hypothalamus.

PKC *see* protein kinase C.

plasma cell cell arising from the terminal differentiation of a B lymphocyte which synthesizes, stores and secretes immunoglobulin. Ultrastructurally it is recognizable by the preponderance of rough endoplasmic reticulum in its cytoplasm, arranged concentrically around the nucleus. The nucleus itself is often eccentrically positioned with the typical 'clockface' arrangement of chromatin.

plasminogen activators enzymes that convert plasminogen to plasmin by hydrolysis of an arginine-valine bond.

***Plasmodium* species** sporozoan red blood cell parasite. The genus includes four species that cause malaria in humans. The sexual phase of the life cycle takes place in the mosquito vector and the asexual phase in the liver and bloodstream of the human host.

platelet derived growth factor (PDGF), growth factor normally found in high concentrations in platelets, which is released after wounding and stimulates proliferation of cells involved in healing. Part of the gene that codes for PDGF has been captured by a simian sarcoma virus and is known as v-*sis*.

plating efficiency   in production of cell colonies *in vitro*, the number of macroscopic cell colonies formed to the total number of cells initially plated, expressed as a percentage.

platinum compounds   e.g. cisplatin, carboplatin, efficacious anti-tumour drugs usually used in combination with further anti-cancer drugs. Cisplatin behaves like an alkylating agent; reacts with nucleophiles and inter- and intrastrand cross-links are formed with DNA; highly nephrotoxic.

PLC   *see* phospholipase C-γ1.

pleomorphic tumours   tumours of a mixed cell phenotype with variable cell morphology with respect to shape and size.

pluripotential stem cell   a stem cell which produces progeny that differentiate into more than one terminally differentiated cell type.

pocket proteins   pRb, p107 and p130 that bind E2F transcription factors at various stages of the cell cycle.

point mutation   mutation at one single base in a gene, resulting in coding for a different amino acid at this location, thus producing a different protein.

pol . one of the three essential genes of retroviruses, *pol* encodes the reverse transcriptase, polymerase, enzyme.

poly (ADP-ribose) polymerase   (PARP), nuclear DNA repair enzyme; (target of cysteine protease enzymes such as apopain) whose destruction is associated with cell death by apoptosis.

polyclonal antibody   antibodies produced from a number of antigen-activated B cells which recognize different epitopes of the challenging antigen. Many B cells will have undergone clonal expansion and differentiation, so the antibodies will be the products of many clones – polyclonal.

polycyclic hydrocarbon   compound consisting of hydrogen and carbon only arranged in resonance-stabilized ring structures.

polymerase   an enzyme that facilitates polymerization, e.g. DNA polymerase.

polymerase chain reaction   (PCR), *in vitro* technique for rapidly providing many copies of a relevant sequence of DNA. A pair of primers directs a reaction in which a heat-stable polymerase repeatedly synthesizes a strand complementary to a single strand DNA template in the 5′ to 3′ direction.

polyp   exophytic growth arising from mucosal surfaces, forming pedunculated (stalked) adenomas. NB, not all polypoid masses are tumours.

positron   short-lived, positively charged subatomic beta particle (β^+).

positron emission tomography   (PET), method of detection, by a body scan, of positrons emitted from administered radioactive isotopes.

potential doubling time of a tumour   (t_{PD}), predicts how fast the tumour will double its cell number, based upon cell production alone, $t_{PD} = \log_e 2/K_B$. (t_{PD}, potential doubling time; K_B, cell birth rate). This is not an indicator of the *actual tumour growth* rate.

pp55$^{c\text{-}fos}$ nuclear protein product of *fos* gene expression, can form transcription factor, AP-1, in combination with *jun* protein product.

pp60$^{c\text{-}src}$ protein product of the cellular *src* gene, non-receptor protein tyrosine kinase which is located on the inner surface of the plasma membrane.

precipitative fixative   fixative solutions for routine histological/pathological tissue preservation, e.g. acetone, methanol, chloroform, with properties that contrast with those of cross-linking aldehyde fixatives.

preinvasive states   changes that occur at a cellular level in a tissue, which are the antecedents of development into a malignant tumour.

preneoplastic conditions circumstances (usually inflammatory), which pose an unpredictable but increased risk of neoplastic development.

primary tumour the original tumour in contrast to secondary tumours, which are metastases from the primary site.

progenitor tissue parent or ancestral tissue.

progesterone hormone produced by the corpus luteum, placenta and adrenal cortex. In the menstrual cycle it prepares the endometrium for implantation of the fertilized egg, and in pregnancy it plays a central role in the maintenance of the uteroplacentofoetal unit. It is also an essential precursor in the biosynthesis of corticosteroid hormones.

prognosis informed judgement of the course and probable outcome of a disease, based on understanding the clinical and pathological features of each case.

proliferating cell nuclear antigen (PCNA), 37 kDa non-histone nuclear protein, specific to proliferating cells and immunoreactive from late G_1 phase, which can be detected, in paraffin wax-embedded tissue, by appropriate antibodies. PCNA immunolabelling provides an index estimate, slightly lower than the growth fraction, of proliferating cells in a tissue.

proliferation associated antigens native cellular antigens (proteins) that are immunoreactive in proliferating cells only; specific labelling of such antigens facilitates proliferation cell kinetic studies without the need to administer such potential labels as bromodeoxyuridine or tritiated thymidine.

promoter (sequence/region) the regulatory region of a gene, very close to the start site of transcription, where binding of transcription factors occurs: this is crucial for the induction of transcription by RNA polymerase II.

proopiomelanocortin common precursor to pituitary polypeptides β-lipotropin, melanocyte-stimulating hormone (MSH), endorphins and enkephalins.

prophase first stage of mitosis, preceded by the G_2 phase of the cell cycle and followed by metaphase of mitosis.

prophylactic substances or actions taken to prevent disease.

prostate gland conical-shaped organ that surrounds the proximal region of the male urethra producing a major contribution to the seminal plasma. Glandular epithelium is normally simple columnar or pseudostratified but histological integrity depends on presence of testosterone. Extremely high incidence of occult prostatic carcinoma in elderly men.

prostate specific antigen antigen specific to prostate epithelium, thus facilitating immunolocalization, and potentially immunotherapy, of tumours of prostate cells.

prostatic acid phosphatase form of the enzyme acid phosphatase specifically found in prostatic epithelia and prostate tumours.

protein kinase C (PKC), family of enzymes activated by growth factors and promoters such as TPA, phosphorylates serine and threonine residues on intracellular substrates.

protein tyrosine kinase (PTK), enzyme which facilitates catalysis of phosphorylation of tyrosine residues on cytoplasmic proteins and glycoproteins – there are receptor and non-receptor PTKs. Cross/autophosphorylation of dimerized receptors is an important mechanism.

proteoglycan component of connective tissue and cartilage in which the protein is glycosylated with many glycosaminoglycan polysaccharide chains. These chains are made up of alternate, often sulphated, hexosamine and uronic acid residues.

proton positively charged nuclear particle with atomic mass of one (1^+).

proto-oncogene normal cellular gene encoding for a cytoplasmic or nuclear protein which participates in the cell's normal proliferation and differentiation programme – thus bestowed with 'potential' oncogenic activity.

protozoan unicellular organism. Can be causative agents of human disease, e.g. *Plasmodium* spp. (malaria), and *Entamoeba* spp. (dysentery).

provirus a viral genome that is integrated into the genome of its host cell. In the case of RNA retroviruses, a double-stranded DNA copy is produced by the virion reverse transcriptase using the virion single-stranded RNA as a template. This DNA becomes incorporated into cellular DNA and can serve as a permanent template for replication of viral RNA and/or a heritable gene capable of transforming cells.

PTK   *see* protein tyrosine kinase.

purine   with reference to DNA, the bases adenine and guanine.

pushing edge/margin   perimeter of benign tumours in a solid organ, having both fibrous and compressed normal tissue components, rendering a benign tumour readily distinguishable from a malignant tumour, which *invades* the surrounding normal tissue.

pyrimidine   with reference to DNA, the bases cytosine and thymine; also uracil of RNA.

radiation   high energy beam, either particulate or electromagnetic. Particulate radiation commonly consists of alpha particles, beta particles or positrons, and electromagnetic radiation occurs across the whole range of the electromagnetic spectrum – gamma rays, X-rays, ultraviolet, visible light and infra-red.

radiograph   a processed film taken during radiography.

radiography   diagnostic (as opposed to therapeutic) radiography, is the process of recording on film, body images produced by X-rays for the purpose of diagnosing disease or damage.

radio-opaque dyes   substances that might be applied or consumed for diagnostic X-ray investigatory techniques, that reflect or absorb (as opposed to transmitting) X-rays. This permits an image to be formed on a photographic plate or fluorescent screen, using differential transmission of the rays by various body structures and outlining of soft tissues by the radio-opaque substance (e.g. drinking of a barium suspension for gastrointestinal investigation).

radiotherapy   the use of ionizing radiation for therapeutic purposes, e.g. killing proliferating malignant cells.

radium   naturally occurring radioactive element, Ra, with atomic number 88, atomic mass of 226 and half-life of 1620 years; a breakdown product of uranium 238, it has several isotopes and itself decays into radon gas. If consumed, radium tends to be a bone-seeking element.

radon gas   naturally occurring radioactive gas, Rn, with atomic number 86, atomic mass of 222 and half-life of 3.83 days; a breakdown product of radium 226, itself decays into solid unstable radioactive isotopes.

***ras* family of proto-oncogenes**   originally identified from v-*ras* of retroviruses which caused rat sarcomas. The 21 kDa protein product finally attaches to the inner surface of the plasma membrane and is activated by growth factors binding to their receptors. Activated Ras binds GTP and also Raf. There are three genes in mammals, Harvey-, Kirsten- and N-*ras*; all belong to a multigene family which is ubiquitous and highly conserved. Point mutations or gene amplifications occur which render them oncogenic.

Rb1   tumour suppressor gene whose protein product is a transcriptional regulator. When missing or damaged it conveys susceptibility to the development of retinoblastoma, osteosarcoma, small cell lung carcinoma.

RBE   *see* relative biological efficiency.

recruitment   repopulation of a tumour, by previously quiescent cells re-entering the proliferative pool, after the original cells have been destroyed.

relative biological efficiency   (RBE), dose ratio of different quality LET beams to produce the same biological effect.

renewing populations   normal tissues where continuous cell production is matched by cell loss, ensuring no net growth. Examples are: skin, gastrointestinal epithelium and haemopoietic tissues.

resection   surgical removal of part of a body structure.

restriction fragment length polymorphism   (RFLP), a DNA polymorphism which results from loss or creation of a site at which a particular restriction enzyme cuts. DNA carrying different allelic forms will generate different sized DNA fragments on digestion with the appropriate restriction enzyme.

reticuloendothelial system diffuse system of phagocytic cells involved in the body's defence against foreign matter e.g. proteins, immune complexes, cells, and/or subcellular agents. In more modern terminology known as the mononuclear phagocyte system.

retinoblastoma malignant tumour derived from retinal cells, which occurs almost exclusively in children. Can occur in familial or sporadic forms, in the former case there is a tendency to bilateral tumours; it is highly radiosensitive.

retinoic acid vitamin A (retinol) metabolite which can induce differentiation and/or suppress cell proliferation in malignant cells.

retrovirus virus whose genome is in the form of single-stranded RNA and requires the activity of reverse transcriptase to produce the appropriate DNA before it can complete its intracellular life cycle by becoming incorporated into the DNA of the infected host cell for replication.

reverse transcriptase an RNA-dependent DNA polymerase which synthesizes DNA using RNA as a template, essential in the life cycle of viruses. In the laboratory, reverse transcriptases are used as tools to prepare complementary DNA copies (cDNA).

rhabdomyoma benign tumour of striated muscle, cells are generally polygonal in shape, and may have glycogen containing vacuoles, cross-striations may be visible.

rhabdomyosarcoma malignant tumour of rhabdomyoblasts of striated muscle with varying stages of differentiation. There may, or may not, be intracellular fibrils and may or may not be cross striations; when highly disrupted thick and thin filaments occur in the cells, whose presence are diagnostic.

RNase enzyme with the ability to cleave RNA

Rous sarcoma virus (RSV), a retrovirus which induces tumours when injected into chickens and transforms chicken fibroblasts in culture. The first viral oncogene to be characterized was the v-*src* gene of RSV.

ruggae folds of mucous membrane typical of stomach (and scrotum) which greatly increase the surface area of the organ.

S-100 protein widely distributed protein that does not conform to a single histogenetic pattern; present in tumours of the nervous system and normal cells of the nervous system. Also may be present in lesions of melanocytic origin.

Sam68 Src-associated molecule 68 kDa, binds to Src and is tyrosine phosphorylated by it.

Sandostatin® *see* octreotide. Pharmaceutical used in management of benign and malignant neuroendocrine tumours of the intestine.

sarcoma malignant tumour of connective tissue.

SCF *see* stem cell factor.

Schistosoma spp. liver flukes; parasites of humans associated with the initiation of bladder cancer as well as other abdominal cancers.

scintigraphy method of imaging the distribution of radioactivity with the aid of a gamma-camera.

scirrhous description of observable macroscopic condition of tissue, which has the feel of an unripe pear when cut. Scirrhous carcinoma – epithelial tumour accompanied by prominent fibrosis.

secondary tumour metastasis, tumour at a distant site derived from the primary, original tumour.

semilogarithmic scale graphic representation in which each increment along one axis (e.g. abscissa) is a logarithmic, not an arithmetic increase, while the other (e.g. ordinate) remains arithmetic. Drawn on a semilogarithmic scale, an exponential curve becomes a straight line.

seminoma malignant germ cell tumour of the testis; cells tend to be uniform with well defined borders resembling primitive germ cells. It is the most common malignant tumour of the testis and is usually highly radiosensitive.

serosa   tunica serosa is the membrane that covers the surfaces of the pleural, pericardial and peritoneal cavities and is reflected on to the outer surfaces of the organs of these cavities. It is made up of dense areolar connective tissue covered with a single layer of mesothelial cells.

sessile   attached by a broad base and not pedunculated, flat.

SH1 domain   Src-homology-1, kinase domain of protein tyrosine kinases (PTKs),

SH2 domain   Src-homology-2 region present in many enzymatic plasma membrane-associated proteins. Distinctive domain of around 100 amino acids which recognizes short peptide motifs bearing phosphotyrosines, particularly on growth factor receptors.

SH3 domain   Src-homology-3 region present in many proteins involved in signal transduction. Domain of around 60 amino acids which recognizes short peptide motifs ($\sim$10 amino acids) that are rich in proline residues.

sigmoidoscopy   direct examination of the interior of the sigmoid colon.

signal transduction pathway   the means by which information is passed to the genome of a cell after binding of the appropriate messenger (growth factor, hormone) to its specific receptor.

simian virus 40   (SV40), oncogenic DNA polyomavirus originally isolated from apparently normal monkey kidney cells; gives rise to the 'large T antigen' transforming protein.

sinusoid   spacious blood channel, particularly of spleen, liver, bone marrow, adenohypophysis, adrenal and parathyroid glands; lined with endothelium but lacking the complex wall structures of venous and arterial blood vessels, and being involved in the specific physiological functions of the organ in which they are found.

slow transforming viruses   viruses, lacking v-*onc* sequences, which do not readily transform cells, but which, nevertheless can cause tumours after a long latent period.

SOD   *see* superoxide dismutase.

somatic   'of the body', with reference to somatic cell mutation; mutation in genome of diploid cells that are not cells of the germ line and thus do not undergo meiosis to form gametes, thus the mutation is *not* inherited.

somatostatin   hormone synthesized in the hypothalamus and delta cells of pancreatic islets; governs release of thyrotropin, corticotropin, insulin, glucagon and gastrin from their respective sites of synthesis.

Sos   intracellular protein which plays a role in the activation of Ras proteins through being a guanine nucleotide exchange factor.

Southern blot   technique developed by E. Southern in which denatured DNA is transferred from agarose gels, in which fragments have separated by electrophoresis, to a nitrocellulose or nylon membrane laid over the gel. Hybridization with a complementary nucleic acid probe is then possible

spermatogenesis   full development of the sperm from the spermatogonium through all stages to the spermatozoon.

spermiogenesis   sequence of events in which the spermatozoon develops from the spermatid.

squame   scale or flake. Anuclear, terminally differentiated (dead) surface cell of the epidermis.

squamous carcinoma   malignant tumour of squamous epithelium with large cells joined by numerous, evident (at electron microscope level) desmosomes; well differentiated examples contain typical keratin 'pearls'.

Src   family of non-receptor protein kinases whose prototype is the membrane-associated pp60$^{c\text{-}src}$ protein.

stage   semi-quantitative assessment of the extent of local invasion of a tumour and thus of the clinical gravity of disease. There are several widely used systems of classification such as TNM staging (particularly lung), Clark's levels (malignant melanoma), Dukes' stages (large bowel cancer) and Jass classification (rectal carcinoma).

static cell populations those tissues in which there is no appreciable ability to repopulate, after damage for example, by cell proliferation. Cardiac muscle and neurones fall into this group.

Stat proteins signal transducers and activators of transcription. Chief targets for tyrosine phosphorylation by Jaks which themselves are activated by cytokine receptor occupancy. Stats form dimers and act as transcription factors.

stem cell progenitor cell in renewing tissue systems from which all other cells are derived. Stem cells are present in tissues throughout the life of the individual, i.e. long enough to accrue sufficient mutations to produce a malignant tumour. In tumours they are the most important targets for chemotherapy.

stem cell factor (SCF, c-*kit* ligand), early acting growth factor – when alone is a survival factor for stem cells; alternatively synergizes with other growth factors such as GM-CSF, G-CSF, EPO; promoting the growth of myeloid and erythroid progenitors.

stochastic susceptible to random influences and thus subject to the laws of probability, the opposite of deterministic.

stoichiometrical binding binding in a numerical relationship dependent on the proportions of constituents in the chemical formula of the compound.

stroma connective tissue supporting the functional cells of an organ.

submucosa tissue found beneath the mucosal covering, typically made up of connective tissue and blood vessels.

superoxide dismutase (SOD), protective mechanism in free radical scavenger system.

synatophysin (p38), calcium-binding, glycosylated polypeptide (38 kDa), integral component of pre-synaptic vesicles. Also exists in a range of normal and neuroendocrine cells and their derivative tumours.

tamoxifen synthetic steroid analogue which recognizes and binds to the oestrogen receptor thus blocking binding of oestrogen and inactivating the dependent stimulatory system; used to treat oestrogen-dependent tumours typically of breast (primary and metastatic).

tannic acid one of the simplest of the family of tannins, formerly used as an antidote for alkaloid poisoning and treating burns. In histochemical techniques fixation of tissue with tannic acid added to the fixative solution protects membranes which otherwise would not survive the rigours of tissue processing prior to microscopy.

Tax protein transactivating protein encoded by the HTLV-I RNA virus

taxol from *Taxus* species (yew trees and hedges), used in chemotherapy; promotes the stabilization of microtubules which are resistant to depolymerization, thus leading to mitotic arrest and cell death.

T-cell clone thymic lymphocytes developed by proliferative response of a single stimulated T cell, thus all having the same properties as the parent cell.

T cell receptor (TCR), definitive T cell marker (TCR-1 or TCR-2), which enables T cells to recognize antigen presented by antigen presenting cells; the T cell receptor is unique to any given T cell and its progeny. T cell receptor chains, TCRα, TCRβ, TCRγ, TCRδ, are coded for by the *TCR* genes.

telophase final stage in mitosis in which the two daughter sets of chromosomes complete their journey away from each other and form the nuclei of two daughter cells, with the division of cytoplasmic contents and formation of new plasma membranes. Preceded by anaphase and followed by the G_1 phase of the cell cycle.

teratoma tumour of germ cells, generally benign in the ovary, but often malignant in the testis, which typically contains diverse cell types representative of all three germ layers.

12-o-tetradecanoyl phorbol-13-acetate (TPA), non-mutagenic tumour promoting phorbol ester, stimulates PKC activity.

TGFα *see* transforming growth factor alpha.

TGFβ *see* transforming growth factor beta.

6-thioguanine   (6GT), antimetabolite analogue of guanine, and similar in its activity to 6-mercaptopurine. Cancer chemotherapeutic agent active in the S phase of the cell cycle, frequently used in the treatment of myeloid leukaemias.

thorium dioxide   compound of radioactive thorium which in colloidal suspension (Thorotrast®) was formally used as a positive contrast agent in diagnostic radiography, before the dangers of very low doses of radiation were appreciated.

thymidylate synthase   enzyme catalyzing conversion of dUMP (uridylic acid) to dTMP (thymidylic acid) through methylation.

thyroglobulin   protein produced by the follicular cells of the thyroid gland, whose tyrosine residues can be converted into thyroxine.

tissue section   preserved and strengthened tissue block then cut into sections thin enough ($\sim$ 4–5 μm) to transmit light, for observation under the microscope. In the case of sections for electron microscopy, they are around 100 nm thick which is thin enough to differentially transmit electrons to form an image.

TNM system   diagnostic/prognostic descriptive staging system of the tumour condition – tumour, node, metastasis.

TNF   *see* tumour necrosis factor.

tomography   imaging method that produces a three-dimensional pictorial representation of cross-sections of the body, usually *via* summation of many two dimensional images.

topoisomerase   enzyme that converts one topological isomer of a macromolecule (usually DNA), into another; has cyclic activity finally rejoining the DNA strands. When prevented from completing its cycle (e.g. by anthracyclins or epipodophyllotoxins) leaves DNA fragmented.

totipotent   a stem cell whose progeny have the ability to differentiate into any cell type of the organism, e.g. the fertilized egg.

TPA   *see* 12-o-tetradecanoyl phorbol-13-acetate.

trabecular   pattern of tumour cells in wide strands or tracts which is characteristic of that tumour class, e.g. hepatocellular carcinoma.

transactivation   mechanism of cellular transformation of slow transforming viruses in which viral proteins activate distant cellular genes.

transcoelomic spread   metastatic tumour dissemination across a body cavity by cells breaking off from the primary tumour, passing across the cavity and then establishing a secondary tumour at the new site.

transcription   the process by which a strand of RNA is synthesized using its complementary strand of DNA as its template.

transcription factors   proteins with DNA-binding motifs (e.g. zinc finger) which bind to specific nucleotide sequences, 'promoters' and 'enhancers', close to the initiation codon of each gene thus controlling transcription.

transfection   gene transfer in which DNA, e.g. from a recombinant plasmid, is introduced into cultured cells which may then express the gene transiently or permanently.

transformation   conversion of a cell from a normal state to one with the capacity for unlimited proliferation and the ability for anchorage-independent growth in culture.

transforming growth factor-alpha   (TGFα), member of the epidermal growth factor (EGF) family, recognizing the EGF receptor. The gene protein product (6 kDa) was initially found in mixture with TGFβ in virally transformed cells whose conditioned medium could confer properties of independent growth on normal cells. TGFα mimics EGF in biological activity and has similarities in amino-acid sequence.

transforming growth factor-beta   (TGFβ), growth factor initially discovered in a mixture with TGFα but subsequently found to be a separate substance. Virally transformed cells produced a conditioned medium containing TGFα and TGFβ which conferred properties of independent growth on normal cells. TGFβ is multipotential, promoting growth in some cell populations but inhibiting it in others, particularly in epithelia. TGFβ cell cycle arrest correlates with an increase in the expression of proteins p15^{Ink4B} and p27^{Kip1} which are both cyclin-dependent kinase inhibitors.

transgenic animals of or pertaining to, two different genomes, especially with respect to a DNA sequence from one genome introduced into another genome, e.g. animals in which a modified gene was inserted into the pronucleus of a fertilized oocyte.

transglutaminases members of a group of cytoplasmic Ca^{2+}-dependent enzymes, activated in apoptosis, whose function is to cross-link proteins to form the 'shell' of apoptotic bodies, thus preventing leakage of intracellular components.

tritiated thymidine DNA nucleoside precursor with radioactive hydrogen (tritium), used as a proliferation marker when taken up into DNA in the S phase of the cell cycle.

trophoblast tissue contribution to the placenta from the blastocyst in mammals. After implantation of the embryo, the trophoblast develops three layers, the outer syncytiotrophoblast, inner cytotrophoblast and an internal mesenchymal layer, all three making up the chorion.

tubular adenoma benign large bowel tumour composed of cells arranged as branching tubules, often forming polypoid mass.

tumorigenic a substance or procedure that leads to tumour formation.

tumour neoplasm: expanding lesion resultant from a cell production rate which exceeds the cell loss rate. Benign tumours remain localized and the cells' phenotype resembles the tissue of origin; malignant tumours invade locally and/or give rise to distant metastases. The cell phenotype and arrangement in a malignant tumour may resemble the tissue of origin (well differentiated tumours) or be so lacking in differentiation that the tissue of origin can not be readily recognized (anaplastic).

tumour angiogenic factors factors that provide the signal for development of new blood vessels to supply the increasing tissue in neoplasms.

tumour doubling time (t$_D$), tumour growth parameter, e.g. time taken for the tumour to double in volume, when the volume is calculated after direct measurements of its size.

tumour growth rate (K$_G$), tumour growth parameter calculated from the volume changes, or weight changes and expressed for example, as g/100g/day.

tumour necrosis factor multipotential cytokine produced principally by activated macrophages/monocytes (TNF-α) and activated lymphocytes (TNF-β); causes tumour cell death indirectly by destruction of the vascular endothelium and directly by receptor-mediated apoptosis.

tumour suppressor genes anti-oncogenes. Genes whose protein products are commonly involved either in mechanisms of cell cycle arrest or cell adhesion. Single or more usually double allelic loss/mutation of such genes appears to be crucial to neoplastic development.

Tyk2 member of the Janus kinase (Jaks) family of PTKs.

tyrosine kinase enzymes catalysing the phosphorylation of tyrosine residues in substrate proteins.

ubiquitin a 76 amino acid protein involved in binding to damaged proteins marking them for destruction. Accumulations of ubiquinated proteins include Mallory bodies in alcoholic liver disease and neurofibrillary tangles in Alzheimer's disease.

ultrasonography method to exploit the differing properties of tissues to absorb or reflect ultrasound waves, and thus produce a visual image of the tissues.

ultraviolet (UV) light electromagnetic radiation not visible to the human eye, whose wavelength is just shorter than that of visible light.

unipotential stem cell a stem cell whose differentiated progeny are of one phenotype only.

urokinase a plasminogen activator, excreted in urine. Enzyme which converts inactive plasminogen to the active plasmin (a broad spectrum protease); inhibitors of this enzyme might thus impede tumour invasion and metastasis.

uterine cervix narrow cylindrical portion of the uterus which projects into the upper vagina.

valine essential amino acid metabolized by transamination and oxidation of the oxoacid, ultimately to proprionic acid.

vasoactive intestinal polypeptide (VIP), hormone produced principally in the pancreas that causes smooth muscle relaxation and stimulates pancreatic bicarbonate secretion.

v-*erbA* viral oncogene of avian erythroblastosis virus (AEV), coding for mutated cytosolic thyroid hormone receptor.

v-*erbB* viral oncogene of AEV, associated with erythroid leukaemia, encodes a protein corresponding to truncated EGFR.

V-CAM vascular cell adhesion molecule, member of the immunoglobulin superfamily (Ig-SF); functions as an endothelial cell receptor for cells of malignant melanoma and others that express $\alpha4\beta1$ integrin.

villiform projections finger-like projections of an epithelial surface.

villous adenoma adenoma with finger-like processes of stroma covered with dysplastic epithelium; large bowel preinvasive lesion.

villus finger-like projection; term often applied to folds in the intestinal epithelium.

vimentin intermediate filament found in mesenchymal cells such as fibroblasts and macrophages also in endothelial cells, melanocytes and lymphocytes.

vinblastine sulphate derivative of a vinca alkaloid causes the arrest of cells in metaphase. Experimentally used for the metaphase arrest technique, used clinically as an anti-cancer agent, typically against lymphomas and Hodgkin's disease, in combination with other drugs.

vinca alkaloid mitotic spindle poison from the periwinkle plant; arrests cells in metaphase, by binding to tubulin and preventing formation of microtubules.

vincristine sulphate like vinblastine sulphate, a derivative of the vinca alkaloid used both experimentally and clinically. Vincristine has found favour in the treatment of leukaemias.

VIPoma neuroendocrine tumour whose cells produce vasoactive intestinal polypeptide.

virus subcellular organism which is an obligate intracellular parasite as it lacks its own means to generate adenosine triphosphate (ATP). Composed of proteinaceous capsid that covers the organism's genome (which may be composed of either DNA or RNA) plus necessary transcriptase enzymes.

VM 26 teniposide, plant derived cancer chemotherapeutic agent active in G_2 phase of the cell cycle, epipodophyllotoxin (from the mandrake plant). Interrupts breakage/reunion reaction of topoisomerase II.

v-*myb* viral oncogene associated with chicken myeloblastosis (acute myeloid leukaemia).

v-*myc* viral oncogene associated with chicken myelocytoma (chronic myeloid leukaemia).

v-*onc* an oncogene identified as part of a viral genome. Homologues of normal cellular genes previously adopted by viruses during evolution.

von Willebrand factor the large, non-coagulating portion of factor VIII complex which is necessary for platelets to adhere to damaged endothelium.

VP16 etoposide, cancer chemotherapeutic agent active in the G_2 phase of the cell cycle, epipodophyllotoxin (from the mandrake plant). Interrupts breakage/reunion reaction of topoisomerase II.

v-*sis* viral gene responsible for the transforming activity of simian sarcoma virus.

v-*src* viral gene responsible for the transforming activity of the Rous sarcoma virus.

Western blotting by analogy with Southern and Northern blotting, technique of protein transfer on to a nitrocellulose membrane after separation by SDS-PAGE electrophoresis, followed by its visualization using specific monoclonal antibodies, which themselves are labelled with an enzyme or radioisotope. SDS (sodium dodecyl sulphate) is a negatively charged ionic detergent which gives the proteins an identical charge density so that in the gel they separate according to molecular weight (tissue equivalent: immunocytochemistry).

WT1 transcriptional regulator lost or mutated in Wilms' tumour.

X-protein   transactivating protein associated with hepatocellular carcinoma (HCC), coded for by the HBV viral *X* gene: may interact with either AP-1 or CREB transcription factors. (Not to be confused with the X region of HTLV, activation of which leads to the synthesis of a different protein – the Tax protein).

X-rays   short wavelength electromagnetic radiation emitted from sources bombarded with electrons.

X-region   region of human T cell leukaemia viral (HTLV) genome including that coding for the Tax protein which increases the rate of proviral transcription and initiates transactivation of further host cell enhancers and promoters.

xenograft   tissue of one species grown in a different species which is usually immune suppressed. In cancer research, typically human tumours grown in nude mice.

xeroderma pigmentosum   a group of rare inherited autosomal recessive disorders, concerning defects in DNA repair, in which the skin is readily damaged by ultraviolet light. The condition produces atrophy and pigmentary changes, and predisposes to cancer of the skin.

Zoladex®   *See* goserelin acetate.

Zollinger-Ellison syndrome   severe gastric hypersecretion of hydrochloric acid and intractable peptic ulcers due to excessive secretion of gastrin by pancreatic gastrinoma.

zymogen   inactive precursor form of enzyme.

Index